STOP AUTISM NOW!

A Parent's Guide to Preventing and Reversing Autism Spectrum Disorders

Dr. Bruce Fife

PB

Piccadilly Books, Ltd.
Colorado Springs, CO

Every effort has been made to ensure that the information contained in this book is complete and accurate. However, neither the publisher nor the author is engaged in rendering professional advice or services to the individual reader. The ideas, procedures, and suggestions contained in this book are not intended as a substitute for consulting with your physician. All matters regarding your health require medical supervision. Neither the author nor the publisher shall be liable or responsible for any loss of damage allegedly arising from any information or suggestion in this book.

Grateful acknowledgement is given to Wikimedia Commons for the use of photographs on pages 52, 60, 75, 158, 201-203, 226, 224, 232, and 249-250 and to Heidi Carolan for the photos on page 146 and Elizabeth Wangari Gachiri for the photos on page 147.

Piccadilly Books, Ltd.
P.O. Box 25203
Colorado Springs, CO 80936, USA
info@piccadillybooks.com
www.piccadillybooks.com

Library of Congress Cataloging-in-Publication Data

Fife, Bruce, 1952-
  Stop autism now! : a parent's guide to preventing and reversing autism spectrum disorders / by Bruce Fife.
      p. cm.
  Includes bibliographical references and index.
  ISBN 978-0-941599-92-4 (pbk.)
  1. Autism spectrum disorders—Popular works. 2. Autism—Nutritional aspects—Popular works. 3. Autism—Diet therapy—Popular works. I. Title.
  RC553.A88F534 2012
  616.85'882—dc23
                                    2011047426

Published in the USA

Table of Contents

1 | Is There a Cure for Autism?

AUTISM SPECTRUM DISORDER

While still just a toddler, David's parents became concerned by his abnormally slow development, lack of speech, and disconnect from normal social interaction. Other children David's age were learning to speak in full sentences and possessed vocabularies consisting of dozens of words. They also showed emotion and interest in things around him, traits foreign to David. Lacking were the smiles of delight seen in the faces of other children when they saw their parents and interacted with them. David looked at his parents with an emotionless blank stare, he never smiled, and at the slightest provocation threw uncontrollable temper tantrums.

Doctors diagnosed David with autism spectrum disorder (ASD), often simply referred to as autism. His parents were told there is no cure. Autism is a lifelong diagnosis. Afflicted individuals fail to ever reach normal function. The only treatment available, they were told, is extensive educational intervention to help achieve some measure of daily functioning.

According to conventional medical wisdom there is little hope for those diagnosed with autism. A diagnosis of ASD is considered a life sentence. Statistically, 75 percent of autistic individuals become institutionalized as adults. Autism affects children of all races and ethnicities. However, four times as many males are affected as females.

Today there are over 1 million people with autism, and this number continues to grow. Over the past several years autism has increased to epidemic proportions. Thirty years ago it affected about 1 in 2,500 children. Today 1 out of every 91 children in the United States and 1 out of 64 in the UK are affected. Rates are similar in many other Western countries. Each year the number of children affected increases by 10-17 percent.[1]

Over the past 12 years there has been a 17 percent increase in childhood developmental disabilities of all types including autism, attention deficit hyperactivity disorder (ADHD), epilepsy, mental retardation, and others. Currently in the US, 4 million children have attention deficit hyperactivity disorder, the most common learning disability, and an incredible one in six children are classified as learning disabled.[2]

Autism can often be identified as early as 18 months. Most cases of autism are diagnosed within the first 3 years of life. However, there have been cases of late-onset autism in individuals who where were 11, 14, and 31 years of age. In families with one autistic child, there is a 20 percent chance of having a second child with the same disorder.

Autism is a neurodevelopmental disorder characterized by impaired communication, poor social interaction, and abnormal repetitive behaviors. The most obvious characteristic is difficulty with both verbal and nonverbal communication. About 40 percent of autistic children never learn to speak. Many seem to have no understanding of facial expressions or body language such as a smile, a wink, or a wave. Those who can speak may do so with difficulty. Others may not learn to speak until later in childhood. Some develop a seemingly unconscious habit of repeating words or phrases spoken by others—a condition called *echolalia*. Between 25-40 percent develop normally for the first 12 to 18 months of life and then rapidly lose their language skills.

Autistic children often have difficulty interacting with other people. They may appear disinterested and aloof, avoiding eye contact and shying away from physical or emotional interaction. They are often painfully sensitive to certain sounds, tastes, and smells. They may cover their ears and scream when the phone rings or wince at the smell of a banana, yet may be less sensitive to physical pain than other children and may pay no attention to a cut or injury.

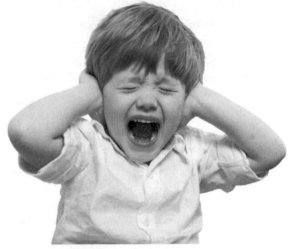

Autistics may develop fixations with specific objects and often display repetitive, ritualistic behavior such as continuously waving their arms, banging their heads on the wall, or obsessively lining up or stacking toys or other objects. Changes to their daily routine—even something as simple as cutting a sandwich straight across rather than diagonally—can lead to a temper tantrum.

Children with autism may also experience motor function disturbances, vision or hearing defects, hyperactivity disorder, mental retardation, or epilepsy. As many as 82 percent experience periodic epileptic seizures. These conditions can range from mild to severe.

Clinical diagnosis is based solely on behavior. According to the *American Psychiatric Association's Diagnostic and Statistical Manual of Mental Disorders, Fourth Edition*, children with autism meet at least six of the following criteria:

Social Impairments
Does not properly use nonverbal behaviors such as gestures and facial expressions
Fails to develop age-appropriate peer relationships
Does not spontaneously share objects or interests with others
Lacks social or emotional reciprocity

Communication Impairments
Is slow to speak
Has difficulty sustaining a conversation
Repeatedly uses the same language
Does not engage in age-appropriate make-believe or socially imitative play

Repetitive Behaviors
Is intensely preoccupied with one or more interests
Is inflexible and unwilling to change set routines
Repeats motions or mannerisms (such as waving arms, flapping, or twisting)
Is preoccupied with parts of objects

In order for a physician to diagnose autism the child must be old enough for the above conditions to become clearly evident. Parents, however, are in close contact with their children every day and can recognize developmental delays long before a formal diagnoses can be made. Some of the early warning signs include:

- Absence of smile by six months of age.
- Lack of non-verbal exchange of facial expressions by nine months of age.
- No babbling, or discontinuation of babbling, by 12 months.
- Lack of gesturing, including pointing, reaching, or waving, by 12 months.
- No words by 16 months.
- Any termination or change in communication or social interaction after they have been developing normally.

Autistic symptoms occur along a spectrum varying in symptomatology and severity; this is why it is referred to as autism *spectrum* disorder. The symptoms are grouped into five diagnostic subtypes that include autism (classical autism), Rett syndrome, Asperger's syndrome, childhood disintegrative disorder (CDD), and pervasive developmental disorders not otherwise specified (PDD-NOS).

Unlike other forms of autism, Rett syndrome affects girls more often than boys. More than half those affected develop seizures. Infants with Rett syndrome generally develop normally for the first 6 to 12 months of life. After that, symptoms start to appear. The most pronounced changes generally occur between 12 to 18 months of age. Symptoms include slowed growth, including smaller than normal head size, loss of communication skills and cognitive abilities, and loss of normal movement and coordination. The first sign is often a decrease of hand control and decreasing ability to crawl or walk normally. They become disinterested in other people, toys, and their surroundings. As the disease progresses, children with Rett syndrome typically develop their own particular odd behavioral characteristics such as hand wringing, squeezing, clapping, tapping, or rubbing; erratic eye blinking or closing one eye at a time; periods of crying or screaming that begin suddenly and may last for hours; and odd facial expressions and long bouts of laughter or screaming that occur for no apparent reason.

Asperger's syndrome is a somewhat less severe form of autism, characterized by significant difficulties with social interaction, repetitive patterns of behavior and interests, but may exhibit relatively normal language and cognitive development.

Children with childhood disintegrative disorder (CDD) will develop normally until about the age 3 or 4, then over a period of just a few months dramatically lose the motor, language, social, and other skills they had already learned.

Pervasive developmental disorder-not otherwise specified (PDD-NOS) shares many of the same symptoms with autism such as communication and social delays and repetitive behaviors, but symptoms are less severe. Children with PDD-NOS meet most but not all the criteria for a full diagnosis of autism.

Up until the 1980s doctors believed that autism was caused by bad parenting. According to the medical opinions of this time, children became autistic because their parents, especially mothers, were uncaring and cold. This was referred to as the "refrigerator mother theory." Young children receiving no love or proper nurturing became aloof and disconnected from family and society. This theory seems absurd now as many loving parents have autistic children.

Most medical professionals still do not understand why autism occurs despite evidence that environmental and immunological factors play important roles in its development. Autism is viewed as a hopeless lifelong condition. There is no medically recognized cure. The only treatment available is designed to manage the disorder through educational programs and behavioral therapies structured to teach children to cope with their disorder by improving communication, physical, and social skills. While there are no drugs designed specifically to treat autism, medications such as antidepressants, antipsychotics, and stimulants may be prescribed to treat specific symptoms.

According to conventional medical wisdom, there is little hope for autistic children. These children are condemned to a lifelong sentence of behavioral therapy, drugs, and torment.

THERE IS HOPE

A diagnosis of autism, however, is not a life sentence. There is a cure. You can stop autism now using dietary intervention and coconut ketone therapy. This new approach is proving to be highly effective at stopping the progression of the disease cold in its tracks, significantly improving symptoms, and even bringing about complete recovery.

What is coconut ketone therapy? Ketones are energy producing molecules made from fats. Our bodies can make them from stored fat or from special fats known as medium chain triglycerides (MCTs) found in coconut oil. Ketones are produced specifically by the body to feed the brain. Richard Veech, MD, a long time ketone researcher and senior scientist with the US National Institutes of Health describes ketones as "superfuel for the brain." Ordinarily, glucose powers our brain cells. However, when the brain is plagued with chronic inflammation, irritation, and immune over-activation, as is seen in all autistic children, brain cells have difficulty processing glucose. The lack of sufficient fuel causes the brain to downshift into a lower rate of performance. Normal growth and development are stifled and learned skills may become lost as the brain's cells are starved for energy and struggle for survival.

Ketones act as an alternative fuel to glucose—a much more potent and efficient fuel. When ketones are available it is like putting high performance gasoline into the tank of your car. You get better gas mileage and higher performance with less wear and tear on the engine and less pollution. Ketones bypass the defect in glucose metabolism and provide the brain with the energy it needs to function and develop properly.

Ketones not only supply a superior source of energy to the brain but trigger the activation of specialized proteins called *brain derived neurotrophic factors* (BDNFs) that function in brain cell maintenance, repair, and protection. They also stimulate the growth of new brain cells to take the place of dead or dying cells. This allows healing and repair to take place.

Ketones are ordinarily produced when blood glucose levels become low. Since glucose is the body's primary source of energy, when glucose levels fall, the body starts mobilizing stored fat to produce ketones in order to maintain adequate energy levels. Medical science has learned how to alter blood ketone levels by manipulating the diet. Ketogenic diets, which boost ketones to therapeutic levels, have been used successfully for decades for the treatment of other neurological disorders, most notably epilepsy.

Another way to elevate blood ketone levels to therapeutic levels is to consume a source of MCTs. However, there are very few dietary sources of MCTs. The richest dietary source by far comes from coconut oil, which is composed predominately of MCTs. Eating coconut oil can raise blood ketones to levels that can have a pronounced effect on brain growth and development.

Feeding your child coconut oil or MCTs is not as strange as it might seem. MCTs are a normal and natural source of nutrition for infants and small children. Another source of MCTs is human breast milk! This isn't some accident of nature—they are there for an important reason. They are essential for proper brain development. In fact, MCT-derived ketones provide the basic building blocks for new brain tissue. They are required to build baby's brains as well as to provide necessary energy. In fact, coconut oil or MCTs are added to all commercial and hospital infant formulas to assure proper brain growth and function. In this book you will learn how to use dietary intervention and coconut ketone therapy to stop autism now.

A MOTHER'S STORY

"In February 2007 we discovered one of our children had Asperger's syndrome, an autism spectrum disorder," says Renee Osterhouse of DeLand, North Carolina. "It was a blessing in a way, because it answered many of the questions we had regarding our daughter's behavior." This discovery also opened the door that lead to her recovery and started the entire family's journey down a path to better health.

"Her list of symptoms went on forever," says Renee, "brain fog, lethargy, sinusitis, headaches, stomach aches, repetitive speech patterns, eyes darting, at times unresponsive, and hearing difficulties. She also had gross and fine motor skill difficulties.

The worst though, were the meltdowns. They were like emotional breakdowns that she clearly couldn't control and which would occur at least every other day."

The Osterhouses were told that the disorder was incurable. Treatment amounted to specialized education and little else. Children don't recover from autism, they were told, they can only manage it. However, Renee felt there had to be something they could do.

"Instinct told me something in her personal environment was causing or at least aggravating her symptoms," says Renee. "She had fleeting moments of clarity I could not explain." All foods containing preservatives, artificial colorings, and hydrogenated oils were removed from the family's diet. Refined sugar and sweets were radically reduced. The air conditioning ducts were updated to lessen the possibility of mold and an air purifier was put in their daughter's bedroom. They threw out all of their non-stick cookware and started drinking water free of fluoride and chlorine. The entire family started taking whole food dietary supplements to assure they received all the nutrients they required.

When Renee started researching autism it didn't take long before she learned about wheat and milk allergies and their possible effects on autism. "At the age of seven, we removed most dairy which seemed to help temporarily," says Renee. "However, her symptoms soon returned."

She found a book titled *Feast Without Yeast: 4 Stages to Better Health* and learned about the effects that yeast (candida) overgrowth can have on health, especially digestive function. Autistic children often have digestive problems. Armed with this new information she put her daughter on an even more restricted diet, removing all sources of yeast including all grains and dairy. All refined carbohydrates were essentially eliminated. "Within a few days we started to notice a difference," says Renee. It wasn't a cure, but there were definite improvements.

"Already pleased with our success with this dietary intervention, it was difficult to hope our daughter could get much better," says Renee. "Then I found Bruce Fife's book *Coconut Cures: Preventing and Treating Common Health Problems with Coconut*. I learned of coconut oil and its healing benefits, as well as its ability to restore balance in the gut by controlling candida.

"With this new information we added 3-5 tablespoons of coconut oil to our daughter's diet…Within a week we noticed a new level of clarity. It seemed to clear away the rest of the cobwebs. Her speech improved rapidly, her vocabulary

---

Ketone Therapy Sweeps the Dust Out of His Head

A couple months into the diet, I was trying to tune in the kitchen radio and Michael said, "That's what my head was like, mom. It was fuzzy before and now it's getting tuned in to the channels." We were elated that the diet had stopped his seizures and he was on no drugs, but we had no idea the diet was as Michael said later, "sweeping dust out of my head."

www.charliefoundation.org

skyrocketed, and her physically painful symptoms became intermittent and controllable. Her hearing is now normal. She initiates conversations and people are able to engage her in conversations as well."

Prior to adding the coconut oil Renee's daughter couldn't read two pages without extreme effort. "When she would read," says Renee, "her eyes would dart all over the page picking up words that were at the bottom and inserting them where they didn't belong. It naturally wouldn't make any sense so she would have to re-read each sentence. After two pages she was exhausted and confused. Dietary intervention along with coconut oil has given her a new life. Now, she will read for hours if we let her…I am pleased to say that our little author has written a 15 chapter book. For the first time in her life, she was able to complete homework on her own and was an honor roll student throughout the school year."

In the following chapters you will learn what causes autism and how to prevent it and successfully treat it using a proven dietary approach. We will examine the controversy surrounding vaccines and what importance they might play in this mind-numbing disorder. You will also discover what affect the mother's health and lifestyle habits can have on autism as well as the role industrial and environmental toxins, diet, food additives, drugs, infections, and other factors may play. You will learn who is at greatest risk for developing autism and why digestive health is a critical issue. But most importantly, you will learn what steps you need to take to prevent autism and how to successfully beat it.

2 | The Vaccine Controversy

A MOTHER'S NIGHTMARE

When she brought her son Evan to receive his scheduled vaccinations, Jenny McCarthy had concerns. She questioned her pediatrician about the possible link between the measles, mumps, and rubella (MMR) vaccine and autism. "I have a very bad feeling about this shot," she said. "This is the autism shot, isn't it?"

"No, that's ridiculous," the doctor replied indignantly. "It's a mother's desperate attempt to blame something."

Although abrupt, he was the doctor and should know if there was any connection between autism and vaccines. We're always told to trust our doctors—after all, they have the training and experience to know what's best for us, right? As the nurse gave Evan the shot, Jenny could not help but feel a little uneasy, "I hope he's right," she said to herself.

Early in the morning Jenny awoke with an uneasy feeling. The clock read 7:45 a.m. Evan always got up at 7:00 a.m. sharp every morning. Worried that something might be wrong she dashed to the nursery. "I opened the door and ran to his crib and found him convulsing and struggling to breathe. His eyes were rolled back in his head."

The paramedics arrived and after about 20 minutes managed to get Evan's body to stop convulsing. At the hospital the doctors said Evan had a febrile seizure, which is caused by an excessively high fever. Fevers are common after vaccinations and sometimes trigger seizures.

"He doesn't really have a fever," she responded, "so how does that play in the scenario?"

"Well, he could have been getting one," the doctor replied dismissively.

That didn't make sense to her at all. She brought Evan home from the hospital thinking something was very wrong.

About three weeks after the initial seizure, Evan had a second episode while they were visiting his grandparents.

"I noticed a kind of stoned look on his face," says Jenny. "I passed him off to Grandma thinking he was just tired, but moments later his eyes rolled into the back of his head and I knew it was happening again. I frantically called 911."

This seizure was different. His body wasn't convulsing, nor was he trying to breathe. Foam was drooling out of his mouth and he began to turn pale.

"I put my hand on his chest and kept saying, 'Stay with me, baby, stay with me.'"

Then to her horror, she watched as his eyes dilated and felt his heart stop. She fell to her knees in anguish as she held his lifeless body. The paramedics rushed in and began CPR. After two minutes Evan started breathing again. He was whisked away by ambulance to a Los Angeles hospital. It was a three hour drive and in that time Evan had another seizure. At the hospital he experienced seven more seizures within a seven–hour period. After two days in the hospital the doctors told Jenny her son had epilepsy.

Not satisfied with this diagnosis Jenny decided to get a second opinion and made an appointment with a neurologist. After the examination he gently put his hand on Jenny's shoulder and said, "I'm sorry, your son has autism."

"I died in that moment but my instincts told me that this man was right," she says.

Was Evan's MMR vaccine the cause of his autism? The CDC, doctors, and media all proclaim that there is no hard scientific proof to support the connection between vaccines and autism. However, Jenny responds, "Who needs science when I'm witnessing it every day in my own home? I watched it happen."

Jenny isn't the only parent who has watched a healthy child who was progressing normally suddenly slide into autism immediately following a vaccination.

"I am a parent of a 6-year-old boy who has autism spectrum disorder (ASD)," says Craig Willoughby. His son was walking, he was talking, he was following all the normal progression steps for a child his age, and he was even a little bit ahead in some areas. "Then he had the DPT shot." says Craig. "That same night, his fever was at 105 degrees F (40.5 C) and he could do nothing but scream. When we brought him to the ER, they asked us if he had received a vaccination, and we said yes. Their reply was, 'Oh, this is normal.' How can something like that be normal? The next day, his fever was gone, and he was listless. He hasn't spoken since. He quit walking until he was two and a half, and it's almost like he isn't my son anymore."

Thousands of parents of autistic children can relate similar stories. While the vaccine-autism connection is hotly denied by drug makers and their friends at the Center for Disease Control and Prevention (CDC), parents have time and time again witnessed firsthand their children's descent into autism following routine vaccinations. Relying on the credibility of the CDC and the vaccine manufacturers, most doctors and public health officials deny any link, claiming scientific evidence does not support such a connection. Is this really true?

THE STORY OF ANDREW WAKEFIELD

If you follow the news you no doubt witnessed the media blitz surrounding the vaccine-autism controversy over the past few years. For a period of time headlines and news anchors loudly proclaimed, "New study shows no link between vaccines and autism." Another blared, "Study linking vaccine to autism was fraud." And still another, "Andrew Wakefield found guilty of fraud in vaccine scandal."

The stories all condemn Dr. Wakefield as a charlatan and absolved vaccines from any perceived connection to autism. The media also reported on a rash of recent studies that allegedly removed all blame from vaccines. One such study consisted of a "scientific review of *select* studies" and found "no credible evidence" linking measles, mumps, and rubella (MMR) vaccinations to autism. Dr. Tom Jefferson, one of the authors of this study stated, "We don't think there is any point in further investigating the association…The controversy should be put to bed."

According to the news accounts, the link between vaccines and autism was just a big hoax. There is no need to worry. The author of the assumed link has been exposed as a fraud and his research discredited. The public is reassured that vaccinations are safe for one and all. Parents should continue with their children's vaccinations as scheduled.

But what about the thousands of parents who swear that their normally developing children mysteriously developed autism immediately following vaccination? Are they all hallucinating? And who is Andrew Wakefield? Why was he singled out as the perpetuator of this grand hoax?

Andrew Wakefield, MD, is a gastrointestinal surgeon and researcher. Most of his research was done while employed at the Royal Free Hospital and School of Medicine, in London—one of the most prestigious hospitals in the world. His specialty is Crohn's disease, ulcerative colitis and related disorders. He has published over 130 peer-reviewed studies in medical journals looking at the mechanism and cause of inflammatory bowel disease and is considered one of the world's leading experts on inflammatory bowel disease. He was the first researcher to demonstrate a link between vaccines and autism.

In the early 1990s he discovered a connection between the measles virus and Crohn's disease. This relationship was verified by other researchers. Measles is highly contagious and is usually passed by exposure to an infected person. Children are most susceptible. However, if the virus is passed in another fashion, it could seriously affect the digestive tract leading to inflammatory bowel disease. For example, children exposed to the measles virus in utero often develop Crohn's disease later on. Another unusual route of exposure is through vaccinations.

In 1995 Wakefield and colleagues published a paper suggesting a possible link between the measles vaccine and the later development of inflammatory bowel disease. After this study was published he began receiving calls from parents who said their children were normal until they received their MMR vaccination. However, immediately following the vaccination they began to lose their communication skills and became autistic.

At first, he thought the callers had contacted the wrong department because he had said nothing about autism in his paper. The parents would explain that their children also developed terrible bowel problems. They had severe diarrhea, bloated abdomens, and were failing to thrive. Growth was stunted. They would often walk around in the middle of the night. The children lost their ability to speak, were banging their heads against the wall, and flying into screaming rages.

It is important to point out that the parents of these autistic children were not anti-vaccine. They took their children to be vaccinated according to schedule. But they saw a rapid decline in their children soon afterwards. The children developed fevers, experienced bowel disturbances, became delirious, and then started losing their ability to speak and interact with others. The parents watched these events unfold before their eyes. They weren't hallucinating. It wasn't a coincidence.

After numerous parents had contacted him, all describing similar symptoms, Wakefield began to wonder if there might be a connection. An investigation was begun. He assembled a team of pediatric gastroenterologists, child psychiatrists, neurologists, and pathologists at the Royal Free Hospital to study the issue. Over the next few years the team examined over 170 children who had developed autism soon after being vaccinated and in every case they had a subtle but definite inflammatory bowel disease.

When the clinicians treated their bowel disease, not only did bowel symptoms improve but so did the behavioral symptoms. The children would smile. They would sleep through the night. Some of them started speaking again; picking up where they had left off years before.

Their primary treatment was anti-inflammatory medication used to treat Crohn's or colitis. Another thing that they found was effective was a gluten- and casein-free diet. This was something the parents had instituted but it had dramatic effects in many cases.

Many people couldn't understand the brain-gut connection. How could the health of the digestive tract affect the brain? However, gastroenterologists see it all the time. It is seen in celiac disease—a digestive problem caused by an intolerance to gluten. One of the features often associated with celiac disease is dementia and seizures.

In 1998 Wakefield along with 12 colleagues published a peer-reviewed study in the *Lancet*, one of the world's leading medical journals, suggesting a possible link between autism and the MMR vaccine.[1]

In this study, the researchers examined 12 children, 3 to 10 years of age, who had a history of normal development until receiving the MMR vaccine. Following the vaccination they lost acquired mental skills, including language, and developed diarrhea and abdominal pain. With the permission of the parents the children underwent gastroenterological, neurological, and developmental assessments. All 12 children had intestinal abnormalities. Nine were diagnosed with autism, one with disintegrative psychosis, and two with vaccine-induced encephalitis. The conclusion of the investigators was that the gastrointestinal disease and associated loss of mental skills was likely associated with vaccination.

Wakefield knew that when the paper was published he would be in for a fight. But he wasn't going to back away. "I decided that I was going to review all the safety studies about measles and measles containing vaccines because if I was going to get into a fight, I needed to know what I was talking about. If I was going to challenge the status quo and say things that might have an adverse effect on vaccine uptake, I had to know what I was talking about. So I read all the papers, and I was appalled. I was absolutely appalled that the quality of the safety studies of the single and combined MMR vaccine in particular, and then I wrote to my colleagues in advance of the paper coming out and I said this is going to attract a lot of attention in the media and I have to tell you that I have now read all these studies. I have written a 250 page report which I'm very happy for you to read and I cannot support the continued use of the MMR vaccine. I will continue vigorously to support the use of the single vaccine but I cannot support the use of the MMR."

Wakefield was not arguing against vaccination in general: he still recommended that children receive the measles vaccine. He was warning against the dangers of the combined measles, mumps, and rubella (MMR) vaccine.

THE DRUG EMPIRE STRIKES BACK

Over the next six years Wakefield and colleagues published 19 more papers in various medical journals on the relationship between gastrointestinal health and developmental disorders. Yet it was the 1998 *Lancet* paper that suggested the connection between vaccination and autism that got Wakefield into trouble.

After the publication of this paper, many parents fearful that their children may develop autism refused vaccinations. In 1995 before Wakefield's paper was written, 95 percent of children in London received the MMR vaccine. After the publication of the 1998 paper, the number of MMR vaccines declined to as much as 50 percent in some parts of London. Vaccine sales plummeted. The drug companies started to worry as vaccine sales began to decline.

Something had to be done about Wakefield, drug company executives all agreed. His work must be stopped and this study discredited. A clandestine plan was set into motion to stop Wakefield from doing any further research on the subject and to destroy his reputation.

Apparently, after experiencing significant pressure from drug companies, the UK's Department of Health contacted the dean of the medical school at Royal Free and tried to close down Wakefield's research, including the clinic caring for autistic children. The reason they gave was that it was unethical to have children with autism undergoing treatment that was still controversial. It didn't matter that children were improving and regaining the ability to speak and interact with others. The research had to be shut down.

Rumors circulated that Wakefield was only using these children so he could act as an expert witness in litigation against vaccine manufacturers. Critics claimed that no other researchers were able to verify Wakefield's findings, implying that his work was flawed. This was a lie perpetuated by drug company pitchmen and their cohorts to deceive the public, discredit his work, and tarnish his reputation. In fact, Wakefield's work was verified by independent researchers in the United States, Canada, Venezuela, and Italy.

To counter Wakefield's findings, the drug companies sponsored new studies to prove that vaccines did not cause autism. His *Lancet* paper was carefully examined for any possible flaw. These investigations provided further (questionable) evidence that Wakefield's work was flawed or even intentionally misleading. He was charged with professional misconduct for fabricating the data in the *Lancet* study.

A freelance journalist by the name of Brian Deer took up the cause of the pharmaceutical industry and began an investigation resulting in a series of vicious public attacks against Wakefield and his colleagues. Deer claimed that the children in Wakefield's study were abused by invasive medical diagnostics and examinations. He fabricated a story in which Wakefield plotted to create a legal case against the vaccine manufacturers in order to destroy the public's trust in the safety of their vaccines and then launch his own vaccine onto the market. In the process, innocent children were abused in order to bring about this diabolical plan. The allegations were ridiculous.

There was a great deal of pressure put on Royal Free Hospital to stop Wakefield's work. Because of the allegations against him, Wakefield was dismissed from Royal Free and eventually his license to practice medicine was revoked. The editors of the *Lancet* retracted his article, branding it a fraud. It is interesting that the article never actually stated that vaccines caused autism—it only suggested the possibility. Yet that was enough to irk the pharmaceutical companies to pressure the journal to remove it. Discredited and unlicensed, Wakefield was unable to find suitable employment in the UK and was forced to move to the United States.

The pharmaceutical industry was successful in destroying Wakefield's credibility, his work, and his career and even drove him out of the country. This is what they do to those who pose a threat to their profits. It serves as a warning to other physicians who are tempted to blow the whistle on the pharmaceutical industry. Of the 13 co-authors of the *Lancet* study, 10 were coerced into admitting the study was flawed and renounced their involvement. Wakefield and two others remained steadfast despite the severe persecution and threats.

PERSECUTION OF TROUBLEMAKERS

This wasn't the first time a physician's credibility and career was destroyed by the pharmaceutical industry. Recently pharmaceutical giant Merck was brought to court for concealing evidence that showed that their now withdrawn painkiller Vioxx caused fatal heart attacks. Confidential company emails leaked to the public were presented as evidence. In these emails Merck identified certain doctors who had criticized the painkiller. The company emails described plans to "neutralize" and "discredit" these doctors. The memos go on to say, "We may need to seek them out and destroy them where they live." Thirty-six physicians were targeted for neutralization with recommended tactics to accomplish the task.[2]

Neutralizing, discrediting, and destroying the creditability of those who pose a threat to profits appears to be a standard practice in the drug industry. In another case, Pfizer was sued for $2 billion over unethical and illegal testing of their meningitis drug Trovan. To block the lawsuit the company tried to discredit and blackmail the attorney general who was prosecuting the case.

In 1996 Pfizer began testing the unproven drug at a field hospital in Nigeria where children were taken to be treated for meningitis. The company never obtained authorization from the Nigerian government to test the new drug. Pfizer never told the children or their parents that they were part of an experiment. The parents assumed they were receiving proper medical care for their children. Testing experimental drugs on anyone without their knowledge or consent is unethical and illegal. Pfizer's experiment turned out to be a disaster. The drug killed 11 children and left dozens disabled. Ironically, Trovan was approved by the FDA for use in the United States in 1998, but for adults only. However, after reports of liver failure quickly surfaced, its use was promptly restricted to only emergency cases in adults. The European Union banned it entirely in 1999.

When investigators uncovered the Tronvan testing on children, parents were outraged and a lawsuit was filed by Nigeria's Attorney General Michael Aondoakaa. In an attempt to avoid the lawsuit Pfizer hired private investigators to uncover corruption links to the Attorney General in an attempt to blackmail him and force him to drop the case. If he didn't stop the lawsuit, they were determined to discredit him and destroy his life. The lawsuit was not dropped. Investigators hired by Pfizer passed their information to the media damaging Aondoakaa's character. Whether the allegations were true or not isn't known. However, such accusations don't have to be true to destroy a person's reputation. In response, Nigerian President Goodluck Jonathan removed Aondoakaa from his post. Pfizer's plot to discredit and destroy Aondoakaa was later uncovered in company memos leaked to the public.

No one is safe from drug company vengeance regardless of academic achievement or honors, as evidenced in the case of Australian obstetrician Dr. William McBride. In the 1960s McBride achieved fame for exposing the bad side of the drug thalidomide, which was used by women to treat nausea and vomiting during pregnancy. He showed that thalidomide caused severe birth defects. Because of McBride's research, thalidomide was taken off the market. During his career he received many honors including being named Man of the Year (1962), Australian of the Year (1962), Commander of the Order of the British Empire (1969), Father of the Year (1972), and Officer of the Order of Australia (1977)—Australia's highest honor given to civilians for meritorious service. Despite his honors, he was looked upon as a troublemaker by the drug industry and someone to keep an eye on.

In 1981 McBride published a study suggesting another morning sickness drug Bendectin (Debendox) also caused deformities in infants. The drug maker didn't want this product to end up the same way thalidomide had and wasted no time in protecting its interests. McBride received a surprisingly harsh backlash. His paper was heavily criticized as being full of methodological flaws and in some cases even fraudulent. Other researchers came forward and claimed they could find no link between the drug and birth defects. They said the drug was harmless. McBride was accused of falsifying his data and was eventually discredited as a fraud. His medical license was revoked.

Disgraced, his voice of warning was permanently silenced. Why would someone with his spotless reputation and high achievements suddenly stoop to fraud? What would he gain? It doesn't make sense unless his downfall was a carefully orchestrated plan. Who would stand to gain the most if McBride were silenced? Obviously, the drug company had a lot at stake. Privately, McBride asserted that big international drug companies were behind his downfall, and that he was a victim of a conspiracy. "It's all very well to talk about perfect scientific protocol," he once said. "Drug companies have a vested interest in keeping their drugs on the market. I have a vested interest in protecting unborn babies. It's as simple as that."

DISINFORMATION CAMPAIGN

After the publication of Wakefield's paper people everywhere started to question the safety of vaccinations. The pharmaceutical industry launched a disinformation campaign to brainwash the public and coerce government policy makers into believing vaccines have no effect on autism and are completely safe. They are even pushing to get vaccines mandated by law, forcing everyone to be vaccinated and removing the freedom of choice from parents. The first step was to attack Wakefield and discredit him. The second step was to sponsor studies that would exonerate thimerosal, a mercury-based preservative used in vaccines, as well as the MMR vaccine from any role in causing autism. The pharmaceutical companies and their allies in government and medicine found a number of scientists willing to produce these studies for the right price.

One of the central figures behind the vaccination debate was Danish psychiatrist Dr. Poul Thorsen. Thorsen headed up a research center at Aarhus University in Denmark called the North Atlantic Neuro-Epidemiology Alliances (NANEA) specifically to study issues such as vaccines and autism. Under Thorsen's direction the NANEA produced two major studies that purported to show that mercury used in vaccines and the MMR vaccine itself did not cause autism. These studies formed the foundation for reports from the pharmaceutical industry and governmental agencies concluding that neither thimerosal nor MMR were responsible for causing autism. In one of his papers he showed that removing mercury (thimerosal) from the vaccines actually increased the incidence of autism. One might conclude from this study that the use of mercury in vaccines protects against autism! This is an absurd conclusion since mercury is a known neurotoxin. Nevertheless, his studies were used as proof to refute Wakefield's claims. The Centers for Disease Control and Prevention (CDC) relied on Thorsen's studies as the principal evidence for the safety of mercury-laced vaccines.[3]

However, it turns out that after closer examination these studies were found to be seriously flawed. In fact, the data was purposely misrepresented to produce a fraudulent outcome favorable to vaccine manufacturers.

Thorsen's dubious character was further unveiled by officials at Aarhus University who disbanded the NANEA and charged him with theft and breach of contract. Thorsen, it was discovered, forged documents supposedly from the CDC to obtain the release of $2 million from Aarhus University. Thorsen then abruptly resigned in March 2009 and disappeared with the money. Also, while working fulltime at Aarhus University, Thorsen held a full time position at Drexel University in Philadelphia, collecting salaries from both universities. This was a direct violation of his contract with Aarhus which forbade outside employment. Drexel University has since severed their relationship with Thorsen and removed all references to him from their website.

Despite his questionable character and the fact that his studies on vaccines and autism were found to be fraudulent, they are still cited by the media and drug company spokespersons as reassurance that vaccines are safe. Based on a handful of questionable studies, including those from Thorsen, officials at the US Institutes of Medicine have stated "the evidence now favors rejection of a relationship between thimerosal and autism."[4]

One of the world's most outspoken vaccine promoters is Paul Offit, MD, with the Children's Hospital of Philadelphia. Dr. Offit has taken upon himself the unofficial title of spokesperson for the vaccine industry. He also serves on the advisory board of vaccine manufacturer Merck and holds a patent for his own vaccine. If your children have been vaccinated in the last few years, they probably have his vaccine coursing through their veins right now. He has written numerous papers on vaccines and a number of books debunking the association between vaccines and autism.

Offit's quest to counter fears of vaccination is so extreme that at times his statements defy reason. For example, he has stated that vaccines are "safer than vitamins." How could a mixture of viruses, mercury, formaldehyde, and other toxic chemicals injected directly into the bloodstream be safer than a vitamin? He also claims that vaccines are so safe and that an infant can receive 10,000 vaccines in a single day without risk of side effects! He later modified that statement by saying it was probably "closer to 100,000."[5] He wasn't joking, nor was he intentionally exaggerating. This statement is based on a theoretical study he did looking at the genes responsible for antibody production and the number humans should be able to produce. This is entirely mathematical connivery. In the real world if you take MMR, for example, and add just one other vaccine, such as the chickenpox (varicella) vaccine, you *double* the rate of serious adverse reactions.[6] So the idea that a child could receive 10,000 or 100,000 vaccines in one day without harm is ludicrous.

Some parents refer to Offit as Dr. Proffit, suggesting financial interests in his own vaccine and his position with Merck are the real motivating forces behind his attacks on Wakefield and his staunch campaign for vaccination, including his push for mandatory vaccination of all children. He earns a royalty from his vaccine and has admitted that "it's like winning the lottery," but has not disclosed the precise amount.[5] We do know, though, that the Children's Hospital of Philadelphia where he works received $182 million in royalties from Merck for Offit's vaccine.

Offit not only encourages vaccination, but is working to have the government force children to be vaccinated by law—no exceptions. If parents don't comply, their children will be forcibly taken away and vaccinated. Parents could even be charged with child abuse or child endangerment, and their children could be sent to live with foster parents appointed by the state. The parent's right to raise their children as they see fit would be taken away. Parents would have no choice but to comply.

Too shocking to believe? Think again. This type of thing is already beginning to happen. In ten states, if a teacher feels your child has ADHD and wanted your child put on Ritalin, if you refuse to allow this, the state could come into your home, take away your child, and charge you with child neglect. Forced vaccinations are also beginning to take place. New Jersey has passed a law requiring all children attending daycare or preschool to get flu shots every year, in addition to all the other childhood vaccines. In Prince George's county Maryland children are not allowed to attend school unless they are vaccinated for chicken pox and hepatitis B. If parents do not get their children vaccinated, they are not allowed to attend school—but if they don't go to school, the parents face the risk of going to jail for breaking truancy laws. While the county has no legal right to force vaccinations, they can accomplish the same end through their truancy laws. The Children's Hospital of Philadelphia, where Dr. Offit works, has mandated that all its employees must receive annual flu shots. Every employee—doctors, nurses, orderlies, secretaries, kitchen staff, and janitors—are required to be vaccinated or face termination.

These types of things aren't just happening in the US but in Europe as well. Recently two sets of parents in Belgium were given a five month prison sentence for failing to vaccinate their children against polio. Each parent was also fined 4,100 euros ($8,000). The parents were offered the option of avoiding prison if their children were vaccinated. In addition to Belgium, France also has strict mandatory polio vaccination laws.[7] Where is it going to end? This can only be viewed as a prelude to a much larger campaign that, in the future, may end up forcing dozens of vaccines on your children whether they attend public school or not and may dictate whether they will be allowed to enter college, get a job, or even travel.

Can you imagine the billions of dollars drug companies and vaccine patent owners, such as Offit, would stand to make if all children were forced to be vaccinated? Offit claims his motivation is for the good of the children. It's not about the money, he says, it's all about the children.

Because many educated parents are now opting not to vaccinate their children, Offit warns this will lead to a dangerous resurgence of infectious disease. He believes parents should be compelled to vaccinate regardless of personal convictions or beliefs. Offit also contends that unvaccinated children pose a risk not only to themselves but to everyone. He and other vaccine promoters criticize parents who opt not to vaccinate their children by labeling them "unfit parents," "a danger to society," and even "baby killers." Actress Amanda Peet, who works as a spokeswoman for the vaccine advocacy group Every Child by Two, calls parents who refuse to vaccinate their children "parasites," implying they rely on the other children's immunity to protect their own.[8] Such words are used by vaccine proponents to depict concerned parents as selfish, ill-informed, and even evil in an apparent attempt to sway public sentiment against them. Name-calling is always easier than presenting the facts, especially when the facts are not on your side.

What about all the parents who claim their children developed autism right after vaccination? Offit says it's just a coincidence. It is just a coincidence that thousands of normally developing children digress into autism immediately after being vaccinated. Offit says that autism normally shows itself between the ages of 1-3 and this just happens to be the time when many children are being vaccinated. There is no link, he says, it's just a coincidence. If that's true, why doesn't autism ever occur just *before* the vaccination? Is that just a coincidence too?

When parents say they've reversed their children's autism using diet, dietary supplements, and other natural therapies, Dr. Offit claims that this too is just a coincidence. He himself admits he has never successfully treated any child with autism. He doesn't think it can be done and criticizes parents for even trying! "Instead of helping," says Offit, "these therapies can hurt those who are most vulnerable…They undermine childhood vaccination programs that have saved millions of lives."[9] According to Offit, parents of autistic children should not seek treatment but just accept their fate and continue getting vaccinated.

Based on a mere handful of studies by such people as discredited researcher Poul Thorsen and others, Offit contends that there is no need for further discussion on the matter. The idea that vaccines cause autism has "been clearly disproved," he says, and we should put the matter to rest. How can a few questionable studies, some of which are known to be fraudulent, provide clear proof? It is impossible to prove a negative—that is, it is impossible to conclusively prove that vaccines or thimerosal do not cause autism. Statements implying that no further safety studies are necessary are made by those who are afraid that continued research will eventually uncover the truth and prove them wrong. Real seekers of truth welcome any additional information.

Where do the studies that seem to exonerate vaccines come from? The answer is simple. They come from the vaccine makers and their allies. Drug companies can't be directly associated with the research themselves, as this conflict of interest would be too obvious. So they have ways around it, ways to produce studies with results to their liking that still appear to be published by independent researchers. One way is for the university professors and researchers to simply not disclose their relationship to the vaccine industry, though many actually work as paid consultants. Several of the published pro-vaccine articles were written by these "independent" consultants. Another method is medical ghostwriting. While it is no secret, few people outside the medical establishment are aware of this dishonest practice.

Here is how medical ghostwriting works. Drug companies hire people with scientific backgrounds, often PhDs, to stay in the shadows and, using data supplied by the companies, crank out glowing reports for their products. The drug companies then find physicians and university professors who are willing to put their names on the studies as the authors. This is good for the doctors because it not only pays well but also helps boost their prestige and advance their careers without actually doing any work.

Medical ghostwriters are given an outline from the drug companies telling them what to write and what data to use. Negative data is not provided. The purpose of these articles is to make the study sound as positive as possible in order to gain favorable media publicity, encourage doctors to prescribe the drugs, and, in the case of vaccines, ease people's fears and convince government bodies to mandate their use. Adverse side effects are often completely ignored, and safety studies can be grossly distorted. This is how dangerous drugs such as Phen-fen, Baycol, and Vioxx were given approval by the FDA. Safety studies for these drugs were all peer-reviewed, approved, and published in leading medical journals. Only after hundreds of users suffered permanent damage or died were these drugs taken off the market.

Medical ghostwriters typically make over $100,000 a year. Drug companies may pay as much as $20,000 for a single article that makes its way into a prestigious medical journal like the *Lancet*, *British Medical Journal*, or the *New England Journal of Medicine*.

As many as a dozen coauthors may sign their names to these bogus studies. Some of these "authors" may not have even read the studies they supposedly have written. Drug companies prefer high-profile authors; the more renowned the writer, the greater the credibility for the article. This explains why some doctors can be listed as authors or coauthors to a dozen or more studies in a single year. In reality, he or she may not have done any actual work on the articles or the studies.

"What appear to be scientific articles are really infomercials," says Dr. David Healy of Cardiff University School of Medicine, Wales.[10] Unfortunately, universities get entangled with the drug companies as well. Drug companies fund research. Universities thrive on the prestige and money generated from this research. Consequently, researchers are pressured to produce favorable results and minimize unfavorable results. The consequences of publishing the facts, regardless of the sponsor, can have drastic repercussions. Dr. Healy lost his position at the University of Toronto after he criticized the drug company Eli Lilly for suppressing evidence that its drug Prozac leads to increased deaths from suicide.

Dr. Healy is a high-profile researcher with 110 peer-reviewed papers and 13 books to his credit. For this reason, he is a prime candidate as an author for ghostwritten studies. He was approached by one company to write an article based on his previous studies, which he was willing to do. "To my big surprise," says Healy, "I had an e-mail shortly afterwards." It stated: "In order to reduce your workload, we have had our ghostwriters produce a first draft based on your published work. I attach it here..."

Healy wasn't comfortable with the glowing review of the drug, so he crafted his own article. The drug company wrote back and said he'd missed something key. In the end, the drug company put someone else's name on the article.

Healy was spooked by the deception. He says it goes beyond being misleading—it can be dangerous. He's seen a lot of articles on drugs, like anti-depressants, that don't mention serious problems. "People and children, for instance, that have been put on these drugs, actually committing suicide or becoming suicidal. But the finished articles actually don't reflect this at all."

Essentially *all* of the major drug companies hire medical ghostwriters to produce favorable journal articles on their products. Healy has seen internal drug company documents containing lists of scientific papers that were written up, ready to go. The only thing missing were the names of high-profile doctors to be listed as the authors. This is routine practice in the pharmaceutical industry. Healy estimates that 50 percent of the drug studies published in medical journals are ghostwritten. You can't tell which ones are legitimate and which are not. Although authors must declare if they have any competing interests that would influence their results, doctors who sign their names to ghostwritten articles do not reveal their relationship with the drug company, so they appear to be impartial researchers.

Whenever a drug receives unfavorable press, drug makers are quick to crank out favorable studies written by ghostwriters to counter the bad publicity. For example, Wyeth Pharmaceuticals flooded medical journals with some 40 ghostwritten articles penned by prominent physicians who sold their name for cash in an all-out effort to offset the scientific evidence linking its female hormone replacement drug, Prempro, to breast cancer.

The sudden flood of studies that mysteriously surfaced immediately after Andrew Wakefield had his medical license revoked appears to be just another drug company sponsored misinformation campaign bent on deceiving the public and health care professionals.

How can you tell which studies are legitimate and which are not? Simple, just follow the money. When a study comes out that shows a relationship between vaccines and autism or some other health problem, there is nothing to gain. Money can't be made by discouraging the use of medicines, unless other costly options are recommended. But when a study shows vaccines and other drugs to be essentially harmless, beware. The drug companies, patent owners, pharmacies, and others who stand to profit are standing in the shadows smacking their lips.

This doesn't mean that all studies that evaluate the safety and effectiveness of drugs are fraudulent or misleading. Yet, the vast majority probably are. Those studies that purport to find no link between autism and vaccines are highly questionable. And when anyone says something like "No further studies need to be done" you know for sure further studies are definitely needed.

The drug cartel can't be trusted and they have the criminal history to prove it. AllBusiness.com's Top 100 Corporate Criminals includes 19 drug companies. Bribery, fraud, price-fixing, kickbacks paid to doctors, cover-ups of fatal side effects, environmental violations, and illegal sales activities are all just a part of doing business for the pharmaceutical industry. From 1991 to 2010 drug companies have been involved in 165 cases of criminal wrongdoing resulting in $19.8 *billion* in penalties. Four companies (GlaxoSmithKline, Pfizer, Eli Lilly, and Schering-Plough) accounted for more than half of all the financial penalties imposed on drug companies over the past two decades.[11] Would you trust your child's health to a corrupt industry that blatantly disregards people's health for the sake of profit?

The vaccine controversy still rages. Drug companies are among the richest in the world. They have the money and power to manipulate "medical" studies, buy politicians, and influence public health policies. They have succeeded in flooding the media and the Internet with pro-vaccine propaganda and in discrediting Andrew Wakefield and others who have stood up to corporate corruption and deceit. You will see both pro and con arguments about vaccines in the media. The arguments can be convincing and cause confusion and doubts, especially when high-profile public health officials or celebrities promote one side or the other. However, the controversy boils down to drug companies versus parents. How do you tell who is right? First, use common sense. Is injecting virulent viruses, bacteria, mercury, and other toxins directly into the bloodstream healthy? Does it improve health? Second, follow the money. Who stands to benefit the most from the information presented—the drug companies or the children?

3 | Do Vaccines Cause Autism?

ARE CERTAIN PEOPLE PREPROGRAMMED TO BE AUTISTIC?

Most doctors and public health officials claim that autism is a "genetic" disorder. This is the excuse they give when they have no idea what causes an illness. This is the position loudly espoused by drug makers in an attempt to divert attention away from vaccines.

As proof, they point to studies of identical twins: if one is autistic, the likelihood that the other twin will have some form of autism is about 60 percent.[1] However, if autism is genetic, then 100 percent of identical twins would become autistic since they share the exact same genes. So this is actually proof that autism is *not* genetic.

Vaccine promoters continue to argue that autism is caused by genetics and claim that it has always existed. They argue that the perceived increase in recent years is actually the result of better diagnosis. This argument is ridiculous seeing that the symptoms of autism are unmistakable, especially to parents who witness normally developing children suddenly regress socially, verbally, and developmentally. Most cases of autism are clustered within a single generation of children. If autism is genetic and therefore has always been around, then where are all the 50- and 60-year-old autistics? Even with better diagnosis, these older autistics would be identified.

After decades of intense research, no clear autism gene has ever been found.[2] Some researchers have claimed to have found genes that might possibly be related to autism, but less than 1 percent of those with autism have these genes. So what causes autism in the other 99 percent?

Despite the drug industry's push to convince the world genetics are to blame, the history of the disorder does not support this assumption. If it were genetic, there would be evidence of the disorder in previous generations, yet most parents of autistic children have no history of autism in their families. The incidence of autism is increasing so rapidly it cannot possibly be explained by genetics. If there were an "autism gene," why has it suddenly burst on the scene out of nowhere? Only one generation ago the disorder was virtually unknown. Today 1 in every 68 families in the US has an autistic child. It is now one of the most commonly diagnosed childhood disorders. Geneticists point out that genetic disorders do not suddenly increase in such astronomical proportions. Autism has come out of nowhere and is now at epidemic proportions. Its appearance is more like that of a plague, indicating some environmental cause. In fact, an environmental cause is the only sensible explanation.

This is the position of most geneticists. The Director of the US National Human Genome Research Institute, Francis S. Collins, MD, PhD, testified to the US House of Representatives Committee in May 2006: "Recent increases in chronic diseases like diabetes, childhood asthma, obesity, or autism cannot be due to major shifts in the human gene pool as those changes take much more time to occur. They must be due to changes in the environment."[3]

What are those environmental changes? Environmental conditions include diet, drugs and vaccines, infections, lifestyle habits, and exposure to natural and manmade toxins. One of the biggest changes over the past couple of decades is the dramatic increase in childhood vaccinations. Do vaccines cause autism? Let's look at their safety record.

HOW SAFE ARE VACCINES?

Sunil Sharma, a textiles merchant from Ghaziabad, India, couldn't believe what happened. Sunil took his nine-month-old twin daughters to a local nursing home for a routine MMR vaccination. Fifteen minutes after the shots both children began gasping for breath. Their eyes rolled back and their bodies wrenched violently from seizures. Within minutes both girls were dead. After several more children died following the vaccination, once again the country's immunization program ground to a halt. This wasn't the first time a series of deaths occurred during a vaccination program. In India this was the third vaccine disaster that year. The other two disasters involved deaths and adverse reactions accompanying the Pneumococcal (HPV) vaccine and the Haemophilus influenzae type b (Hib) vaccine, two routine childhood vaccines.

That same year Australian officials suspended flu vaccinations for children under the age of five after 99 children suffered dangerously high fevers and convulsions (severe seizures) following the immunization. Although seizures are a known side effect, the vaccine was causing 50 times more than would be expected. An analysis published in the journal *Eurosurveillance* calculated that this vaccine caused two to three times more illness than it might have prevented.

A very similar flu vaccine was used later that year to vaccinate tens of thousands of children throughout North America. Despite the warnings from Australia, the vaccine was still used. It was no surprise when the Food and Drug Administration (FDA) started reporting a high number of seizures in children. The seizures occurred within 24 hours after receiving the vaccination. The maker of the vaccine, Sanofi Pasteur, issued a statement emphasizing that there was no clear link between the flu shot and the seizures. In other words, all the seizures immediately following the vaccinations were coincidences. The package insert prepared by Sanofi Pasteur that accompanies the vaccine specifically listed seizures as a possible adverse effect of the drug. They were very aware of the potential problem. Despite the rash of seizures, the FDA refused to stop the vaccination program as was done in Australia, but continued to encourage parents to have their children vaccinated according to schedule.

In Finland and Sweden the flu vaccine program was suspended because it was linked to narcolepsy, a sleep disorder. In Finland a staggering 300 percent increase in cases of this rare brain disorder was reported, all in children who had received the vaccine.

In the UK after an 18-year legal battle, damages were finally awarded to a mother whose son suffered severe brain damage after receiving an MMR vaccine. Robert Fletcher was 13 months old when he received the vaccination. Eighteen years later he is still unable to talk, stand unaided, or feed himself. While not autistic, he is severely mentally retarded, endures frequent epileptic seizures, and requires round-the-clock care from his parents. A medical assessment panel consisting of two physicians and a barrister (lawyer) concluded that MMR was to blame.

"My husband John and I have battled for 18 years for the cause of Robert's disability to be officially recognized," says Robert's mother. "We were told the vaccine was perfectly safe. Like most people, we trusted what the doctors and nurses were putting to us…what matters is the recognition that MMR was the reason this happened."

The above events are just a small sampling of the many vaccine related stories reported in the news during a single year (2010). Unfortunately, stories like these are not unusual but repeat themselves year after year.

Many parents view vaccinations as just a routine part of childhood and don't think much about it. They are conditioned to believe that vaccines are totally safe and even necessary in order to avoid illness.

No vaccine is completely safe. Every time a child is vaccinated there is a risk of adverse reactions. It is not uncommon for a child to become ill after getting a shot. If the child is relatively healthy the reaction is minor and only temporary—a fever and slight discomfort for a few days. However, in some cases it can lead to severe complications, including death. According to the manufacturer's package inserts, vaccines given to infants can cause any number of adverse side effects including encephalopathy (brain damage), thrombocytopenia (hemorrhaging or bleeding in the brain), and hyporesponsive episodes (muscle limpness and unresponsiveness). After all, 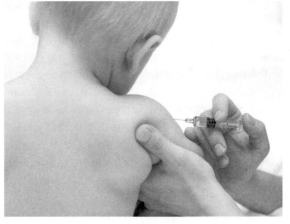 vaccines contain disease-causing viruses and an assortment of other microorganisms and chemicals to purposely activate the immune system into a feverish state of intensity. Injecting these toxins into the bloodstream is bound to have some effect. Unfortunately, the brain is one of the most affected organs.

We are repeatedly told that vaccines are safe even for infants. Let's look at the officially recognized and documented side effects acknowledged by the drug industry for just the MMR vaccine. This data was obtained from the www.drugs.com website:

Immediately following a MMR vaccination a child could expect to experience one or more of the following: redness, pain, swelling or lump at the sight of the injection as well as headache, dizziness, fever, joint or muscle pain, nausea, vomiting, diarrhea, sore throat, cough, and irritability. These are the most common reactions and are even expected to one degree or another.

Less common but more serious reactions, which may occur anytime within 30 days of the vaccination, include:

Encephalitis. Brain swelling and inflammation.

Encephalopathy. Brain damage with symptoms ranging from mild alterations in mental state to dementia, seizures, and coma.

Subacute sclerosing panencephalitis. Infection in the brain caused by the measles vaccine virus.

Guillain-Barre syndrome. Autoimmune disease in which the body's immune system attacks its own nervous system causing nerve damage (tingling or numbness, muscle weakness, and paralysis).

Convulsions (seizures). Abnormal electrical activity in the brain that causes violent uncontrolled muscle spasms and shaking.

Ataxia. Loss of coordination due to the brain's failure to regulate the body's posture and movements.

Polyneuritis. Inflammation of nerves in many parts of the body accompanied by pain, muscle wasting, and paralysis.

Polyneuropathy. Chronic inflammation and swelling of the peripheral nerves leading to loss of strength and sensation.

Ocular palsy. Nerve disorder that causes paralysis of the muscles that coordinate eye movement and position. Causes visual difficulties including double vision.

Paresthesia. Nerve disorder resulting in a burning, prickling, itching, or tingling sensation in the skin.

Aseptic meningitis. Inflammation of the linings of the brain (meninges), usually caused by a virus from the vaccine.

Vasculitis. Inflammation of the blood vessels.

Erythema multiforme. A disease of the skin and mucous membranes that causes a rash accompanied by blisters and ulcers.

Urticaria. Another name for hives—raised, itchy areas of skin.

Pancreatitis. Inflammation of the pancreas. Causes severe abdominal pain. May be accompanied by nausea, vomiting, and fever.

Diabetes type 1. Autoimmune disorder of the pancreas which destroys cells that secrete insulin.

Orchitis. Inflammation of the testis.

Thrombocytopenia. Blood disorder associated with abnormal bleeding.

Purpura. Bleeding within the skin.

Regional lymphadenopathy. Disease of the lymph nodes.

Arthralgia/arthritis. Joint pain, inflammation, and swelling.

Myalgia. Muscle pain.

Retinitis. Inflammation of the retina of the eyes manifested by night blindness and gradual loss of peripheral vision.

Optic neuritis. Inflammation of the optic nerve which may cause partial or complete blindness.

Conjunctivitis. Inflammation of the conjunctiva—the thin membrane covering the white of the eye.

Otitis media. Inflammation and pain in the middle ear usually caused by an infection. Commonly referred to as an earache.

Deafness. Partial or complete hearing loss.

Pneumonitis. Inflammation of the lungs. Causes difficulty breathing and is often accompanied by a cough.

Rhinitis. Inflammation of the nasal passages. Usually associated with nasal discharge.

Panniculitis. Inflammation of fat tissue, especially in the abdominal wall.

Atypical measles. Measles infection caused by vaccination.

Syncope. Partial or complete loss of consciousness caused by a reduction of blood flow and lack of oxygen to the brain.

Death. Many of the above conditions can become serious enough to cause death.

This list does not include the various allergic reactions which may also cause additional symptoms.

Note the multitude of symptoms that affect the brain and nervous system. It is apparent that vaccines can wreck havoc on brain and nerve tissue. It doesn't take a brain surgeon to recognize a possible link to autism. In fact, Dr. Julie Gerberding, the president of Merck Vaccines and former director of the CDC, has admitted that autistic conditions can result from encephalopathy following vaccination.[4]

As a side note, it's interesting that executives of the major drug companies are often former employees of the CDC, as is the case with Dr. Gerberding. When CDC officials retire they are often given high paying positions with drug companies as a means to reward them for their faithful (and industry friendly) service in the CDC. The reverse also happens. Drug company executives are hired to take high ranking positions in the CDC. Some of these executives jump from the drug industry to the CDC and then later hop back to a plush job in the drug industry. This close relationship between the drug industry and the CDC makes one wonder whose interests are these CDC directors looking out for—the public's or the drug makers'? As the controlling force in the CDC, they wield enormous power in influencing government policies concerning vaccinations. This may explain why children in the United States receive more vaccines than any other country in the world—some 12 to 18 more vaccinations than children in most European countries. It may also explain the senseless vaccination of all newborns for hepatitis B—an adult disease transmitted by unprotected sex or sharing of dirty needles. What's next, childhood vaccines to treat menopause, osteoporosis, or male pattern baldness?

As you look at the many adverse side effects listed above, keep in mind that this list is only for the MMR vaccine. Each of the different vaccines is associated with a similar list of adverse symptoms. In addition, there are many more symptoms associated with each of the vaccines that are not listed but have been reported by parents and doctors. Since 1990 the CDC has collected reports of adverse reactions resulting from vaccinations. This database is called the Vaccine Adverse Event Reporting System (VAERS). You can access the database yourself at http://vaers.hhs.gov/index. On this website you can report adverse reactions or look up those reported by other parents and doctors. Understanding how to navigate around this website is a little confusing, so you will need to invest some time if you go there.

A look at the VAERS database shows thousands of reported events every year involving hundreds of symptoms, most of which are repeated in case after case. Many of the symptoms listed—such as attention disturbance, abnormal behavior, personality change, digestive troubles, and seizures—are all common features associated with autism.

Often children will do well during the actual shot but later develop such excruciating pain that they scream with a high-pitched cry as if being tortured. The crying continues unceasingly for several days. No amount of attention or coddling will ease the pain. The children periodically fall asleep out of sheer exhaustion, but wake up screaming again. If you ask your pediatrician about this he will say it's a "normal" reaction after a vaccination and not to worry about it. They even have a name for it. It's called an *encephalitic cry*, meaning it is caused by inflammation and swelling in the brain. The swelling causes so much pressure to build up in the brain that the pain is excruciating. The child is literally being tortured. Encephalitis isn't harmless! It can lead to serious brain damage.

This list of recognized adverse reactions is limited to symptoms occurring within 30 days of vaccination. But some adverse reactions may not become evident until months or years later and may appear to be totally unrelated to the vaccination. If a vaccine left a child with ADHD or a learning disability, it may not be diagnosed until he or she was old enough to enter school. Vaccines could also set a child up to develop an autoimmune disorder such as type 1 diabetes, asthma, celiac disease, rheumatoid arthritis, or multiple sclerosis, which may not be diagnosed for years. If the vaccine contained live viruses (e.g., chicken pox, measles, mumps, and rubella) the infection could remain in the body for years. These organisms could set up residence in certain areas of the body such as the intestinal tract, the joints, or the brain where they could lie undetected or cause local chronic irritation and inflammation. For example, one healthy 3½ year old girl developed encephalitis 20 months after a chicken pox vaccination. Molecular analysis confirmed the virus strain from the vaccine was the cause.[5] If the virus takes up residence in the digestive tract it could lead to chronic irritable bowel disease.[6] In the joints it can cause chronic arthritis.[7-23]

Every time a child is vaccinated he or she is at risk of developing any one or more of these side effects. Is it any wonder that an infant could cry incessantly for days after a vaccination? Is it worth the risk? Doctors say yes because the risk of harm is very small, but when parents complain that their son or daughter had a serious adverse reaction, such as convulsions, autism, or SIDS, these same doctors claim it's only a coincidence. They brush aside serious consequences, refusing to acknowledge the obvious and admit that the risk is actually far greater than they lead us to believe.

WHAT'S IN VACCINES?

We are led to believe that vaccines merely contain dead (meaning "harmless") viruses or other microorganisms in a saline solution. When the body detects the inactive virus our immune system reacts as if the virus is alive and starts producing antibodies against the "invader." This way the body builds a natural immunity to the virus without experiencing an actual infection. Years ago that may have been the case, but today vaccines are mass-produced, usually months or even years in advance of their use, and are primed to evoke a more hardy immune reaction to assure a longer lasting effect. This requires the addition of a number of other ingredients that can have very serious consequences on our health.

The list of ingredients in the vaccines used today would turn anybody's stomach. The most crucial component in any vaccine, of course, is the disease-causing virus for which immunity is desired. Viruses are obtained from body fluids (blood, urine, pus, etc.) from infected individuals and grown in animal tissues such as rat brains, monkey kidneys, and chicken embryos. Sometimes live viruses are used. Whether live or dead, the virus is collected and combined with an assortment of preservatives and adjuvants—toxic substances that boost the immune response to the vaccine. The finished vaccine will contain some combination of the following ingredients: formaldehyde (disinfectant), mercury (thimerosal), aluminum (a known neurotoxin), ethylene glycol (antifreeze), benzethonium, methylparaben (fungicide), polysorbate 80, glutaraldehyde, neomycin sulfate, monosodium glutamate (MSG), mycobacteria (bacteria used to trigger a greater immune response), and various other chemicals as well as remnants of dead animal (pig, monkey, dog, etc.) blood and tissues in which the viruses were cultured. The vaccine is then sealed in a sterile package for your protection.

Contamination is another issue. In 2009 drug maker Baxter International shipped their new seasonal flu vaccine to Europe for distribution to 18 countries. Before shipping the vaccine to the various clinics, health officials in the Czech Republic tested a batch on ferrets. To their shock, all the ferrets died. On investigation, they found that the vaccine was contaminated with the deadly avian flu virus (H5N1). Had they sent the vaccine out to the public it would have killed millions of people. Baxter claimed it was a mistake.

You would think that a drug that is going to be injected into the bloodstream of millions of people would be free of all contaminates! Apparently not; as many as 60 percent of vaccines contain miscellaneous viruses and bacteria, both living and dead.[24-27]

This toxic combination is injected directly into your child's bloodstream where it has easy access to the brain, the liver, the kidneys, and every other organ in the body. As a parent, you would never feed your family these substances because of the harm they might do, so why would it be safe to have them injected into your children's bloodstream?

There is no safe level for some of these poisons, and combining toxins increases their toxicity. Multiple vaccinations also increase the chance of suffering from adverse effects. The damage caused by these poisons can vary greatly ranging from no noticeable symptoms to severe brain damage or death. You cannot inject poisons into the body without any effect. It's only the degree of harm that varies.

Of all the ingredients in vaccines, the most questionable is thimerosal. By weight thimerosal consists of 50 percent mercury. Mercury is toxic at any level. After many complaints from both parents and physicians and under overwhelming scientific evidence of its danger, in 1999 the CDC along with the American Academy of Pediatrics (AAP) asked pharmaceutical companies to voluntarily remove thimerosal from their vaccines. By 2001 thimerosal was no longer added to most vaccines, however, stockpiles of mercury tainted vaccines were continually being sold until 2004. While mercury has been removed from most vaccines, the major exception is the annual flu vaccine, which continues to contain thimerosal.

The AAP, which has always supported the vaccine industry and initially opposed the removal of thimerosal, issued a press release stating: "Parents should not worry about the safety of vaccines. The current levels of thimerosal will not hurt children, but reducing those levels will make safe vaccines even safer. While our current immunization strategies are safe, we have an opportunity to increase the margin of safety." After reading this statement you might wonder, if thimerosal was as safe as they claim, how does removing something that is "safe" make the vaccines safer? Sounds like double talk—an attempt to hide the fact that mercury at any level is not safe.

The CDC and the American Academy of Pediatrics continue to tell us that vaccines are safe. They say the mercury, aluminum, viruses, bacteria, and other toxic substances in vaccines are harmless and do not cause autism or any serious harm. But where is the proof?

You might wonder, aren't there any ironclad studies that prove the safety of vaccines? Unfortunately, no. The safety of vaccines has never been established. While there have been some short term studies that monitor patients for a few days, there has never been any long-term, double-blind, placebo-controlled studies establishing the safety of vaccines in humans. Drug companies refuse to do such studies, claiming that it would require them to deny the vaccine to the control group, which would be unfair to those people. Sounds like more double talk to avoid doing a study that could jeopardize the vaccine status quo. Actually, the placebo group would be the lucky ones.

The available evidence as seen by the multitude of reported adverse reactions demonstrates that vaccines can and do cause a variety of brain and nerve disorders. Animal studies have also shown that vaccines affect brain development. When infant rhesus macaque monkeys are given vaccinations in doses equivalent to what human infants receive, they develop abnormalities in areas of the brain that control social and emotional behavior.[28]

THE DRUG CARTEL
Drug Sales Versus Human Lives

The amounts of the various ingredients in vaccines are not as precisely measured or as controlled as we might think. Vaccines are not standardized between manufacturers. And even for a given manufacturer, vaccines are not standard from one batch to the next. The way vaccines are prepared and stored also affects potency and reactivity.

The level of toxic ingredients and contaminants in vaccines can vary greatly from one batch to the next. Vaccine manufacturers recognize this problem and even have a term they use for batches that have been identified as causing a higher number of adverse reactions than others. They call them "hot lots." You would assume that when a hot lot is identified that the manufacturer would recall it, just as is done by the food or auto industries. When a food item has been identified as being contaminated with E coli, for example, it is immediately recalled. Not so with vaccines, if the drug companies can get away with it.

In the UK, GlaxoSmithKline was taken to task for allowing thousands of children to be inoculated with a toxic DTP (diphtheria, tetanus, pertussis) vaccine even though they knew it had failed crucial safety tests.[29] One family sued the drug maker after their son was permanently brain damaged by the vaccine. During the trial the victim's attorney presented to the court an internal memo from the pharmaceutical company acknowledging their awareness of this particular batch of vaccine and the directive by company officials to not send the batch to just one location but to spread it out so there would be no clustering of deaths and other serious side effects. GlaxoSmithKline lost this court case. This was just one of many cases brought against the GlaxoSmithKline and other drug companies over the years from harm caused by a variety of drugs and vaccines.

To avoid lawsuits, drug companies have sought protection from the government. For example, SmithKline Beecham (GlaxoSmithKline) made a deal with the UK government indemnifying them against all litigation arising from adverse effects caused by vaccines. If vaccines are as safe as they claim, why would they do that? Apparently SmithKline knew that their vaccines weren't as safe as they tried to make everyone believe. At the time that they made this deal with the government, their MMR vaccine contained a strain of the mumps virus (Urabe AM9), which was known to cause meningitis.

This MMR vaccine was first introduced into Canada, but after causing a meningitis epidemic was quickly withdrawn. Despite the grave risk it posed to children, it was still introduced into the UK and other countries. However, because GlaxoSmithKline knew they had a liability, they were able to get the government to grant them immunity from any legal action. Their rationale must have been that the few children whose lives would be destroyed by the vaccine would be a small price to pay for the general welfare of the population who would be spared from contracting these diseases. At least that's what was implied. They certainly wouldn't have mentioned the huge profit potential for themselves or the fact that safer alternatives existed. The bottom line was corporate profits. Children's lives are not the issue, although drug companies often pretend to be concerned. But why push a dangerous vaccine onto the public when safer alternatives existed?

Four years later this vaccine with this dangerous viral strain had to be recalled. None of the families received any compensation for the damage the vaccine caused and the company received no reprimand acknowledging their responsibility. Despite causing outbreaks of meningitis in the UK, Canada, Japan, and Australia it was *not* taken off the market. It was put into storage and then sent to Third World countries like Brazil and India to be used in mass vaccination campaigns. The result was epidemics of meningitis in these countries. Apparently company profits are more important than children's lives.

Parents are never told about the real consequences of vaccines, but only that they prevent disease. Vaccines are not as safe or as effective as we are led to believe. The truth is that vaccines cause more disease than they prevent. Vaccine makers know this, which is why they work so hard to obtain immunity from legal action. If vaccines were as safe as we are told, this immunity would not be necessary.

Prior to 1986, if your child were injured by a vaccine you were allowed to file a lawsuit against the drug maker to receive compensation for your injuries. Since then the drug companies have been successful in making it harder to take them to court. In 1982 the four major vaccine makers (Merck, Wyeth, Lederle, Connaught) threatened to stop selling vaccines in the US unless Congress passed a law giving them complete immunity from prosecution. They didn't succeed that time. However, in 1986 an act was passed giving drug companies partial liability protection that made lawsuits much more difficult. Drug companies continued to lobby for complete immunity.

In February 2011 the drug companies finally got what they wanted. The US Supreme Court made a ruling to shield drug makers from being sued by parents whose children have suffered injury from vaccinations. The court decision leaves parents with no way to hold vaccine makers accountable. If your child becomes paralyzed, autistic, epileptic, or mentally retarded due to a vaccination, you are on your own. Supreme Court Justice Antonin Scalia stated that side effects are "unavoidable" when a vaccine is given to millions of children. He explained that if drug makers were forced to pay compensation for devastating injuries, the vaccine industry would go bankrupt. In other words, he is saying that the profits of the drug industry are more important than the safety of our children. Now drug makers have no reason to focus on safety issues. Vaccines are likely to become even more dangerous, and parents have little recourse. The only thing they can do is refuse vaccination, but even that is becoming increasingly difficult as the drug industry pushes for more mandatory vaccinations.

Are vaccines safe? You be the judge.

Supporting Evidence

Vaccine promoters refuse to accept the testimonies of parents who claim that vaccinations caused their children's autism. Personal accounts are referred to as anecdotal evidence. Anecdotal evidence does not establish scientific proof because there are too many unknown variables involved that could have influenced the outcome, such as diet, environment, medications, and genetics. However, when many thousands of people are claiming the same thing, as is seen with autism, it is highly likely that there is some connection.

Vaccine proponents want hard scientific evidence to prove the connection between autism and vaccinations. They loudly proclaim there are no peer-reviewed, placebo controlled, double-blind, randomized studies demonstrating this assumption. And until there are, they refuse to believe in any such association. Yet they quickly cite questionable, poorly designed studies written by ghostwriters and others with ties to the drug industry as definitive proof that vaccines are safe and do not cause autism, and then quickly add that no further studies are necessary. This is ironic since they demand proof that vaccines cause autism, but deny that any additional studies are necessary to provide the proof.

Autism usually surfaces by the age of 6, but can occur at any time prior to that. About 40 percent of parents with autistic children report that their normally developing children suddenly experienced developmental regression after being vaccinated. That amounts to about a half million mothers and fathers stating that they witnessed their children slip into autism as a result of vaccinations. The eyewitness accounts of half a million people holds more weight than statistical data involving 100, 500, or even 1,000 subjects that claim to show no definitive relationship between autism and vaccines.

Some truths are recognized because they are so obvious that they need no elaborate studies to verify their validity. If you strike your hand with a hammer, you are going to feel pain; if you fall from the top of a three-story building, you are likely to suffer injury. These things are obvious because they have been witnessed time and time again. There is no need for a peer-reviewed, double-blind, placebo controlled study to prove them. However, when a half million parents report that their children developed autism immediately following vaccinations, it is brushed aside as a coincidence.

Why is it so difficult to believe that vaccines cause autism? The vaccine makers stand to lose a lot of money if autism is officially recognized as a side effect to vaccination, so they've put up a vicious fight. We've seen this type of thing before. It happened with the tobacco industry when it was claimed that smoking caused lung cancer. For decades the tobacco industry denied the association, even in the face of overwhelming evidence. Their own studies showed that smoking was harmless and employed scientists and celebrities to promote their cause. Yet, after many years, and many additional deaths from lung cancer, they were proven wrong and even taken to task for concealing evidence linking smoking to cancer. Do we have to wait another two or three decades before there is overwhelming evidence to prove the link with autism? Do millions of children need to suffer in the meantime?

According to a recent Nationwide survey:

MORE DOCTORS SMOKE CAMELS THAN ANY OTHER CIGARETTE

CAMELS *Costlier Tobaccos*

Typical cigarette ad of the 1940s and 1950s. The ad's message: "Trust me, I'm a doctor."

Andrew Wakefield's 1998 *Lancet* study struck a severe blow to the vaccine promoters because it provided a high-quality, peer-reviewed study demonstrating a possible link between vaccines and autism. Basically what Wakefield found was that the digestive tract of a certain percentage of autistic children is infected by the measles virus. This virus irritates the lining of the digestive tract causing inflammation, swelling, and ulceration. The measles virus that they found was not the wild type that naturally infects children, but was a strain used only in the MMR vaccine, proving a relationship between vaccines and gastrointestinal disorders, which are common in autistic children. Wakefield did not claim vaccines caused autism, but only suggested the possibility of an association and recommended further research.

The vaccine industry violently lashed out at Wakefield and falsely accused him of fraud and scientific misconduct and succeeded in having him discredited and his paper retracted. Although many charges were filed against him he was only found guilty of acting without the required ethical approval from an institutional review board (which he denies) and "misconduct" for subjecting children to unnecessary medical procedures, such as colonoscopy, even though he had parental consent. These were his only "crimes." Based on this, his paper was retracted. The results of his study were not questioned or disproven: they still remain valid. Prosecutors could find no fault with his research or his conclusions.

Wakefield's "crimes" are greatly overblown by critics and the media making him out to be a charlatan perpetuating an elaborate fraud, thus discrediting him and his research in the minds of the public. Most people mistakenly believe his *Lancet* paper was retracted because it was fraudulent. That's not the case. The paper was retracted for procedural infractions, as noted above, although the real reason was due to pressure from the pharmaceutical industry.

Vaccine promoters would have you believe that Wakefield's study was the only one that has linked vaccines to autism, but that's not the case. In addition to the *hundreds* of studies showing that vaccines can cause brain damage and nervous disorders, there is evidence that shows a direct relationship to autism.

Several studies have shown results similar to those discovered by Wakefield and colleagues.[30-35] For example, a study out of Japan found a measles virus originating from the MMR vaccine in the digestive tract of autistic children with Crohn's disease and ulcerative colitis. However, non-autistic children did not have the virus.[36] These studies suggest that the measles virus from the MMR vaccine can infect the body and contribute to the cascade of events that leads to autism.

A series of papers by neurosurgeon, Russell Blaylock, MD demonstrated a clear connection between vaccinations and autism and other developmental disorders. Blaylock explains in detail exactly how vaccines can cause brain damage that may lead to autism.[37-39] Blaylock shows that the likelihood of a child developing autism or some other developmental disorder increases the earlier vaccines are given to the child, and increase further with the amount administered.

Researchers at Stony Brook University in New York have shown that giving the hepatitis B vaccine to newborn boys more than triples their risk of developing autism.[40] This study demonstrates that vaccines do have a direct influence on autism, confirming the results of an earlier study by the same researchers using a different database of subjects.[41]

Three years after Wakefield's study was published, the *British Medical Journal* (BMJ) published a study meant to refute Wakefield's findings.[42] This study reported that the incidence of autism started to rise in children born in the late 1980s and increased dramatically in those born from 1989 to 1993. The MMR vaccination program was introduced in the UK in 1988, just as the autism epidemic was beginning. By 1989, over 90 percent of the children in the UK were receiving this vaccine. While vaccine coverage remained the same, autism rates continued to rise. Therefore, the authors contend, the MMR vaccine is not to blame for the continued increase in autism during that period of time. This study *does* acknowledge the sudden rise in autism at the same time the MMR vaccine was introduced. How do the authors explain this correlation? They called it a coincidence. It seems that any facts that go contrary to the vaccine promoters' agenda are brushed off as coincidences. There seems to be an awful lot of coincidences regarding vaccines and autism.

Since Wakefield specifically mentioned the MMR vaccine, all the studies written to refute his work have focused solely on the MMR vaccine or thimerosal, which was used in this vaccine at the time. In so doing, the researchers ignore the effect of any and all other vaccines. When information about other vaccines are added to the data in the above BMJ study, it is clear that the number of children developing autism has risen with the *number* of vaccines given, not just the type. Inadvertently this study provides further proof of the vaccine-autism connection.

The authors produced a graph depicting the rise of autism from 1988 to 1993 and tried to show that MMR vaccine rates had no correlation. However, they left out the increase in total given vaccinations during this time (see graph). The graph with the added information shows the initial rise in autism after the introduction of the MMR vaccine in 1988. Autism rates jumped again when the DTP vaccinations were accelerated in 1990, and yet again when the Hib vaccine was introduced in 1992.

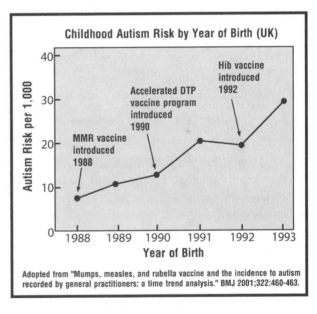

Adopted from "Mumps, measles, and rubella vaccine and the incidence fo autism recorded by general practitioners: a time trend analysis." BMJ 2001;322:460-463.

One of the faults of this and other studies is assuming that autism only results immediately after a vacci-nation. While this is often the case, it is not necessarily so. Some children are more susceptible to the vaccinations than others, so the age and time after vaccination that autism appears can vary widely from one child to the next. Some may develop autism before their first birthday while others aren't diagnosed until they reach six or seven years of age, after they have received many vaccinations.

Sallie Bernard and colleagues have proposed that autism can be caused by mercury poisoning, either from vaccines or other sources. They point out that exposure to mercury can cause the neurological, sensory, motor, and behavioral traits that define autism.[43] Thimerosal has become a major source of mercury in children who within their first two years of life have received quantities of mercury that far exceeds Environmental Protection Agency (EPA) and FDA safety guidelines. The researchers note that genetic and non-genetic factors establish a predisposition whereby some children are more vulnerable to the adverse effects of thimerosal.

A series of studies published by Mark R. Geier, MD, PhD and colleagues have assessed the impact of thimerosal in vaccines on the risk of autism and other neurodevelopmental disorders.[44-47] Using data from the US Department of Education Report on the prevalence of various childhood diseases and the VAERS database, Geier and colleagues have compared the rates of autism and other neurodevelopmental disorders to the amount of thimerosal children receive through the DTaP vaccine. Children receiving thimerosal-containing DTaP vaccines were compared to children

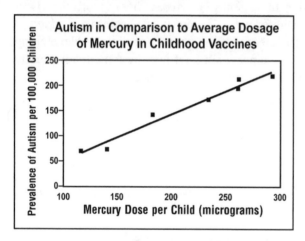

receiving thimerosal-free DTaP vaccines. They found a linear correlation between the amount of thimerosal received and the development of autism (see graph). The evidence shows the appearance of autism "following thimerosal-containing childhood vaccines does not appear to be coincidental." These studies don't conclusively prove that thimerosal causes autism, but they clearly show that it does increase the risk. While thimerosal has been removed from the MMR vaccine, it is still used in most yearly flu vaccines and in some tetanus, encephalitis, and meningococcal vaccines.[48] Interestingly, autism was first discovered in 1943 just a few years after manufacturers began adding thimerosal in to vaccines.

Prior to 2001, a 2-month-old could receive more than 62 micrograms of mercury from vaccines in a single day. The Maximum permissible limit set by the EPA at this age is only 0.262 micrograms. *This is 150 times over the maximum limit!* The influenza vaccine that is recommended annually for children starting at age 6 months still delivers 25 micrograms of mercury, 76 times the EPA limit for children of this age (0.654 micrograms). Geier and colleagues calculate that for every 1 microgram of mercury present in a vaccine, the incidence of autism increases by 1 case per 100,000 children.[44] In addition, the influenza vaccine is encouraged for all pregnant women. This immediate overload of mercury into the mother's bloodstream will have an effect on the developing fetus.

While removing thimerosal from most vaccines may reduce the risk of autism somewhat, it will not eliminate it. Mercury exposure can occur from sources other than vaccines such as fish, mercury dental fillings, and pesticides. Vaccines also contain many other neurotoxins besides mercury. Mercury-free vaccines may be safer, but they still pose a dangerous risk.

Another line of evidence for the vaccine connection is the lack of autism among unvaccinated children. While it is possible for an unvaccinated child to get autism, it appears to be very rare. Prior to mass childhood vaccination programs that began in the late 1950s, autism was extremely rare. It didn't become a major health issue until the late 1980s when aggressive vaccinations programs were initiated. In populations around the world where they still do not have routine vaccinations, autism is practically nonexistent.

Even in the United States, those who are not vaccinated seem to be protected from autism. For example, more than half of Amish children are unvaccinated and the autism rate among them is about 1 in 5,000. In comparison, the autism rate among other children in the United States is 1 in 91. This means Amish children have an autism rate that is 50 times lower than the fully vaccinated non-Amish children who live next door to them!

In a recent survey involving some 8,000 unvaccinated children (none of which were Amish), only four were diagnosed with autism. Among a general population of this size, 80 children would be expected to be autistic. Of those four in this population who were autistic, at least two indicated signs of excessive mercury exposure. Mercury exposure could come from a variety of sources besides vaccines.[49]

It is apparent that vaccines increase the risk for autism, but do they actually cause it? Vaccines clearly contribute to autism and may be the primary factor involved, but there are other important issues that also seem to play a role. Some of those issues will be discussed in Chapter 6.

4 | Should Your Children Be Vaccinated?

VACCINE MANIA

Vaccine proponents like to blame genetics as the cause of autism—an apparent attempt to divert attention away from a more likely cause. If you look at the graph on the following page, you see that a genetic cause would be impossible. Within just one generation autism has risen from being almost unheard of to one of the most commonly diagnosed childhood disorders. The rate of occurrence matches that of a contagious disease or some environmental catastrophe. Obviously, something in the environment over the past three decades has changed. What could it be? The most likely candidate is the dramatic increase in the number of childhood vaccinations over this same time period.

In the 1940s, when autism was extremely rare, children received only four vaccines—diphtheria, tetanus, pertussis, and smallpox. In the 1980s the number of vaccines given to children increased to seven—diphtheria, tetanus, pertussis, measles, mumps, rubella, and polio. Children received 15 doses of seven vaccines by the time they were two years old. At the same time, autism rates began to soar. More vaccines were added in the following years and autism rates continued to climb. Today, 14 different vaccines administered in 37 doses are given to children by the age of two. One in every 68 American families now has an autistic child.

Our children are experiencing an epidemic of neurological and autoimmune disorders. Over the past 30 years, the number of vaccinations our children receive has skyrocketed. During that same period of time the number of children with autism, learning disabilities, ADHD, asthma, bowel disorders, and diabetes has more than tripled! According to the CDC, 796,000 children were learning disabled in 1976. Today one out of every six children in America is developmentally disabled.

An infant receives its first vaccine on the day of birth. At two months of age the infant receives 8 vaccines, all of which may be given at the same time. Eight vaccines injected into a 13-pound, two-month old infant is equivalent to 80 doses in a 130-pound adult! Two months later 7 more vaccines are administered. By the time a child is 6 months old he has been given 25 doses of 9 vaccines. In their first year babies receive 32 doses of 14 vaccines.

What effect do all these vaccines have on a young child? Public health officials tell us that vaccines are safe even when a child receives several doses at the same time. You might think that the safety of multiple vaccinations has been thoroughly studied, yet surprisingly it hasn't. While there have been a number of short-term studies done to examine the risks of multiple vaccinations, there have been no long-term studies. Health officials just assume that the long term effects of receiving one dose is no different from receiving multiple doses. There are no safety studies to confirm this. In order to identify the connection between vaccines and autism or other developmental disorders, long-term studies are required.

When differences in short-term studies are observed, they are ignored. In one study, for example, the safety and efficacy of simultaneous administration of MMR, DTP and trivalent oral poliovirus (OPV) vaccine in a test group of children was compared with the administration of the same vaccines in a control group given MMR followed two months later by doses of DTP and OPV. The rates of *serious* vaccine-associated reactions immediately following the vaccinations were similar in both groups. Less severe side effects, however, were higher in the test group. The researchers discounted these side effects because they were "judged to be related to the study design rather than to differences in the safety of the two vaccine schedules." Their conclusion was that multiple vaccines were safe and effective.[1] This study only evaluated the children for a few days. There was no way to tell what would happen with these "less severe" side effects over time. For that matter, there was no way to tell if the serious side effects would become more serious over time in one group compared to the other, or if new serious side effects would emerge later.

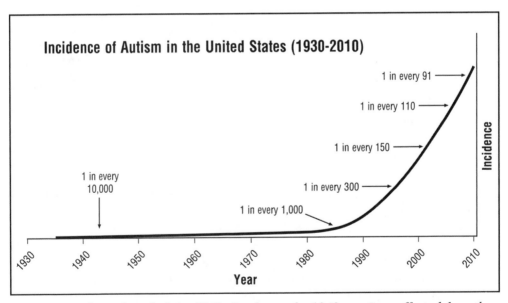

Autism was first identified in 1943. In the early 1940s autism affected less than 1 in 10,000 children in the United States. It remained a relatively rare condition until the 1980s when rates began to climb dramatically. By 1995 that number of children with autism jumped to 1 in every 1,000. By 2009 it had climbed to 1 in every 91 children.

Vaccination Schedule for Children
Age 0 Through 6 Years (United States)

Age	Vaccine
Birth	Hepatitis B
2 months	Hepatitis B, Rotavirus, Diptheria, Tetanus, Pertussis, Hib, PCV, Polio
4 months	Rotavirus, Diptheria, Tetanus, Pertussis, Hib, PCV, Polio
6 months	Hepatitis B, Rotavirus, Diptheria, Tetanus, Pertussis, Hib, PCV, Polio, Influenza
12 months	Hib, PCV, Measles, Mumps, Rubella, Varicella, Hepatitis A
18 months	Diptheria, Tetanus, Pertussis, Influenza, Hepatitis A
2-3 years	Influenza
4-6 years	Diptheria, Tetanus, Pertussis, Influenza (2 doses), Measles, Mumps, Rubella, Varicella, Polio

Hib = Haemophilus influenzae type b. PCV = Pneunococcal conjugate vaccine.

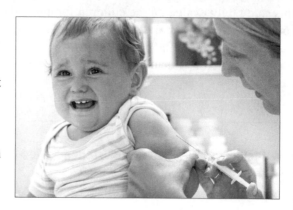

This vaccine schedule is for 2011 (more vaccines may be added in the future). By age six, children receive a total of 48 doses of 14 vaccines. Most children in Western countries are overvaccinated. You can find the schedules for other countries online. For details on select countries see the following:

Canada
http://www.phac-aspc.gc.ca/im/is-cv/
UK
http://www.patient.co.uk/doctor/Immunisation-Schedule-(UK).htm
Australia
http://www.health.act.gov.au/c/health?a=sendfile&ft=p&fid=1265849866&sid
New Zealand
http://www.moh.govt.nz/moh.nsf/indexmh/immunisation-schedule
Japan
http://www.city.shinjuku.lg.jp/foreign/english/guide/fukushi/fukushi_2.html
Europe (Austria, Belgium, Bulgaria, Croatia, Cyprus, Czech Republic, Denmark, Estonia, Finland, France, Germany, Greece, Hungary, Iceland, Ireland, Italy, Latvia, Lithuania, Luxembourg, Malta, Netherlands, Norway, Poland, Portugal, Romania, Slovakia, Slovenia, Spain, Sweden, Switzerland, and Turkey)
http://www.euvac.net/graphics/euvac/vaccination/austria.html

In humans, the most rapid period of brain development occurs during the third trimester of pregnancy and continues through the first two years of life. By age two, brain development is 80 percent complete. Vaccines are loaded with neurotoxic compounds; it is inconceivable to believe that these toxins do not in some way adversely affect the developing brain of a child.

As can be seen from the VAERS database, even one dose can have very serious side effects. When you combine two or more doses, the risk or odds of experiencing an adverse reaction increases proportionally. The toxic contents of the vaccines can even sensitize a child so that a second or third or 48th dose has a greater adverse impact on the body, so a child may have little or no reaction to the first or second dose, a greater reaction to the next, and then experience severe damage from the next.

Are all these vaccinations really necessary? And do they really save lives? In Sweden hepatitis B vaccine is not given to every newborn as is done in the United States. The Swedish are more sensible; this vaccine is only given to infants when mothers test positive for the hepatitis B virus—that is, it is only given to infants who are actually at risk. In the United States children receive up to 32 doses of 14 vaccines by their first birthday. In Sweden one-year-olds receive only half that amount—18 doses of 6 vaccines. The mortality rate of Swedish children under the age of one year is 2.74 per 1,000 live births. In the United States the first-year mortality rate is more than twice that of Sweden (6.06 per 1,000).[2] American children receive twice as many vaccines and experience more than twice as many deaths as the Swedes. The same is true in most other European countries. European children receive fewer vaccinations and have a lower death rate than American children. We are told that vaccines save lives, but the facts say otherwise. Apparently the aggressive vaccination program is not working.

It is interesting that the US spends more money on health care and has a higher child vaccination rate than any other nation in the world. You would think American children would be among the healthiest, yet 45 other countries have lower first-year child mortality rates. The US infant death rate is higher than most other industrialized nations and is not much better than many underdeveloped countries where infectious diseases are still major health problems. Something is definitely wrong.

WHICH VACCINES DO YOU REALLY NEED?

In the United States children receive over 60 doses of 16 different vaccines by the age of 18. Are all these vaccinations really necessary? Are the health risks to our children today any greater now than they were in the 1970s when children received only a fraction of the vaccinations that they do today? Most vaccines are unnecessary. Some do more harm than good. Others are only useful under certain circumstances. However, *all* vaccines carry risks. Before making a decision on which vaccines your children should receive, you need to weigh the benefits against the risks. The following sections discuss the attributes of each of the vaccines commonly administered to children up to age six.

Measles, Mumps, and Rubella (MMR)

Measles, also known as rubeola, is a contagious respiratory infection caused by the measles virus. It is a common childhood disease. There is no specific treatment for measles and most children recover with adequate rest in seven to 10 days. Symptoms typically include rash, fatigue, runny nose, red eyes, and fever.

An otherwise healthy child will recover from a measles infection without problems. The disease can be much more severe in adults and even fatal. Much of the apprehension or fear we feel at the possibility of one of our children coming down with measles is based on what it can do to adults or to children who are already in ill health. If your children are healthy, a measles infection is not a serious matter. Once infection is gone, children are immune for life.

Infants are generally protected from measles for the first 6-12 months after birth due to immunity passed on from their mothers. The measles vaccine is usually combined with mumps and rubella vaccines and administered simultaneously. The MMR vaccine is given twice to children; once at 12 to 15 months of age and again at 4 to 6 years of age.

Currently measles is very rare in the US and in most other industrialized nations. Generally, fewer than 100 cases are reported in the US each year. Death from measles is extremely rare in the US nowadays. According to the CDC, during the three year span 2005-2007 (the most recent years full data was available), in all age groups combined there was a total of only 1 death. In children, there have been no deaths. By comparison, in all age groups there were 20 times more deaths in the US caused by malaria (usually considered a disease of the tropics) than by measles.

Rubella (German measles), also known as "three-day measles," is another common childhood disease. Rubella is not the same as measles (rubeola) described above. They are two separate illnesses caused by different viruses. Rubella is a mild disease in children and symptoms may go unnoticed. However, this virus can cause significant birth defects if an infected pregnant woman passes the virus to her unborn child. This is the only justification for vaccination.

Since the reason for vaccination is to protect newborns, why is this vaccine given to all male children? It is totally unnecessary. Women who have had the infection as children have a natural immunity and their future children are protected while in the womb and for about a year thereafter. However, vaccinated women may not be protected since drug-induced immunity can wear off over time. Vaccinating young girls may actually increase risk since they will not gain the protection of natural lifelong immunity. They might have little protection as adults when pregnancy is likely.

Mumps is a common contagious childhood disease caused by the mumps virus. It can occur at any age but typically affects children ages 2-12 who have not been vaccinated. In children the disease lasts from 10-12 days and clears up on its own. Symptoms include fever, loss of appetite, and swelling of the salivary glands, which causes the cheeks to puff out—the hallmark sign of the illness. In children it is a minor illness and up to 20 percent of those infected show no signs or symptoms.

In adolescents and adults the disease is more serious. Complications may include inflammation of the testicles sometimes leading to atrophy and sterility, swelling and inflammation of the pancreas or the brain, hearing loss, and in women, inflammation of the ovaries and miscarriage during pregnancy.

The mumps vaccine has proven to be almost useless and even harmful. Each year more than 1,000 people in the US come down with mumps and almost all of them have been vaccinated against this disease. Infection with the natural mumps virus passes on a lifelong immunity. However, the immunity gained from vaccination is short lived. Antibody levels decline rapidly, leaving the person vulnerable to infection after a few years. Vaccination must be repeated again and again to maintain immunity. This actually causes a more serious situation because mumps, like measles, is much more menacing when contracted after childhood. Since routine vaccination of children began, a growing number of vaccinated young adults and adults are being infected. What has happened is that an insignificant childhood disease has been transformed into a much more dangerous adult disease.

Measles, mumps, and rubella are diseases almost every child normally gets if not vaccinated. It's been this way throughout history. In fact, if you were born prior to 1957, before mass MMR vaccinations began, you don't need the MMR vaccination because essentially everyone in this age group has had each of these infections as children and is now immune.

We would all be better off getting these diseases as children just as our grandparents did and be over with it, without the necessity of vaccinations. Once vaccinated, you are put at greater risk for the rest of your life because drug-induced immunity can wane over time and these diseases are more dangerous if contracted after childhood. Once vaccinated, a person requires repeated vaccinations to maintain protection. By vaccinating children, they become dependent on vaccines for the rest of their lives—a clever financial strategy for vaccine makers.

Vaccination has reduced the incidence of these diseases in children. In recent years many parents have chosen to forgo the MMR vaccination due to worries about autism. Consequently, the incidence of measles, in particular, has been on the rise. Health care workers and vaccine proponents often cite this fact to instill fear in parents claiming that if their children aren't vaccinated they are at great risk of getting these diseases. Actually, that's a good thing! Children *should* get these infections, just as children have for generations. These children will be much healthier afterword and never have to worry about getting these diseases as adults.

Varicella

Varicella (chicken pox) is another virus that is totally unnecessary. It is generally a mild disease in children but a much more serious one in adults. Here again the vaccine imparts only temporary immunity. Merck now produces a vaccine that combines the MMR and chicken pox vaccines. The four-in-one combination is called ProQuad or MMRV.

Rotavirus (RV)

Almost all children are infected with the rotavirus by the time they reach five years of age. Once a child is infected, he or she is left with lifelong immunity. Rotavirus is one of the most common causes of diarrhea in children. For most children the infection is relatively mild and completely treatable with adequate fluids and rest.

For generations, children have encountered this virus without complications, but now drug companies see it as a grave health threat that must be stopped. Vaccination is their answer. The rotavirus vaccine is given three times at ages 2, 3, and 4 months. The rotavirus vaccine produced by Merck, RotaTeq, is the one invented by Dr. Paul Offit. This is a totally unnecessary vaccine with no real benefit but plenty of risks.

Diphtheria, Tetanus, and Pertussis (DTP and DTaP)

Diphtheria, tetanus, and pertussis vaccine is first given at two months of age followed by five booster shots by age 12. Protective immunity after receiving all the recommend shots only lasts 10 years, so anyone who has not had a booster shot within ten years is susceptible. This would include the vast majority of the adult population.

Diphtheria is caused by a bacterial infection that commonly affects the nose and throat. It can be passed to others. It may be a problem in certain parts of the world where sanitation and personal hygiene is substandard, but in the US and other developed countries it's almost unheard of. In the US the disease is so rare that since 1980, less than one case per 100 million people occurs each year. Some would claim the low incidence of infection is due to vaccinations, yet most adults do not have current vaccinations and are still unaffected. Your chances of encountering this disease is very slim. If you did contract it, however, there are antibiotics available that can treat this disease, so vaccination is still completely unnecessary.

Tetanus (lockjaw) is another bacterial infection. The bacteria that cause the disease live in soils all around the world. An infection can occur when spores enter the body through an open wound—for example, by stepping on a dirty nail. Tetanus is not contagious and cannot be passed from person to person. It too can be treated with antibiotics, so vaccination is not necessary.

Pertussis (whooping cough) is also a bacterial infection. It is a highly contagious respiratory infection that causes uncontrollable, violent coughing. A deep "whooping" sound is often made when the patient tries to take a breath. When an infected person sneezes or coughs, tiny droplets containing the bacteria are expelled into the air, so it can easily spread to others. Although pertussis is potentially more serious than diphtheria or tetanus, especially in infants, it too can be treated with antibiotics. There are less than 10,000 cases of pertussis in the entire US each year and in the majority of these cases the patients have been vaccinated. So there is no guarantee that the vaccine will provide the promised protection. Since pertussis vaccines are known to cause seizures and brain damage, parents must weigh the risks of vaccination against that of the disease.

The whole-cell pertussis vaccine has been in use since the 1940s. Children who receive the whole-cell pertussis vaccine routinely suffer from fevers and seizures which sometimes lead to Dravet syndrome, a severe form of epilepsy. The vaccine requires at least four doses and is considered only 50-80 percent effective in preventing the disease. Some studies show clinical efficiency as low as 36 percent. In other words, between 20-50 percent and possibly as many as 64 percent of those who are properly vaccinated remain vulnerable to the disease.[3] In recent years, concerns about the safety of the whole-cell pertussis vaccine prompted the development of a more purified vaccine that is associated with fewer adverse reactions with about the same efficiency against the disease. The combined DTP vaccine uses whole-cell pertussis vaccine, while the DTaP vaccine uses the purified (acellular) pertussis vaccine.

Inactivated Poliovirus (IPV)

Poliomyelitis (polio) is a contagious disease caused by the poliovirus. It is looked upon with fright because it can cause permanent partial or full paralysis. We've all seen photos of children who have been crippled by this disease. While the risk of paralysis exists, the danger we imagine is greatly exaggerated. For the vast majority of people polio is a mild illness. At least 90 percent of those infected experience no noticeable symptoms; in 4-8 percent of cases symptoms are no worse than a cold or mild flu. In 1-3 percent of cases the virus finds its way into the central nervous system where complications can arise. Out of every 1,000 cases, between 1-5 may end up with some degree of paralysis. In most cases, paralysis is only temporary.

The polio vaccine (IPV) is first given at 2 months of age followed by three booster shots over the next four to six years. Like other vaccines, immunity is only temporary. Most adults who were vaccinated as children no longer have immunity. But they need not worry. If you live in a country with good sanitation and clean water the threat of catching polio is virtually nil. North America, Europe, Australia, and dozens of other countries have officially been declared polio-free. In the US the last natural case of polio occurred in 1979. The only polio outbreaks since then have all been caused by the polio vaccine. You are actually at greater risk of getting polio if you are vaccinated than if you are not. So it may be wise to skip this unnecessary vaccine.

Hepatitis B

The most insane vaccine policy is the practice of giving newborns the hepatitis B vaccine. All infants in the US are routinely given this shot the day they are born. Two additional booster shots are recommended during the infant's first year of life. Hepatitis B is not a children's disease. It is an adult disease passed only through the sharing of tainted hypodermic needles or unprotected sex with an infected person. The only possible way a baby could get the disease is during birth from an infected mother. Mothers generally know if they are infected. If the mother doesn't know, it can be easily determined by a blood test. But that isn't being done. As soon as a baby is born it is taken to the nursery and given the shot. The mother isn't even asked. Whether the infant is a robust 10 pounds or a premature 3 pounder, it receives the same dose. There have been no safety studies done with the hepatitis B vaccine on newborns. So no one knows what affect it has on them. However, there are more reports of serious adverse reactions in children receiving this vaccine than there are cases of childhood hepatitis B.

Influenza

Influenza/pneumonia is listed as the eighth leading cause of death in the US. Prior to every flu season the CDC warns that tens of thousands of Americans will die from the flu that year. Children under 5 and people over 65 years of age are at greatest risk. So yearly flu shots are heavily recommended for these populations and are encouraged for all ages. It is recommended that children get their first flu shot at age 6 months and then once every year thereafter. Regardless of our age we are encouraged to get flu shots every year until we die.

According to the CDC, some 30,000 to 50,000 Americans die each year from the flu. We are led to believe that getting a flu shot is the only way to assure ourselves protection. However, a report published in the *British Medical Journal* says the mortality figure the CDC cites each year is greatly exaggerated and is meant to frighten people into getting flu vaccinations.[4] The CDC combines the deaths from the flu and pneumonia into one category, and that's the figure that is reported annually. For example, in 2007 the CDC lists a total of 52,717 deaths caused by influenza/pneumonia. However, when you separate the two, you find that the flu actually caused only 411 deaths for all ages over the entire year. Pneumonia caused the remaining 52,306 deaths. The number of deaths in small children was only 13! According to the data on the CDC website, the number of flu deaths in small children is usually less than 20 every year. Considering the millions of children in the country, the risk is rather small. To put it into perspective, nearly four times this number of children die from cancer each year. Your child is at greater risk of dying from cancer than from the flu!

Despite what you may hear in the media, flu shots have never been proven to be very effective. Numerous studies have even shown flu vaccinations to be essentially worthless for children. Researchers at Strong Memorial Hospital in New York evaluated the effectiveness of flu vaccination in children under the age of 5 and found no benefit whatsoever.[5]

Researchers at Oxford University reviewed 51 studies to evaluate the effectiveness of vaccines in protecting against influenza. They found that in children under 2 years of age flu shots were no more effective than a placebo.[6]

The CDC recommends influenza vaccination for women who will be in their second or third trimester of pregnancy during the influenza season. However, according to a five-year study by researchers at Kaiser Permanente Vaccine Study Center in Oakland, California, unvaccinated women are no more susceptible to the flu than vaccinated women are. Their infants also have no greater incidence of influenza whether their mothers are vaccinated or not.[7]

For young children flu vaccination provides no useful protection. For people who are 65 and older flu vaccines appear to be just as useless. Over the last two decades in the United States, vaccination rates among the elderly have increased from 15 to 65 percent, yet there has been no decrease in influenza deaths. In fact, both hospital admission rates and mortality in those 65 years and older have *increased* with increasing vaccine coverage over time.[8-10]

One of the reasons why flu vaccination has limited success is because the vaccines provide only temporary protection against a few specific strains of influenza. Other strains are not affected. Manufacturers make a guess at what strain of influenza will dominate the coming flu season and produce vaccines against it months in advance. If they guess wrong the vaccines don't do any good. Numerous strains of influenza can be in circulation simultaneously and new ones are continually arising, so immunization against only one or two provides very limited protection.

Even if a person were given the correct vaccine it wouldn't do any good. Dr. J. Anthony Morris (former Chief Vaccine Control Officer at the FDA) has stated, "There is no evidence that any influenza vaccine thus far developed is effective in preventing or mitigating any attack of influenza. The producers of these vaccines know that they are worthless, but they go on selling them, anyway." [11]

The vast majority of people who catch the flu each year do not experience any complications and within a few days are over it. Unlike those who are vaccinated, those who are affected by a wild strain of influenza are left with a life-long immunity. When the swine flu (H1N1 virus) of 2009 was in full bloom, doctors were bracing for a pending pandemic, which fortunately never materialized. Despite the potential threat, seniors over the age of 65 were told that they did not need a flu shot. Virtually everyone in this age group had been exposed to epidemics of a similar strain of influenza back in the 1930s and 1940s, before mass immunization programs were initiated. Most seniors had a natural immunity to the H1N1 virus and did not need the vaccination. Children who are allowed to develop natural immunity to the various strains of influenza will be protected for life.

Other Vaccines

Currently three additional vaccines (pneumococcal, haemophilus influenzae type b, and hepatitis A) requiring a total of 15 shots are recommended for children under age 6 in the US. Pneumococcal and haemophilus influenzae type b are caused by bacteria. We have antibiotics available that can fight these illnesses, so generally healthy people have little to worry about. As with any of these infections, it's those who are already in poor health who are at greatest risk.

Hepatitis A is a liver disease caused by a virus. It is usually spread through the sharing of dirty needles or unprotected sex. The risk to children is tiny and vaccination only imparts temporary immunity. By the time children reach adulthood, when this disease is more likely to be of concern, immunity has worn off. So what's the point?

In most cases, a single vaccination is not enough to induce long term immunity. The vaccinations must be repeated over a period of several months or years. One of the reasons for this is that the immunity gained by vaccinations almost always wears off over time. For example, the pertussis vaccine is only effective for three years.[12] Consequently, it is given to children six times by the time they are 12 years of age. Many of the outbreaks of childhood diseases such as whooping cough and measles are not caused by unvaccinated children. They affect those who are vaccinated just as often as those who are not. We tend to believe those who are vaccinated are protected, when this may not be the case. As a result, most people who are vaccinated have a false sense of security.

You are likely to see new vaccines added to the "Recommended Immunization Schedule" in the future. Drug companies are currently working on over 100 new vaccines. Vaccines are being cranked out for just about every illness imaginable whether they pose any real threat or not. As these new vaccines become available, more and more will likely find their way onto the "Schedule."

Following current medical recommendations, by the time a person reaches his 70s, he will have received at least 130 vaccinations. At the rate we are going, this number may double or triple by the time your children reach this age, if they live that long.

DO VACCINES IMPROVE HEALTH?

The entire purpose of vaccinations is to prevent disease. But do vaccines really make us any healthier? The evidence suggests not. Often vaccinated children are just as prone to the diseases they are vaccinated against as unvaccinated children, and perhaps even more so as vaccines often cause the illnesses they are meant to prevent. As you've seen above with the flu vaccine, there is no measurable benefit. This is probably true for most vaccines. In fact, a recent survey shows that vaccinated children suffer two to five times more disease and disability than unvaccinated children. The survey covered the health history of over 8,000 unvaccinated children. The incidence of numerous health problems were recorded including asthma, ADHD, autism, epilepsy, diabetes, sleep disorders, ear infections, sinusitis, allergies, and more. In every case vaccinated children displayed a higher incidence of these conditions than unvaccinated children.[13]

This survey confirms the results of other studies. For example, in a study published in the *British Medical Journal* children of 15,000 mothers were observed for 5 years from 1990 to 1996. The death rate in vaccinated children against diphtheria, tetanus, and whooping cough was found to be more than twice as high as unvaccinated children (10.5 percent versus 4.7 percent).[14]

A study out of New Zealand also showed unvaccinated children to be significantly healthier.[15] The study involved 254 children, 133 were vaccinated and 121 remained unvaccinated. The results are shown below.

Condition	Vaccinated (%)	Unvaccinated (%)
Asthma	15	3
Eczema or allergic rashes	32	13
Chronic ear infections	20	7
Recurrent tonsillitis	8	2
Sudden infant death syndrome	7	2
Hyperactivity	8	1

Another study in the US showed that unvaccinated children were healthier than the general population. The study involved 1,004 unvaccinated children and compared them with the general population (including both vaccinated and unvaccinated children).[16]

Condition	General Population (%)	Unvaccinated (%)
Asthma.	8-12	0
Atopic dermatitis.	10-20	1.2
Allergies	25	3
ADHD	5-10	0.79

Because of aggressive marketing tactics by vaccine makers and government mandates, most children today are subjected to a barrage of vaccinations starting on the day of birth. Is it any wonder why one out of every two children has chronic health problems and one out of every five is developmentally disabled?[17] These are the latest statistics coming from separate studies published in the journals *Pediatrics* (June 2011) and *Academic Pediatrics* (May-June 2011). Our children are becoming sicker and sicker. As more vaccines are added in the near future this situation is sure to get worse.

"By over-vaccinating our children" says Russell Blaylock, MD, "public health officials are weakening their immune system, making them more susceptible to a number of infections, and less able to combat infections. This provides these officials an endless source of 'horror stories' to justify additional vaccines.[18]

DECLINE OF INFECTIOUS DISEASE

A century ago infectious diseases were the leading cause of death in young children. Today, the leading causes of death in children under five years of age are accidents, genetic disorders, developmental disorders, sudden infant death syndrome (SIDS), and cancer. The reason for the decline in deaths from infections is generally attributed to vaccinations.

The incidence of mumps, diphtheria, polio, Whooping cough (pertussis), and other contagious diseases has fallen dramatically. Vaccine proponents proudly point to this fact as proof that vaccinations work. This fact is also used to justify their efforts to force vaccinations on everyone, claiming that if people choose not to be vaccinated these diseases could once again rise to epidemic proportions.

However, that's not the case. Vaccinations were not the cause of the dramatic decline in disease rates. All of these diseases were sharply declining *before* the vaccination programs even began. For instance, in the US the death rate for measles declined by 97.7 percent during the first 60 years of the 20th century. In 1900 the mortality rate was 133 deaths per million people but by 1960 it had dropped to 0.3 deaths per million. This drop in deaths occurred before there was a vaccine for this disease.

The same thing has happened with whooping cough, mumps, diphtheria, polio, and other diseases. Even for diseases such as scarlet fever, tuberculosis, and typhoid, for which there have been no vaccination programs, death rates have fallen. Death rates from all infectious diseases have dropped more than 90 percent during the first half of the 20th century, before vaccines to any of them were introduced. Obviously, vaccines are not the reason why infectious diseases have declined so drastically over the past century.

The real reason for the decline in disease is due to the increased availability of food and clean drinking water, improved sanitation, and better living conditions. In 1900 the streets were crowded with horses and carriages. Manure littered the streets. Trash and kitchen scraps were often dumped in the street. Flies, mosquitoes, and rats were everywhere, spreading disease. Sewage and animal waste often contaminated drinking water. People didn't wash their hands or their clothes as often as they

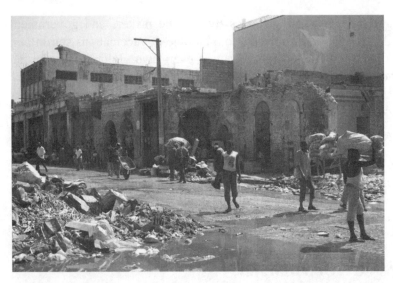

In areas of the world where sanitation is a problem, they still have a high incidence of infectious disease.

should. Even in the late 1800s, doctors didn't wash their hands between patients. After performing autopsies on cadavers of diseased victims or surgeries on critically ill patients, they would often merely wipe their hands off on a towel before attending to another patient or delivering a baby. For this reason, childbed fever was one of the most common causes of death in both infants and mothers after childbirth. During the early 1900s sanitation and personal hygiene greatly improved and along with it came a sharp decline in disease rates. Vaccines appear to have contributed very little, if anything, to the overall decline.[19-20]

If you look at the graphs on the following pages you will notice that the curves showing the average rate of decline do not change when vaccines were initiated, indicating they had little overall effect. Currently the annual death rates in small children for measles, mumps, rubella, chicken pox, tetanus, diphtheria, polio, and most other childhood diseases are essentially zero. More children die from candida (yeast infection) overgrowth each year than from *all* these other diseases combined! These current rates would be the same whether vaccinations were given or not.

Mothers who have had these diseases transfer antibodies to their children who are then protected for the first 6-12 months of their lives. This allows the infant's immune system time to mature. When children do get a childhood infection naturally the response is different from that induced by a vaccine. Not only is the immunity longer lasting, but it primes the immune system so that it becomes more effective in fighting off other infections and destroying cancerous cells. For example, it has been found that women who have had mumps during childhood are less likely to develop ovarian cancer then women who did not have this childhood infection.[21]

Vaccine proponents often attempt to intimidate and bully parents who choose not to vaccinate their children. They try to make them feel guilty by claiming that the parent's actions will be the cause of a new epidemic that will put everyone in danger. Well, if their own kids are vaccinated what do they care? They're protected, right? That's what they keep telling us—vaccines provide adequate protection. Only those who have chosen not to be vaccinated would be at risk, and they are willing to take that risk.

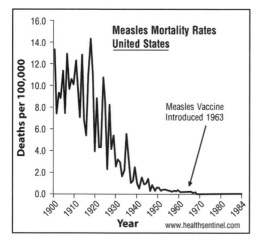

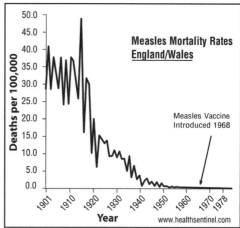

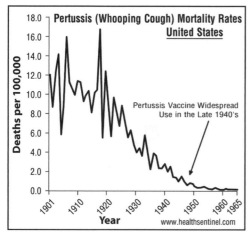

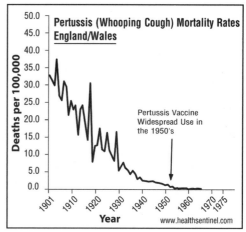

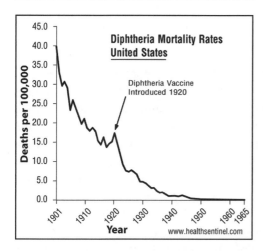

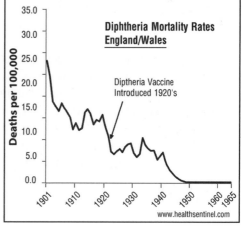

Death rates due to infectious disease in the US and UK began dropping rapidly during the 20th century long before vaccines were introduced. This decline in infectious disease corresponds with the improvements in sanitation not with the introduction of vaccinations.

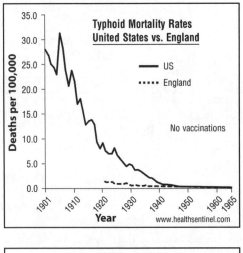
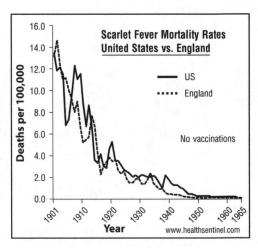
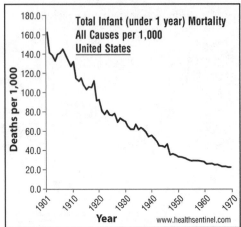
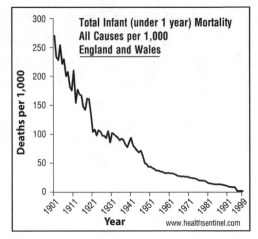

The death rate from all infectious diseases declined during the 20th century even for diseases for which there were no vaccines.

A new epidemic of childhood diseases is not likely. The high death rates we saw from infectious diseases a century ago will never return even if everyone refuses vaccination, as evidenced from the graphs. Modern sanitation practices have guaranteed this. Disease incidence may increase to some degree, but this is not necessarily a bad thing. The reason children died in the past was because they were in poor health to begin with due to malnutrition and filthy living conditions. Children nowadays are far better off and are not likely to suffer any lasting harm from most childhood diseases. Catching these illnesses is actually a good thing as it allows children to strengthen their resistance to infection and cancer and become immune to the disease for life. In times past, parents expected and even welcomed these infections as a rite of passage through childhood. It was not unheard of for mothers to purposely expose their children to those with an infection in order for them to catch the illness while young so they could build a lifelong immunity to the disease.

Instead of preventing disease, vaccines may be the cause of much of it. Since vaccines have come into widespread use, once rare or previously unheard of disorders have burst onto the scene. One of these is sudden infant death syndrome (SIDS). SIDS is the leading cause of death in infants under 1 year of age. Researchers have ruled out suffocation, vomiting or choking, birth defects, and infection as the cause. Exactly why SIDS occurs remains a mystery. However, the more vaccinations a child receives, the greater the risk. Following the immunization schedule recommended by the CDC, an infant receives as many as 18 vaccinations within the first 6 months of life—the period of time SIDS usually occurs. Again, safety studies have never been done to know how all these vaccines affect newborns.

BOTTOM LINE

Which vaccines should your children receive? In most cases, none of them. Healthy children have little to fear from the diseases for which vaccines are used. These children are strong enough to mount a robust defense and overcome these infections. Those children whose immune systems are not functioning at par or whose health is compromised in some way are the ones who will suffer the most if they catch one of these infections. These are the ones who could benefit the most from immunization, however, they are also the ones who will experience the greatest adverse reactions. They are the ones who will end up with autism, epilepsy, or developmental disorders. Ironically, the ones who can benefit the most from vaccinations are also the ones who are hurt most by them.

It is not always easy to tell which children have health concerns that would put them in danger from vaccinations. Any child that has obvious health or developmental problems is at high risk. If your child has had a serious illness of any type, even if the illness is now under control, he or she is at increased risk. It's not always easy to identify if an infant's health has been compromised and is vulnerable to vaccinations. Children with compromised health can appear to develop normally. So how can you tell? Here are some possible clues:

Infant
Has or ever has had colic, jaundice, ear infection, thrush, allergies
Frequent illnesses
Bottle fed in place of breast fed
Cries frequently
Premature birth
Low birth weight
Suffered a bad reaction from a previous vaccination

Mother
Vaccinated when pregnant
Sick often
Poor lifestyle habits (smoking, alcohol, caffeine, drugs, etc.)
Poor diet or malnourished
Diabetic/insulin resistant
Gestational diabetes

Autoimmune disorder (asthma, allergies, lupus, etc.)
Numerous amalgam dental fillings
Exposed to environmental or industrial toxins during pregnancy
Serious illness during pregnancy

For most children it is probably best not to receive any vaccination. Healthy children usually don't need them and less healthy children are the ones who are harmed the most by them. The only exceptions would be if there is an immediate and direct threat. For instance, if a mother has hepatitis B, the newborn should be vaccinated.

If you do choose to have your children vaccinated, wait until they are at least two years old before they receive any of them. Make sure the vaccine does not contain thimerosal or a live virus (except for smallpox if an outbreak ever occurs). Get only one vaccine at a time, not a combination (i.e., MMR, MMRV, DTaP), and space them six months apart to give the immune system enough time to recover. Live viruses are often contained in the following vaccines:

Flu
Polio
Smallpox
MMR
Pneumococcual Polysaccharide (PPSV)
Varicella
BCG (tuberculosis)

Normally by age 15 most unvaccinated children have had measles, mumps, and rubella and have acquired a natural immunity to them. This is the way it has been for generations of children. When infected as children these diseases are relatively mild and often asymptomatic and can go completely unnoticed. As a person gets older, these diseases can cause more trouble. If you are worried about your unvaccinated children catching one of these diseases later in life, you might consider waiting until they are 15 or 16 and have them tested. If blood tests show they have not been exposed to these diseases then you might consider having them vaccinated at this time. If possible, get each vaccine separately, six months apart.

HOW TO AVOID UNWANTED VACCINATIONS

Once you have made a decision to forgo a vaccination you will be confronted with naysayers who will try to convince you otherwise. They will feed you the half-truths and misconceptions the drug industry has perpetuated for years. They may even ridicule you in an attempt to make you feel guilty or stupid.

Some will counsel you by saying things like, "Talk to your family doctor, and follow his recommendations. He has the training and expertise to know what's good for you." While this may sound logical, it isn't true. Doctors are trained to follow the recommended vaccination schedule. Unless they have taken the time to research the issue on their own, which most do not, their sole reservoir of knowledge about vaccines comes straight from the vaccine makers who write the literature they read and sponsor the educational seminars they attend. Parroting the drug makers, doctors will tell you that vaccines are completely safe and that you put your children at greater risk by not having them vaccinated. Well, you know better.

If you are pregnant, get tested for hepatitis B. If you are infected, your baby should receive this vaccine. If not, there is absolutely no reason for it. If you don't want your newborn to receive this vaccine, you can amend the "consent for medical treatment" forms you sign upon entering the hospital before delivery. Write on the form that you do not give consent for your baby to receive the hepatitis B vaccination. Then make sure the doctors and nurses are aware of this after delivery so they don't forget.

After delivery, you will be expected to bring your baby to the doctor for periodic checkups. This is when infants normally receive hepatitis B booster shots and other vaccinations. If your doctor insists your child get a particular vaccination, simply tell him "no." Stand firm. Despite his possible objections, you have the right to decide what is injected into the bodies of your children. No one can force your children to be vaccinated.

Your next hurdle will be when your children are old enough to enter school. All 50 states in the US require children to be immunized against measles, diphtheria, haemophilus influenzae type b (Hib), polio, and rubella in order to enroll in daycare or public school. Forty-nine states also require vaccination against tetanus; 47 against hepatitis B and mumps; and 43 states require vaccination against chicken pox. If your children are homeschooled then there is no problem. If not, you will need to get an exemption before they can attend.

There are three types of exemptions: medical, religious, and philosophical. All 50 states allow the medical exemption. For example, if your child is allergic to an ingredient in the vaccines, you will be granted a medical exemption. You will need a signed letter from your doctor.

All states, with the exception of Mississippi and West Virginia, allow a religious exemption. The exemption is only allowed for religions which have a written tenet opposing vaccinations. A letter from your church leader is required. California doesn't specifically allow a religious exemption, however, the philosophical exemption can encompass personal religious beliefs which essentially confers a religious exemption.

Eighteen states allow a philosophical, personal, or conscientious belief exemption. The following states allow this exemption: Arizona, Arkansas, California, Colorado, Idaho, Louisiana, Maine, Michigan, Minnesota, New Mexico, North Dakota, Ohio, Oklahoma, Texas, Utah, Vermont, Washington, and Wisconsin.

Requirements and exemptions are different in each state and laws change periodically. You should become familiar with the specific vaccine requirements in your state. You can find details for each state at: http://www.nvic.org/Vaccine-Laws/state-vaccine-requirements.aspx. For information in Canada go to: http://vran.org/exemptions/. Additional information is available at www.vaclib.org. For Australia go to http://www.vaclib.org/exempt/australia.htm. In the UK and New Zealand, vaccination is not compulsory.

There is no guarantee that vaccines will protect against any infectious disease or that the injection will not cause complications, injury, or death. If your child is injured by a vaccine, it is your responsibility. You will have little recourse and will be left to deal with the consequences on your own. You have the right to make an informed decision regarding your children's health. Parents should be the only ones who make that decision, not government officials, drug companies, school administrators, or doctors following some predetermined vaccine schedule. It is each parent's responsibility to investigate the pros and cons of vaccination before making a decision. In fact, it is irresponsible not to investigate the consequences of exposing your children to potentially life threatening pharmaceuticals. You cannot rely on other people's opinions, especially when these people stand to profit from your child's vaccination. If you still have questions or concerns about vaccinations, before making a decision you may want to check out some of the following websites:

National Vaccine Information Center (NVIC), www.nvic.org
The Age of Autism, www.ageofautism.com
The Coalition for Safe Minds, www.safeminds.org
Dr. Mercola, http://vaccines.mercola.com
Think Twice, http://www.thinktwice.com
Vaccine Injury Info, www.vaccineinjury.info

5 | The Underlying Cause of Autism

BASIC STRUCTURE OF THE BRAIN

The nervous system consists of the brain, spinal cord, and peripheral nerves. At the center of this network are the brain and spinal cord, which function as the control center for the body and together are referred to as the central nervous system.

The three main structures of the brain are the *brain stem*, the *cerebellum*, and the *cerebrum*. Every area in the brain has an associated function, although many functions may involve a number of different areas. The brain stem is an extension of the spinal cord and monitors involuntary activities such as breathing and digestion. The cerebellum coordinates muscular movements and monitors posture and balance. The cerebrum, which occupies the topmost portion of the brain, is by far the largest of the three, comprising 70 percent of the weight of the entire nervous system. Its appearance is that of being convoluted and folded. Its outer surface is called the *cerebral cortex* and contains most of the master controls of the body. In the cortex, sensory data is analyzed; we think, remember and reason; and impulses originate that control the entire spectrum of muscle and gland activity. Beneath the cerebral cortex and deep within the cerebrum is the seat of emotions and learning.

Compared to other cells in the body, nerves contain a disproportionately high amount of lipids (fat and cholesterol). Ignoring the water content, the brain consists of about 60 percent fat. This gives the brain a soft consistency similar to gelatin. Because it is a delicate and vital organ, it is encased within the hard protective shield of the skull, wrapped in a tough fibrous membrane called the *dura mater* (Latin for "hard mother"), and surrounded by a liquid called the *cerebrospinal fluid* that acts as a cushion to absorb the impact from falls and bumps.

Blood vessels in the brain provide another form of protection. The brain is very sensitive to chemical and microbial insults. Toxins and microorganisms which are often carried in the blood could cause a great deal of harm to sensitive brain tissues if no defenses were in place. To screen out harmful substances, the cells in the blood vessel walls of the brain are joined tightly, forming what is called the *blood-brain barrier*. This barrier keeps out most unwanted substances.

The brain consists of several thousand miles of interconnected nerve cells (about 100 billion in all) with innumerable extensions that control every movement, sensation, thought, and emotion that encompasses the human experience. Nerve cells come in different varieties with varying functions. Some relay sensory information from peripheral nerves throughout the body to the brain, others deliver commands from the brain to the rest of the body, and still others function as scaffolding for the support of other nerves. Despite being composed entirely of nerve cells, the brain itself does not feel pain. The nerves there have no pain receptors. A headache is felt due to sensory impulses coming chiefly from the tissues surrounding the skull.

The brain contains two types of nerve cells: glia and neurons. Glia (Latin for "glue") are the most numerous of the brain's cells and provide the structural support, the glue, so to speak, that holds all the brain cells together. There are a number of different types of glial cells, each of which performs different critical functions including nutritional support, insulating neurons from one another, fighting off pathogens, removing dead neurons, and regulating the environment of the cerebrospinal fluid surrounding the brain. Glia, however, do not relay signals: that is the function of the neurons. Neurons transmit signals by means of electrochemical impulses which allow us to think, act, and perceive our environment. A single neuron can be directly linked to tens of thousands of other neurons, creating a totality of more than 100 trillion connections, each capable of performing hundreds of calculations per second. This forms the basis of the brain's capacity for memory and thinking.

Neurons consist of three basic parts: (1) the cell body, which contains most of the cell's organelles (cell organs), (2) the axon, a long cable-like projection of the cell that carries electrochemical messages (nerve impulses) along the length of the cell, and (3) dendrites or nerve endings that branch out like a tree to make connections to other cells and allow the neurons to "talk" with each other or sense the environment.

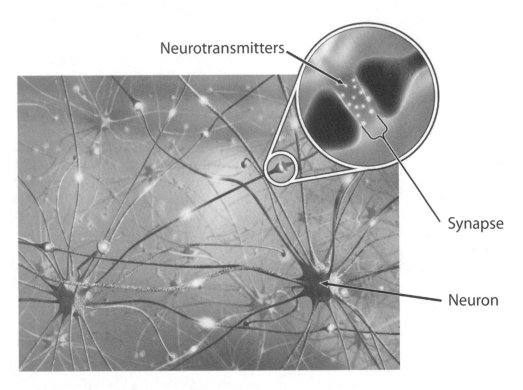

Neurotransmitters

Synapse

Neuron

Neurons send messages at lightning speed in the form of electrochemical pulses. There is no partial pulse—that is, they either fire a transmission or they remain silent. Intensity is expressed by how many neurons fire and how rapidly. A strong reaction results from many neurons firing in rapid succession. Neurons fire pulses whenever instructed to do so. A pulse can be triggered by sensations from peripheral nerves or commands or thoughts in the brain. Neurons relay electrochemical signals from one nerve cell to the next, and send signals in only one direction. The signals are picked up by the dendrites and transported along the cell through the axon, then branch out to the many axon terminals and are passed to the dendrites of connecting neurons.

The axon terminals do not actually touch the dendrites of neighboring neurons. The electrochemical signal must "jump" from one cell to the next. The gap between an axon terminal and a dendrite is called the synapse. Each neuron typically has between 1,000 to 10,000 synapses. The synapse is an incredibly narrow space—only about two millionths of a centimeter in width. When a nerve impulse reaches the end of an axon, it transfers the signal to the next neuron by releasing chemicals called *neurotransmitters* into this fluid-filled space. These neurotransmitters cross the synapse to the next neuron, triggering an electrochemical impulse that is passed along in a like manner to the next neuron.

Neurotransmitters are the means by which neurons communicate with each other. There are a number of different neurotransmitters. Endorphins, epinephrine, melatonin, glutamine, and dopamine are some of the most recognized ones. Specific neurotransmitters are used by specific neurons in different parts of the brain. Psychoactive drugs exert their effects by activating neurotransmitter receptors in neurons. For example, addictive drugs such as cocaine, amphetamine, and heroin trigger neurons sensitive to dopamine.

HUMAN BRAIN DEVELOPMENT

The brain, much like a computer, relies on an intricate system of circuits to store, process, retrieve, and transmit information. However, unlike a computer, we are not born with this circuitry hardwired. The billions of circuits and connections gradually assemble and arrange themselves in response to life's experiences. Through repeated neurological activity this circuitry is reinforced and soldered together.

Using magnetic resonance imaging (MRI) and positron emission tomography (PET) scans, researchers have been able to observe how the brain matures and develops over time. The most rapid period of brain growth and development occurs during the last trimester of pregnancy (i.e., the final three months) and the first two years after birth. During this time the brain more than quadruples in size. This is referred to as the brain growth spurt and is the most critical stage of brain development. During this time there is an overdevelopment of synaptic connections. Approximately 1 million of these connections are formed in the brain each day. During early childhood and even up into adolescence, excess connections, which can interfere with proper brain function, are gradually removed or "pruned." The cerebral cortex, which regulates

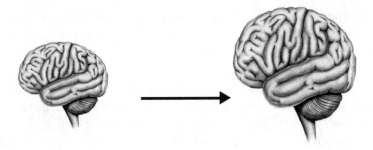

A normal infant's brain increases in weight from 350 g to 1200 g by age two.

higher brain functions such as emotions, emotional control, problem solving, and language, is the last part of the brain to mature.

The pruning process is essential in order to streamline and organize the brain's circuitry. In people with autism, the pruning process has been disrupted. The brain's wiring is faulty, causing misfiring in the communication between the brain cells.

Imaging studies have revealed that the nerve fibers in autistic children are disorganized, which cause a jumbled array of conflicting and competing signals, muddling the mind. This jumble of electrical signals essentially causes "static" that interferes with proper brain function affecting understanding, attention, reasoning, and language.

It is like tuning into a radio station. If you don't get the frequency just right, the signal is drowned out by the static. Depending on the amount of static, it could be very difficult to understand and make any sense of what is being broadcast. The same is true with an autistic child. The signals he receives are jumbled and incoherent making it impossible for him to understand what is going on around him and how to respond appropriately. Some sounds may even be painful or annoying. This can cause a great deal of frustration for the child, resulting in outbursts and inappropriate behavior.

Anything that interferes with the normal differentiation and development of the brain can lead to defects in circuitary. The most critical time for a child's brain development is during the first 26 months of age. However, since the brain continues to mature for many years, developmental disorders can occur throughout childhood.

IMMUNE FUNCTION

The immune system protects against infectious organisms and toxins; recycles old, diseased, or renegade cells (cancer); and promotes tissue repair and healing. The backbone of the immune system is the army of white blood cells which constantly patrol the body. There are many varieties of white blood cells, all with different functions. Some white blood cells act as phagocytes and eat foreign invaders, while some secrete lethal substances on them, and still others produce antibodies—proteins created to neutralize specific microorganisms.

The immune system is normally capable of providing adequate protection against infection. However, due to the blood-brain barrier, the central nervous system is generally inaccessible to the white blood cells and antibodies. Therefore, the brain has its own immune system, separate from the rest of the body. Specialized glia cells called *microglia* act as the brain's primary defense system.

Normally, microglia are in a resting state and rather inconspicuous. When activated by an intruder or an injury they spring into action, quickly proliferating, enlarging, mobilizing, and going on the attack, engulfing foreign substances and removing damaged cells. Essentially, they take on the duties and character of white blood cells. In the process, they send signals that increase blood flow, stimulate inflammation, and rally various substances to their aid. After the crisis is over, the microglia gradually return to the docile existence they led before the insult.

Ordinarily, this process protects the brain from insults due to infections, injury, and toxins while stimulating cleanup and repair. However, in the process of fighting an infection or removing dangerous toxins, some collateral damage is sustained. It's somewhat like firefighters putting out a fire. As they flood the burning building with water and break out windows for air circulation, they cause some damage themselves. However, this damage is necessary in order to save the building from total destruction and to prevent the fire from spreading. Once the fire is out, cleanup and repair restores the building to its former use.

When the microglia are activated, they initiate the release of a variety of substances to aid in the brain's defense. While beneficial in the short run, some of these substances, such as proinflammatory cytokines and chemokines, nitric oxide, excitotoxins, proteases, and free radicals, are potentially harmful to brain tissues.

Frequent exposure to stressors like heavy metals, drugs, toxins, or infections can keep the microglia continually activated, stoking the flames of inflammation and promoting tissue damage. Inflammation also disrupts the blood-brain barrier, causing it to become leaky. White blood cells, blood proteins, bacteria, and other substances that were once locked out of the central nervous system are now allowed to enter, stirring up more trouble and activating more microglia and producing more inflammation, creating a vicious cycle. As long as inflammation is present, collateral damage to brain tissue continues and the cleanup crew is unable to complete the job of repairing and rebuilding. In adults, brain function is lost, leading to Parkinson's disease, Alzheimer's disease, and various forms of dementia.[1-3] In a small child, not only is brain function lost but normal development is disrupted also, giving rise to epilepsy, autism, and other learning and developmental disorders.[4-6]

CHRONIC IMMUNE ACTIVATION: THE ROOT CAUSE OF AUTISM

A newborn's immune system is immature and incapable of fighting off a serious infection. Infants depend on their mother's antibodies for protection for the first few months of life. At birth they have a high level of their mother's antibodies circulating in their bloodstream. Breast milk supplies additional antibodies along with other germ-fighting substances.

During the first few months of life the antibodies passed from the mother to the infant steadily decrease. When a healthy baby is about two to three months old it starts to produce its own antibodies. At this time, the infant's blood levels of antibodies are at its lowest because the initial antibodies passed on by the mother are nearly depleted and the infant's immune system produces antibodies at a much slower rate than in adults. It takes about six months for the baby's immune system to reach a point where it is capable of defending itself. The immune system continues to mature for several years. Consequently, the immune response is dramatically different among infants, toddlers, adolescents, and adults. A fetus is the most vulnerable. This is why even relatively minor infections, such as rubella, can be devastating for an unborn child. Maternal rubella can lead to severe birth defects and is a known cause of autism, though any infection is potentially dangerous to a fetus.

In 2003 neurosurgeon Russell Blaylock, MD, proposed the idea that autism was caused by the over-activation of the brain's immune system. Repeated immune stimulation from vaccines, infections, and toxins (including mercury and aluminum) could result in severe disruption of proper brain development. He also predicted that removing mercury from vaccines would help reduce the problem, but would not eliminate it.[7] Everything he said has proven to be accurate.

Two years after the publication of Blaylock's paper, researchers at Johns Hopkins University published a study that supported his hypothesis. The researchers examined brain tissues from 18 people with autism, aged 5 to 44 years, who had died from accidents or injuries. They also measured levels of inflammatory proteins in the cerebrospinal fluid (the fluid that surrounds the brain and spinal cord) in six living autistic patients, ages 5 to 12 years. In each case, they found extensive activation of the microglia and widespread elevated inflammation. The evidence indicated that brain immune activation had persisted for years.[8] Their conclusion was that overstimulation of the brain's immune system plays a major role in the pathogenesis of autism. They suggested the use of therapies that would modify immune responses in the brain as a way to treat autistic patients. These findings have been confirmed by a number of other researchers.[9-13]

It is apparent that a chronic inflammatory state exists in the brains of autistic patients. The high levels of neurotoxic compounds generated from this process interferes with proper brain development, causing autism.[14]

What causes microglia activation and chronic neuroinflammation? Vaccines, disease-causing microorganisms, toxic metals, environmental pollution, neurotoxins in food, head trauma, mind altering drugs, and allergic reactions can all contribute to neuroinflammation. Autism can result when a child or fetus is exposed to a combination of these factors over an extended period of time. The next chapter explores the various conditions that can lead to neuroinflammation.

6 | Causes of Neuroinflammation

VACCINES

Vaccines infuse a mixture of germs and toxins directly into the bloodstream purposely to elicit an immune reaction. The younger the child is when he or she receives the shot, the more turmoil it causes. An infant's immature immune system will be unable to mount a normal controlled defense. The response will be slow and inefficient in ridding these poisons from the body. Booster shots are often needed to induce a strong enough response to make it effective. Each shot causes a prolonged period of inflammation in the immature brain that could last for one to six months.

Giving vaccinations to very young children is bad enough, but the repeated administration of vaccines creates an even bigger danger. Never in any time in history have children received so many vaccinations. During this same period of time developmental disorders have risen to epidemic proportions. This is not a coincidence.

Following the recommended vaccination schedule, children receive their first shot on the day of birth. Between one and two months of age, six more shots are given. Two months later another six shots. After another two months, four more shots. Over the next four years another 18 shots are administered. Since microglia activation can persist for up to six months with each shot, the brain could be in a continual state of intense immune hyperactivity for the child's first few years of life. During this time the brain will be under constant assault from runaway inflammation, destructive free radicals, and harmful excitotoxins created by the immune response. Microglia become more sensitized with each additional vaccine. Each succeeding vaccine intensifies the brain's immune response, increasing the likelihood of serious brain damage.

Another problem with vaccines is that they can overburden the immune system, weakening its ability to fight off natural infections.[1-5] While vaccines may help defend against some infections, they may lower the body's ability to fight off others. Natural infections such as the flu, colds, earaches, or candida overgrowth (i.e., diaper rash, thrush) promote more inflammation, making the situation even worse.

At some point the intense immune activity can become self–perpetuating, leading to autism. In some cases, this may occur very early in life before the child is old enough to communicate in any meaningful way. In others, the child will develop normally for the first year or so before regressing into an autistic stupor.

INFECTIONS
Brain Infections

Infections are a common cause of neurodegenerative and neurodevelopmental disorders. If bacteria, viruses, or fungi penetrate the blood-brain barrier they can cause a local infection in the brain. In some cases, this leads to an acute infection— encephalitis. In other cases, the immune system may be capable of preventing the infection from progressing to encephalitis, yet not completely eradicate it. In this situation, a low-grade chronic infection may occur that could persist for years. As long as the brain's immune system is activated, harmful byproducts continually eat away at the brain. More damage is actually caused by the brain's overactive immune system than by the infection itself.

Many cases of dementia, Parkinson's disease, and other neurodegenerative disorders are caused by chronic brain infections.[6-11] In the vast majority of these cases, the infection is not discovered until an autopsy is performed.

In a child or fetus, infection can destroy brain tissue and interfere with normal brain development, thus leading to autism. As far back as the 1970s, infection of the mother by the rubella virus during pregnancy was recognized as a cause of autism.[12-13] The virus can spread to the fetus causing a number of birth defects including blindness, deafness, heart and muscle defects, and autism.[14] The rubella virus isn't the only known cause of autism. Infection by *Borrelia burgdorferi* and cytomegalovirus (CMV) during pregnancy have also been linked to autism.[15-16]

Borrelia burgdorferi is the bacterium that causes Lyme disease. Lyme disease is spread by the bite of infected deer ticks. Since the ticks are very small, bites often go undetected. Flu-like symptoms may develop, which may be mistaken as an ordinary flu infection. Left untreated, the disease can affect the joints, heart, and central nervous system.

Cytomegalovirus is a herpes virus. Like all herpes viruses, after the initial infection CMV usually lies dormant within the body, but can be reactivated when the immune system is challenged, such as during an illness or when under heavy stress. The virus is very common, infecting at least 50 percent of the population. In adults an acute infection causes only minor symptoms and lasts only a few weeks. Unborn babies can be infected if their mothers become infected with the virus or a latent virus is reactivated. Infants who are infected before birth usually show no symptoms after they are born, however, over time some develop hearing, vision, neurological, and developmental problems. Some become autistic. In the United States, it is estimated that about 1 percent of all newborns are infected with CMV.

While unborn children are at high risk, any microorganism that infects the brain has the potential to cause autism regardless of the person's age. Encephalitis caused by the common oral herpes viruses (herpes simplex) has been documented to cause autism in older individuals. In one case, a normally developing 14-year-old girl developed autism from a herpes infection that entered her brain.[17] In another case, a healthy

31-year-old man contracted herpes encephalitis and over the following months developed all the symptoms considered diagnostic of autism.[18] Any infectious microorganism that enters the brain can cause brain damage or autism regardless of the person's age. In older people encephalitis usually causes dementia or other related neurodegenerative conditions; in young children whose brains are still growing and maturing, autism or some other developmental defect is often the result.

Infectious microorganisms that have been linked to the development of autism include measles, rubella, herpes simplex virus, human herpes virus-6, mumps, varicella, cytomegalovirus, mycoplasma, and *Chlamydia pneunomiae*.[19-21]

Systemic Infections

An active infection can cause autism without even being present in the brain. That's right. An infectious microorganism doesn't even need to be in the brain to cause neurological damage! This is a very important concept to understand. Infections of any type, whether from the flu, food poisoning, bladder infection, colitis, yeast infection, pneumonia, or even periodontitis (gum infection), release pro-inflammatory cytokines—special proteins manufactured by the immune system to activate inflammation. Any injury or infection causes the release of cytokines into the bloodstream to stimulate inflammation. As the cytokines cross over the blood-brain barrier, they activate microglia, triggering an inflammatory response in the brain. Even though no infectious organisms actually enter the brain, the microglia shift into a heightened level of activity just as if they had.[22-25]

Neuroinflammation triggered by systemic infection can affect behavior and mental function. Physicians are very familiar with delirium—a temporary state of mental confusion accompanied by anxiety, hallucinations, disturbed speech, and impaired cognition associated with someone fighting an infection. If a person is already suffering from a neurodegenerative or neurodevelopmental disorder, a systemic infection can accelerate mental decline.[26]

This process has been documented with various neurodegenerative conditions such as Alzheimer's disease. Like autism, a major problem with Alzheimer's disease is the chronic activation of microglia. In one study, for instance, even a minor infection such as a cold was shown to accelerate mental decline and double the rate of memory loss. This study involved 222 patients with mild to severe Alzheimer's. Over the course of six months, blood samples were taken periodically from each patient to measure cytokine levels. During the study period, about half of the patients had one or more colds or other respiratory or gastrointestinal infections. Those who experienced increased cytokine levels due to these infections had *twice* the rate of cognitive decline than those with normal levels.

Interestingly, some of the patients had elevated cytokine levels at the beginning of the study due to chronic inflammatory conditions like arthritis, irritable bowel syndrome, hemorrhoids, and such. If they got an infection during the study period they experienced *10 times* the memory loss.[27] They started out with elevated cytokine levels, and the infection just increased those levels even more, accelerating their mental decline even further. The higher the cytokine levels, the greater the effect it has on microglia activation and consequently, brain health.

Acute and chronic illnesses that increase inflammation, even outside the central nervous system, may have serious consequences on cognitive function and mental development. The authors of the study stressed that the decline in mental function was not a temporary effect but remained even after the illness and inflammation had passed.

Many children with autism have a very long history of chronic infections and illnesses, indicating subnormal immune function. This makes them highly susceptible to the live viruses contained in the MMR, Varicella, polio, influenza, pneumococcal pneumonia (PPSV), and tuberculosis (BCG) vaccines, as well as infections from natural sources. Live virus vaccines pose a special danger because they can take up permanent residence in the body, hiding out in the kidneys, spleen, liver, lungs, intestines, nerves, or brain. These low-grade or subclinical infections continually stimulate the release of pro-inflammatory cytokines into the bloodstream.

Antibodies to the MMR vaccine (specifically the measles virus) have been found to be significantly higher in autistic children than in normal children, strongly suggesting involvement of the MMR vaccine in the development of autism in these children.[28] It also indicates that the measles virus has taken up permanent residence somewhere in the body, causing a low-grade infection or perhaps a virus-induced autoimmunity that affects the central nervous system. In one study, for example, out of 125 autistic children, 75 (60 percent) had elevated antibodies to the MMR vaccine, but none of the 92 normal children tested had elevated levels.[29] In a similar study involving 88 autistic subjects, elevated antibodies to the MMR vaccine were found in 83 percent of the autistic children, but not in any of the 47 normal children tested.[30]

Studies have shown that the measles virus from vaccines can infiltrate the gut and set up residence, causing chronic colitis (inflammation of the gastrointestinal tract). Any live vaccine virus can potentially do this. Studies show a large number of autistic children have gastrointestinal problems—abdominal pain, bloating, diarrhea, and constipation.[31-32] These issues are often accompanied by mild to moderate degrees of inflammation in both the upper and lower intestinal tracts.[33] There is a strong correlation of gastrointestinal symptoms with autism and the more severe the inflammation, the greater the severity of autism.[34]

It is important to realize that an infection anywhere in the body triggers microglia activation in the brain. Chronic infections, such as colitis, can keep microglia in the brain constantly activated. Frequent acute infections, especially when combined with periodic vaccinations, can do the same. Many minor infections that are normally not given much thought such as sinus, ear, throat, and periodontal (gum) infections can also contribute to the problem.

Maternal Infections

Infections during pregnancy can increase the risk of neurological disorders in offspring. In a series of studies conducted at Rush University Medical Center in Chicago, researchers injected pregnant rats with lipopolysaccharide, or LPS, which is a major constituent of the cell wall of certain bacteria. LPS triggers an immune response in the host without causing an actual infection from living bacteria. They chose this method because bacterial vaginosis occurs in up to 20 percent of pregnant women and can also infect the womb.

Rat pups that had been exposed to LPS while in their mother's womb were born with approximately 25-30 percent fewer dopamine neurons than normal rat pups. This loss of neurons was not noticeable in the rats' behavior because 70-80 percent loss must occur before symptoms become evident. However, over time more dopamine neurons were gradually lost, so that by 17 months of age, these rats had 46 percent fewer dopamine neurons compared to normal rats of the same age.

The rate of neuron loss was accelerated when the pups were exposed to one of two environmental toxins, 6-hydroxydopamine and rotenone, the latter being a commonly used pesticide that is known to damage dopamine neurons. At birth, as well as throughout the animals' lives, the brain tissue of the rats exposed to the LPS showed signs of increased inflammation. LPS initiated inflammation in the womb and exposure to environmental toxins fanned the flames, keeping inflammation alive, leading to an ongoing loss of dopamine neurons.[35-37] This illustrates that a combination of assaults on the brain can greatly accelerate brain damage and interfere with normal brain development.

While the researchers noted the possibility of bacteria reaching the uterus due to bacterial vaginosis, bacteria or their toxins could also come from other types of infections. Another common source is from oral infections in the mother. Studies show that the bacteria commonly found in the mouth and associated with periodontal (gum) disease can find their way into the amniotic fluid of pregnant women.[38] In fact, gum disease is a well documented risk factor for premature and underweight births.[39] Preterm and underweight deliveries indicate incomplete development and potential health problems in the future, including a greater risk of autism.

Any type of maternal infection can adversely affect the fetus whether it is actually passed to the fetus or not. A mother's immune response to infection includes the release of pro-inflammatory cytokines that pass through the placenta and cross the blood-brain barrier of the fetus, triggering neuroinflammation.[40] It has been reported that during pregnancy, mothers of autistic children commonly have a higher number of fevers and bacterial and viral infections.[41-43] In one study, for example, it was reported that 43 percent of mothers with an autistic child experienced upper respiratory tract, influenza-like, urinary, or vaginal infections during pregnancy compared to only 26 percent of mothers with normal children.[44] In another study, women were more likely to have an autistic child if they had been admitted to the hospital with a viral or bacterial infection during pregnancy.[45]

ALLERGIES

Food and environmental allergies also cause systemic inflammation that can trigger microglia activation. An allergy is an inappropriate hypersensitive reaction to an ordinarily harmless substance. Substances that cause allergic reactions are called antigens. An antigen triggers an immune response, producing antibodies and pro-inflammatory cytokines, just as if fighting an infectious microorganism. Allergies, although common, are not a normal reaction. They are a result of an imperfectly functioning immune system—a situation common among autistic children.

Some allergies cause only a minor response and may go undetected. Others can elicit a violent response leading to anaphylactic shock, which could result in death.

Common allergic symptoms include abdominal pain, nausea, vomiting, diarrhea, inflamed nasal membranes (stuffy nose), asthma, chest pain, hives, swelling, headache, and low blood pressure. Food allergies may also influence behavior causing irritability, aggression, hyperactivity, and depression.

Allergies can be triggered by just about any type of food. However, some foods tend to be more troublesome than others. The foods that most often cause allergies are wheat, milk, nuts, peanuts, soybeans, eggs, chicken, fish, and shellfish. Allergic reactions to single foods such as milk are common. About 2 to 3 percent of infants in Western countries are estimated to be allergic to cow's milk. Reactions to two or more foods, such as both wheat and milk, are much less common.

Allergies can contribute to autism in some cases.[46] Therefore, removing allergens from the child's diet can bring about noticeable improvement. Milk and wheat have been given the greatest attention in regards to autism. A number of studies have shown improvement in behavior when autistic children are placed on wheat-free and milk-free diets.[47]

Antigens are typically large protein molecules within the foods; in wheat it is gluten that is of most concern and in milk it is casein. A gluten-free, casein-free (GFCF) diet is often recommended to help treat autism. A 2008 survey conducted by the Autism Research Institute showed that out of the 2,500 cases in which a gluten-free, casein-free diet was used in the treatment of autism, 66 percent of children experienced some degree of improvement. However, not all children with autism experience benefits by eliminating milk or wheat.[48] This makes sense, since not all children have allergies to these foods.

Some children have a gluten sensitivity called celiac disease. Celiac disease is an autoimmune disorder in which the lining of the small intestine is damaged by gluten. The damage seriously impairs nutrient absorption, resulting in weight loss as well as vitamin and mineral deficiencies. Exactly how gluten damages the intestinal lining is not fully understood, but an abnormal immunological response is involved. The immune system becomes sensitized to gluten and reacts in the same way it would to an antigen. The proportion of people affected by the disease varies widely among different countries and populations. In the United States it is estimated that 1 out of every 133 people are affected.

The severity of the disease varies, and many people never develop noticeable symptoms. These people can go through life without realizing they are not absorbing nutrients properly and unknowingly experience subclinical levels of malnutrition. Symptoms range from vague tiredness and breathlessness to weight loss, diarrhea, gas, vomiting, abdominal pain, and leg swelling. In children, celiac disease has also been associated with epilepsy, learning disorders, attention deficit hyperactivity disorder (ADHD), and developmental disorders.[49] Although a brain-gut connection may not be obvious, if you understand that inflammation anywhere in the body can trigger inflammation in the brain, neurological symptoms seem reasonable.

The only effective treatment known for celiac disease is complete lifelong abstinence from gluten. All foods containing gluten, which includes wheat (durum, semolina, kamut, and spelt), rye, and barley, must be avoided. Although oats do not contain gluten, they are usually processed with grains that do and become contaminated with gluten, so they should also be avoided. When gluten is removed from the diet, the lining of the intestine has a chance to heal. Within a few weeks symptoms generally clear up and the sufferer starts to enjoy normal health. Although health improves, gluten can never be reintroduced into the diet. Gluten sensitivity is a permanent condition.

ENVIRONMENTAL AND INDUSTRIAL TOXINS

In recent history, mankind has drastically changed the chemistry of the environment in which we live. Since the end of World War II, the world has been flooded with tens of thousands of synthetic chemicals. Many of these are highly toxic. Every year more than 1 billion pounds of chemicals are released into the environment worldwide. As a consequence, we are exposed to an endless variety of toxins in the air we breathe, the foods we eat, and the water we drink. We are also exposed to chemicals in items we come into contact with every day such as synthetic carpets, paints, hair spray, cosmetics, furniture polish, drugs, food additives, toothpaste, detergents, household cleaning aids, weed killers, pesticides, gasoline, etc. Some of the chemicals in these products are potent neurotoxins that can harm the brain of a developing fetus or young child.

We are in the midst of a "silent pandemic," says Philippe Grandjean, MD, PhD, Department of Environmental Health, Harvard School of Public Health. Neurodevelopmental disorders like autism, ADHD, and mental retardation affect millions of children worldwide and, according to Dr. Grandjean, fetal and early childhood exposure to industrial chemicals is largely to blame. He and his colleagues at Harvard systematically examined publicly available data on chemical toxicity and identified over 200 chemicals, in addition to those already known, that have the capacity to damage the human brain.[50] The total number of neurotoxins is thought to exceed 1,000, although no authoritative estimate of the true number is available.[51] Exposure to these chemicals during early fetal development can cause brain injury at doses much lower than those necessary to affect the adult brain.

Many of these chemicals deliver a double whammy in that they are not only neurotoxic but also depress the immune system, increasing vulnerability to infection and accompanying inflammation. Insecticides, herbicides, and fungicides are of this type.

It is obvious that direct exposure to high amounts of pesticides could cause serious health problems to children and adults. What's not so obvious is the effect small doses can have. In one study researchers compared exposure of pesticide drift from nearby farms to autism rates. They found that pregnant women living within 1,600 feet (500 m) of fields that were sprayed with pesticides had 6 times the chance of giving birth to an autistic child. The risk was greater depending on how often the pesticides were applied and how close the mother lived to the fields.[52] Agricultural pesticides aren't the only problem; household pesticides can be just as dangerous.

Phthalates, synthetic chemicals used in plastics (especially PVC), appear to contribute to the problem. Researchers studying a possible link between vinyl flooring and allergies accidently discovered an increased incidence in autism. They found that infants or toddlers who slept in bedrooms with vinyl flooring were twice as likely to develop autism. Vinyl floors often emit phthalates and contribute to indoor air pollution. Poor ventilation in the bedrooms also seemed to contribute to the problem.[53]

Wood and linoleum floors were not associated with autism. The study was conducted in Sweden, where only about 1 percent of homes have carpeted floors. Carpeting contains other contaminants, including pesticides and brominated flame retardants, which have been found to harm brain development in animal studies. Older carpets which have gone through a long period of degassing and multiple cleanings are less likely to cause trouble.

Phthalates are present in a wide range of industrial, household, and consumer products, including vinyl wall and floor coverings, roofing materials, safety glass, car parts, lubricating oils, detergents, food packaging, adhesives, paints, inks, medical tubing, pharmaceuticals, footwear, electrical cables, stationary, nail polish, hair sprays, liquid soaps, shampoos, perfumes, and moisturizers. Phthalates leach into the environment and expose humans through ingestion, inhalation, and absorption through the skin. Children with developmental disorders have been found in general to have higher concentrations of phthalates in their urine than other children.[54]

Prenatal exposure to nicotine has long been known to influence brain development. Autism rates are higher among women who smoke during pregnancy.[55] Even after birth, secondhand tobacco smoke can have an effect. Studies show that children exposed to secondhand smoke are more likely to develop symptoms of a variety of mental health problems.[56]

It appears that air pollution from a variety of sources can have an effect on brain health. In another study researchers found that children born to mothers who live close to freeways are at increased risk of autism. The researchers looked at children in communities around Los Angeles, San Francisco, and Sacramento. They collected data on where the children's mothers lived during pregnancy and at the time of birth as well as the proximity of the homes to a major road or freeway. Children living within 1,000 feet from a freeway at birth had a twice the incidence of autism.[57] The study did not find a link between autism and proximity to other major roads, apparently due to the reduced volume of traffic. In Los Angeles, some freeways carry more than 300,000 vehicles daily.

The type of pollution affects autism rates. A study in the San Francisco Bay area found that five air pollutants correlated with the incidence of autism, with mercury having the highest correlation.[58] Similarly, a study found a strong link between mercury emissions from coal-burning plants and the incidence of autism in counties in Texas.[59]

TOXIC METALS
Heavy Metals

Metals can meddle with the mind. Overexposure to certain metals such as iron, manganese, copper, zinc, aluminum, nickel, cobalt, cadmium, chromium, mercury, and lead can promote inflammation and interfere with normal enzyme action and energy metabolism. In medicine, these elements are loosely referred to as the "heavy metals" and more specifically as "toxic metals." Some are more toxic than others. A few, such as iron, manganese, copper, zinc, and chromium, are required by the body in minute quantities, acting as nutrients in small amounts but toxins in larger amounts. The others have no known purpose in the body and are toxic at any level. Many of these metals are dangerous pollutants in our environment. Exposure to heavy metals can come from industrial, environmental, dietary, or medical sources.

Studies have shown that many neurodegenerative disorders such as Alzheimer's, Parkinson's, and ALS, as well as neurodevelopmental disorders like autism are often associated with heavy metal accumulation in brain and body tissues.[60-67] In fact, studies have shown that the severity of autism can be directly associated with the amount of toxic metals in children's bodies.[68]

While exposure to toxic metals can occur though industrial sources, dietary sources are perhaps of greater concern because they affect many more people and do so without warning. If you live or work around toxic metals, you know there is a risk of exposure. But people consuming foods or medicines may have no idea that they are exposing themselves and their future children to potential harm. Two of the most common toxic metals of major concern are mercury and aluminum.

Mercury

Mercury exposure has been a hotly debated topic among concerned parents, doctors, and vaccine promoters. Many people don't realize how poisonous mercury is. It is the most toxic non-radioactive substance known to science. A minute amount exposed to the skin can cause immediate death. Microscopic amounts can cause brain damage. It is even more deadly if swallowed, inhaled, or injected. To think that exposure to "just a small amount" could be harmless is illogical, yet vaccine advocates continue to claim thimerosal causes no harm. As proof, they point to recent studies that show no connection between thimerosal and autism. These studies have the fingerprints of the vaccine industry all over them. Some even show that thimerosal protects against autism, suggesting that mercury is not only safe but *healthy*, which is absurd. "You couldn't even construct a study that shows thimerosal is safe," says Dr. Boyd Haley who is the head of the chemistry department at the University of Kentucky and one of the world's leading authorities on mercury toxicity. "It's just too darn toxic. If you inject thimerosal into an animal, its brain will sicken. If you apply it to living tissue, the cells die. If you put it in a Petri dish, the culture dies. Knowing these things, it would be shocking if one could inject it into an infant without causing damage."[69]

Studies from drug maker Eli Lilly's own laboratories have shown that thimerosal is toxic to tissue cells in concentrations as low as one part per million—100 times weaker than the concentration in a typical vaccine. Even so, the company continues to promote thimerosal as safe. In 1977 the company produced a topical disinfectant that incorporated thimerosal as a "nontoxic" preservative. In Toronto 10 babies died after having a dab of the disinfectant applied on their umbilical cords.[69] Even when applied topically, thimerosal is a deadly poison.

Large exposures have an immediate effect. But smaller doses, even lethal doses, can have a latency period of months or years. A dramatic example of this occurred in 1996. In August of that year Dr. Karen Wetterhahn, a chemistry professor at Dartmouth College, was working in the lab when she spilled a drop of dimethylmercury onto her latex glove. She quickly removed the gloves and washed her hands. She then cleaned up the lab and went home, thinking no more about the incident. Unknown at the time, the latex gloves she was wearing were not adequate protection against the spilled mercury. Although exposed to only a tiny amount of mercury, it would ultimately prove lethal. Over the next five months Wetterhahn suffered no symptoms from the mercury and continued her life as usual. Then suddenly in January 1997 she began to experience tingly fingers and toes, her field of vision started to shrink, her speech became slurred, and she began to have problems with her balance. After several episodes of bumping into doors, unsteady gait, and falls, she was taken to the hospital. She was diagnosed with mercury poisoning. Tests revealed that she had a blood mercury level 80 times the toxic threshold. After two weeks she slipped into a coma from which she never recovered, dying a few months later.

From hair analysis it was discovered she was exposed to only one, and ultimately fatal, dose of mercury in August, the date when she had the mishap in the lab. What was interesting about this case is that it took five months before the mercury had any effect on her. This incidence demonstrates that mercury poisoning can have a long latency period. If a lethal dose of mercury can go undetected for months, then it may be reasoned that a sublethal dose, such as that found in vaccines, could possibly go unnoticed for a long time before symptoms arise.

Mercury is found in organic and inorganic forms. The inorganic form can be divided into elemental mercury and mercuric salts. The mercury in a thermometer is elemental mercury. Organic mercury is formed when elemental mercury combines with organic compounds. Methylmercury and dimethylmercury are two common and deadly examples. Mercury in any form is toxic, but organic mercury is more toxic than the inorganic. Mercury poisoning can result from vapor inhalation, ingestion, injection, or absorption through the skin.

Mercury has many industrial and manufacturing uses. It is used in bronzing, electroplating, paper manufacturing, photography, silver and gold production, embalming, taxidermy, vinyl chloride production, wood preservation, and in the making of fluorescent lamps, neon lamps, paint, batteries, explosives, fungicides, insecticides, and many other products.

One major source of mercury exposure comes from eating contaminated fish. Pregnant women are cautioned about eating fish because the mercury content may cause birth defects. The FDA estimates that 1 in 6 women in the US have mercury levels that increase the risk of neurological damage to their children.[70]

Another major source of mercury exposure comes from medicine, most notably vaccines and dental fillings. Dental surgeons (dentists) began using a mixture of mercury, tin, copper, zinc, and silver to make amalgam tooth fillings in the early 1800s. These "silver" fillings offered a cheaper alternative to the more expensive gold fillings. The unique feature that made mercury so valuable in dentistry is the fact that it is the only metal that is liquid at room temperature. When mercury is mixed with harder metals, the resulting amalgam is soft and pliable, thus allowing it to be

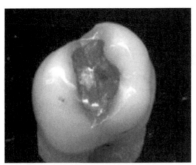

Our greatest exposure to mercury comes from amalgam dental fillings.

molded snugly into the cavity of a tooth. Although mercury was recognized as a deadly poison at the time, those who used mercury amalgams believed that by mixing the mercury with other metals, the mercury was bound tightly in the alloy and posed no threat to health. However, that's not the case.

Amalgam fillings consist of a whopping 50 percent mercury! The amount of mercury in a single filling is more than enough to cause brain damage and even death. As the filling sits in the tooth, mercury vapor is constantly released and absorbed into the body. Once the filling is put into the tooth, mercury vapor will continually be emitted as long as it stays in the mouth. Fillings as old as 50 years have been shown to still give off mercury vapor. Animal studies show that exposure to mercury vapor at concentrations known to be released by dental amalgams in people produce brain lesions identical to those seen in Alzheimer's disease.[71] Mercury also erodes the myelin covering around brain and nerve cells, suggesting a connection to multiple sclerosis.[72]

Elemental mercury, the type in amalgam fillings, emits mercury vapor at room temperature. In the warm and acidic environment of the mouth, mercury vapor is released at a much higher rate. When food is consumed, abrasion to fillings by chewing along with exposure to hot and acidic foods accelerate mercury release. Even the American Dental Association (ADA) acknowledges the release of mercury vapor into the mouth (admitting mercury isn't tightly bound as they once believed); but they contend that the amount absorbed is only harmful to a small number of highly sensitive people and that for most people there is little to worry about. What they fail to acknowledge is that mercury is toxic at *any* level!

In a 2006 FDA hearing on the safety of amalgam fillings, dental experts testified of the deleterious effects of amalgam fillings on health. Among other things, it was brought out that in human autopsy studies the amount of mercury in the brains of the subjects studied was directly proportional to the number of fillings in their teeth. It was not proportional to any other factors, including fish consumption. Thus there is a direct relationship between amalgam fillings and brain levels of mercury. The hearing also revealed that babies whose mothers have amalgam fillings are born with higher mercury levels in the bodies. In fact, the amount of mercury found in baby's hair is proportional to the number of fillings in the mother's teeth.[73] Mothers with amalgam fillings are exposing their unborn children to the damaging effects of mercury and increasing their child's risks of autism without even realizing it.

The ADA Council on Dental Materials advises dentists on how to protect themselves against the hazards of handling scrap amalgams. Amalgams from extracted teeth need to be treated as hazardous waste. Among the many precautions, dentists are told to prevent contact with skin. The fumes coming off amalgam fillings are so toxic that they are instructed to avoid breathing the unseen vapors and to store the amalgam by submerging it under water in unbreakable, tightly sealed containers. The work area must be well ventilated and all employees must be thoroughly advised on the proper way to handle this hazardous material. It is also advised that all employees in dental offices get checked yearly for mercury levels. Despite these precautions, dental workers are still at high risk of mercury poisoning.[74]

This same toxic waste that must be handled with so much caution is exactly the same material that is placed in your mouth. Yet, the ADA says that when it is placed in a tooth in your mouth, it suddenly loses all it toxicity and becomes safe. This just doesn't make sense. With all the evidence against the use of amalgam fillings and with the ADA's own precautions to dentists, it makes one wonder if the royalties* the ADA receives from amalgam fillings has anything to do with their position on the matter. Another reason may be that they have been denying the danger of mercury fillings for so long that if they suddenly admitted that they were wrong, it would be extraordinarily embarrassing and they would lose credibility in the scientific community.

Aluminum

Aluminum has long been known to be toxic to living tissues. In adults it has been identified as a cause of dementia.[75] It is used in vaccines as an adjuvant to boost the body's immune response to the vaccine. Toxic ingredients like aluminum kick the immune system into overdrive boosting the body's production of antibodies. By doing this the vaccine manufacturer can use a smaller amount of the antigen (disease-causing microorganism) which makes production less expensive. Mercury is added to vaccines as a preservative as well as an adjuvant. With the removal of mercury, vaccine makers have increased the amount of aluminum in order to get the same immune response.

One of the arguments against the claim that mercury is involved in the onset of autism is that even though mercury has been removed from most vaccines, autism rates have continued to climb. Vaccine makers shout, "See, it isn't the mercury (or vaccines) that cause autism!" Attempting to exonerate vaccines from guilt by replacing one neurotoxin with another neurotoxin doesn't make vaccines any safer. In fact, increasing the amount of aluminum in the vaccines may have made them even more toxic then the mercury-laden ones.

Vaccine makers continue to reassure the public that vaccines are safe and the amount of aluminum they use poses no danger. This claim was severely challenged by Dr. Chris Shaw and colleagues at the University of British Columbia in Vancouver, Canada. A number of studies have linked aluminum with neurodegenerative diseases such as Alzheimer's, Parkinson's, and amyotrophic lateral sclerosis (ALS). After the first Gulf War in 1991, veterans returned with various neurological problems, particularly

---

*The ADA receives royalty payments from amalgam manufacturers, as well as from makers of toothbrushes, mouthwashes, dental floss, and other products through its "seal of acceptance" program. While receiving funding from manufacturers, the ADA in turn agrees to promote the product to both its members and the public. The ADA claims through its "seal of acceptance" that it has researched the safety of mercury amalgam and found it to be safe. In truth, they have never done a peer-reviewed study demonstrating the safety of mercury fillings.

ALS—a neuromuscular disorder. While many environmental causes were suggested, the role of the anthrax vaccine came under increasing scrutiny. Dr. Shaw and colleagues set out to examine the adjuvant, aluminum hydroxide, which was used in the vaccine.

In the study, young mice were injected with *only* the adjuvant (no bacteria, preservatives, etc.) at a dose equivalent to that given to US military service personnel. All the mice were subjected to a battery of motor and cognitive-behavioral tests over a 6 month period. Afterwards, brain tissues were examined for evidence of inflammation and cell death. What the researchers discovered shocked them. The mice demonstrated significant loss in neuromuscular control consistent with ALS and showed significant defects in water-maze learning compared to the controls. Samples taken of the brain tissue revealed the cells were destroying themselves.[76]

The aluminum adjuvant was causing major inflammation and brain cell death. After witnessing the effects of the aluminum Shaw exclaimed, "No one in my lab wants to get vaccinated…This totally creeped us out. We weren't out there to poke holes in vaccines. But all of a sudden, oh my God—we've got neuron death!"[77]

This level of toxicity was evident from the aluminum used in a *single* vaccine. What damage is done when multiple vaccines are given, as is recommended by the childhood vaccine schedule? Today children are getting concentrations of aluminum that are 10 to 20 times higher than mercury. Aluminum is not only toxic in itself, but it also impairs your body's ability to excrete mercury. As a consequence, aluminum will make whatever amount of mercury you are exposed to (via vaccines, food, dental fillings, etc.) more toxic.

There have been no long term safety studies evaluating the aluminum content in vaccines, but there have been studies on other injected sources of aluminum. Aluminum is a common contaminant in commercial intravenous (IV) feeding solutions. According to the American Society for Parenteral and Enteral Nutrition (ASPEN), injected IV feeding solutions should contain no more than 4 to 5 mcg of aluminum per kilogram of body weight. For a 10 pound (5 kg) infant that would be 20 to 25 mcg per day.[78] ASPEN even requires a warning label to be placed in the product literature of nutritional IV solutions alerting users to the danger of possible aluminum poisoning. Premature and young infants are particularly at risk because their kidney function has not yet matured and is incapable of fully detoxifying certain contaminants, such as aluminum.

These figures and warning were based in part on a study by the Medical Research Council Dunn Nutrition Unit, Cambridge, UK. The researchers compared the neurologic development of 182 children at 18 months of age, who were born premature and had received IV feeding. Half of the infants were given a standard nutritional IV solution that contained aluminum and the other half was given a solution that had been filtered to remove most of the aluminum. They found that the children who received the unfiltered solution were more likely to have "impaired neurologic development." Those who received the unfiltered solution were exposed to 500 mcg of aluminum over a period of 10 days, equating to about 50 mcg per day. The other group received only about 10 mcg of aluminum daily or 4 to 5 mcg per kilogram of body weight per day.[79]

The study originally included 227 premature infants but 45 died before reaching the age of 18 months. An autopsy performed on one infant, who reportedly died from sudden infant death syndrome (SIDS), revealed high aluminum concentrations in its brain.

If aluminum that is injected into the bloodstream with a solution of vitamins, minerals, and other nutrients can cause brain damage, why can't the aluminum injected with a vaccine containing bacteria, viruses, preservatives, and other noxious chemicals do the same?

On average, vaccines contain between 200 to 400 mcg of aluminum per shot. Prevnar (a pneumococcal vaccine) has the least at 125 mcg and Pediarix (DTaP-hepatitis B-polio combination) contains the most with a whopping 850 mcg per dose.

At birth a newborn gets a dose of 250 mcg of aluminum from the hepatitis B vaccine. Keep in mind that according to ASPEN's guidelines a seven pound (3.5 kg) infant should receive no more than 14 to 17 mcg of aluminum at any one time. On day one newborns receive 15 times the maximum limit just from the hepatitis B vaccine! If a child is born premature or with complications he or she may also receive additional aluminum from IV feeding solutions.

The hepatitis vaccine is repeated after one month and again the next month. At two months of age an infant has received at least 6 shots, delivering as much as 1,225 mcg of aluminum on a single day.[80] This is repeated two months later followed by many more vaccinations over the next several years. It's hard to imagine that such a high dose of a known neurotoxin is not doing some harm. Remember, the aluminum in a single vaccine was all that was needed for Dr. Shaw and colleagues at the University of British Columbia to see neuroinflammation and brain cell death, and this was 6 months after the vaccination! Repeated vaccinations can keep this destructive process going continually. Aluminum from vaccines is known to accumulate in the tissues, causing chronic inflammation.[81]

Vaccines and injected medications and feeding solutions are not our only source of exposure to aluminum. We are exposed to varying amounts of aluminum from products we use every day. Aluminum is found in some processed cheeses, baking powder, table salt, antacids (Di-Gel, Maalox, Gelusil, Mylanta, and Rolaids), buffered aspirin (Bufferin), antidiarrheal preparations (Donnagel, Kaopectate and Rheaban), antiperspirants, and in foods cooked in aluminum pots and coffee made in aluminum percolators. Aluminum cans can also transfer significant amounts of aluminum to beverages. Foods wrapped in aluminum foil may absorb the mineral, especially if the food is acidic. Aluminum may also be found as an added ingredient in *some* canned fish and shellfish, liquid or frozen whole eggs and egg whites, dried eggs, beer, and pickles.

You can avoid the dietary sources of aluminum by choosing your foods carefully and reading ingredient labels. Avoid all foods that list any ingredient containing the word "aluminum," such as aluminum ammonium sulfate, calcium aluminum silicate, sodium aluminosilicate, and sodium aluminum phosphate. Baking powder commonly includes sodium aluminum phosphate. Most baked goods containing baking powder will have this ingredient. This includes almost all donuts, muffins, cakes, and similar goods purchased at grocery stores and restaurants, as well as pancake, muffin, and cake mixes. You can purchase aluminum-free baking powder, but most commercial baked goods that list baking powder as an ingredient use the aluminum-containing variety. Table salt typically contains aluminum as an anti-caking agent, but you can buy salt without it. Natural sea salt is a good choice. Some processed (soft) cheese contains aluminum, but real cheese does not. You can tell processed cheese from real cheese because it is labeled as "pasteurized prepared cheese" or some similar term.

DRUGS

Drugs for the most part are synthetic chemicals foreign to the human body. They are also toxic. Some are more toxic than others. Some target the brain. Any drug that affects the brain has the potential to cause disruption and inflammation.

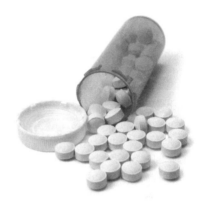

There are many drugs that can affect the brain. Some of these drugs can cross the placenta and affect the unborn baby's brain as well. None of them do the baby any good and some of them can cause serious harm. A few have been directly linked to autism.

Thalidomide is one of these.[82] At one time thalidomide was a popular remedy for nausea during pregnancy until it was discovered that it caused severe birth defects. Although it was withdrawn from general use, it is still used for infections caused by leprosy and some forms of cancer. It has also been recommended for the treatment of lupus and rheumatoid arthritis. However, high rates of neuropathy (nerve pain) have minimized its use.

Misoprostol is another brain-destroying drug that affects unborn infants. It is used for the prevention of gastric ulcers but can also be used as an abortifacient. Autism is known to result following unsuccessful abortion attempts using this drug.

The use of antipyretic drugs (fever reducers) such as acetaminophen, during pregnancy or in young children may interfere with normal immunological development in the brain leading to neurodevelopmental disorders such as autism.[83] Acetaminophen is sometimes given to children to relieve pain and reduce fever. If a child is having a bad reaction to a vaccine, giving him acetaminophen could compound the problem and may even cause autism.[84] Acetaminophen is used as an ingredient in a variety of over-the-counter and prescription pain relievers and cold/flu remedies. Brand names for medications containing acetaminophen include Tylenol, Anacin, Panex, Pain-Eze, St. Joseph Aspirin-Free, Allerest Sinus, Contact Sinus, Dimetapp Cold and Fever, Dristan Cold, NyQuil Cold Medicine, Sinutab, Sudafed Sinus, Sominex Pain Relief, and Alka-Seltzer Cold and Sinus. For a more complete listing of hundreds of acetaminophen medications go online to http://www.ncbi.nlm.nih.gov/pubmedhealth/PMH0000521/.

Ironically, some medications used to treat symptoms associated with autism can actually promote it. Valproic acid is an anticonvulsant used to control epileptic seizures, a common symptom associated with autism. However, valproic acid can make the other symptoms of autism even worse.[85] Likewise with haloperidol, used to treat hyperactivity, behavior problems, and mood disorders, also aggravates autism.[86]

Anticholinergics are a class of drugs that are not specifically linked to autism, but do disrupt brain function and overuse may contribute to the problem. Most sleep aids, allergy medications, and cold remedies are anticholinergic drugs. They are among the most common medications on the market. They work by interfering with the normal functions of the brain. Anticholinergics inhibit the action of cholinergic neurons by blocking the action of the neurotransmitter acetylcholine. Blocking this neurotransmitter prevents nerve transmissions that control involuntary movements of the smooth muscles in the gastrointestinal tract, urinary tract, lungs, and blood vessels.

Nearly all of the antihistamines used for the treatment of allergies and colds are anticholinergics. These drugs are also used to induce sleep. Anticholinergic drugs are used to treat a variety of other disorders such as stomach ulcers, gastritis, heartburn, ulcerative colitis, cystitis, asthma, chronic bronchitis, motion sickness, muscular spasms, and high blood pressure.

As you might expect, any drug that alters brain chemistry and affects so many body systems is bound to have some adverse reactions. Whether taken during pregnancy or given directly to a child, these drugs can disrupt brain function. For a young developing brain, this isn't good. Some of the reported side effects on the nervous system include anxiety, delirium, confusion, disorientation, agitation, memory loss, hallucinations, inability to concentrate, inability to sustain a train of thought, incoherent speech, unusual sensitivity to sudden sounds, illogical thinking, and seizures. Seniors who take anticholinergic drugs experience a rapid acceleration of memory loss and cognitive decline. Some doctors refer to them as "stupid pills" because they accelerate brain aging and degeneration. For this reason, seniors are often cautioned not to use them. These drugs certainly aren't any healthier for children. Some of the brands you might be familiar with include Benadryl, Children's Tylenol Allergy, Contac, Jack and Jill Bedtime, Sominex, Anacin PM, Tylenol Cold Relief Nighttime, and Vicks NyQuil Cold & Flu Relief.

Antibiotics can be a problem because they encourage the overgrowth of certain bacteria that produce brain-altering neurotoxins and can promote and amplify mercury toxicity. Antibiotics are prescribed to fight bacterial infections. They have no effect on viral or fungal (yeast) infections. Therefore, they are of no value in fighting many common illnesses such as colds and flu, most sore throats, sinus infections, upper respiratory infections, and the like.

Doctors often give antibiotics indiscriminately, more to placate the patient or parent than to actually treat a health condition. There is little that can be done for most viral infections. When parents take their sniffling child to the doctor, there is really nothing the doctor can do. The body must fight the virus on its own. Office visits are expensive and when you go, you expect to receive some help. If the doctor spends five minutes in an examination with you and then sends you away with a hefty medical bill and just advice to get plenty of rest, you may feel cheated. So, to placate the patent, doctors routinely prescribe antibiotics which they know will do no good, and in reality can do a great deal of harm.

Antibiotics tend to kill all types of bacteria in the body, including those in the digestive tract. Many of these bacteria are essential for good health. They produce a variety of nutrients that benefit us, and they help to keep harmful bacteria, viruses, and fungi under control. When they are killed by antibiotics, viruses and yeasts are allowed to overpopulate the digestive tract. This is why antibiotic use can lead to candida overgrowth or yeast infections. While the gut is eventually repopulated with bacteria after antibiotics are discontinued, the entire ecosystem of the digestive tract is altered. Without competition from friendly bacteria, unfriendly disease-causing bacteria are allowed to flourish. This can have a dramatic effect on both digestive and overall health.

Several studies have found that children with autism have a much higher usage of oral antibiotics than other children. Autistic children may or may not experience any more infections as other children, but they tend to use antibiotics much more frequently, especially during the first 36 months of their lives. One study showed that by 36 months of age autistic children used antibiotics an average of 11 times compared to only 5 by normal children.[87] The vast majority of the antibiotics were prescribed for ear infections. This is really tragic because studies have shown that antibiotics are not effective for ear infections.

Studies as far back as the early 1990s have shown that antibiotics do not prevent ear infections.[88-89] More recent studies have shown they are not useful in treatment either.[90] So there is no reason to use antibiotics for ear infections. In fact, one of the most popular drugs used to treat ear infections, Augmentin, may even cause autism.[91] Augmentin is a widely prescribed antibiotic used to treat ear infections, sinusitis, pneumonia, bronchitis, urinary tract infections, and skin infections. It is suspected of causing urea poisoning, exerting toxic effects on the brain and corroding the digestive tract.

Autistic children tend to have abnormal gut bacteria (microflora).[92-94] Higher usage of oral antibiotics in infancy may also partially explain the high incidence (approximately 50 percent) of chronic gastrointestinal problems in individuals with autism. One study found that 94 percent of 80 children with regressive autism and chronic constipation/diarrhea had approximately 10,000 times the normal level of *Escherichia coli* (E. coli) in their stools.[95] Other studies have found significantly higher numbers and greater varieties of species of clostridium, which includes the species that causes tetanus and botulism. The measles virus has also been detected in the digestive tract of a substantial number of autistic children.[96] In addition, autistic children are missing or have low levels of many common microflora found in healthy digestive systems.[92]

Some of the unfriendly bacteria, such as clostridium, ruminococcus, and E. coli produce potent neurotoxins. It has been suggested that these neurotoxins are absorbed into the bloodstream and are carried to the brain where they trigger inflammation and microglial activation. Since these bacteria can establish a permanent residence in the digestive tract, they provide a constant source of irritation and inflammation in the brain.

Researchers have speculated that reducing the numbers of these toxin-producing bacteria in the gut may be useful in the treatment of autism. This idea is supported by the fact that some parents have reported that their children's symptoms have temporarily improved after antibiotic treatment. This led researchers at Rush Children's Hospital in Chicago to examine the effect of antibiotic therapy as a possible treatment for autism. Their study showed that some autistic children improved slightly with antibiotic therapy, but the gains the children made were short lived. The investigators concluded that antibiotic treatment was not a useful therapy for autism.[97] Antibiotics work in the short run because they kill all the bacteria, including the troublemakers, but once the antibiotics are discontinued these microbes quickly reestablish themselves, so no lasting benefit is achieved. Antibiotics are likely the *cause* of the abnormal gut flora, so administering more antibiotics isn't going to make the situation any better.

Normal microflora also play an important role in protecting us from mercury poisoning. These friendly bacteria are able to convert organic mercury (such as methylmercury) which is rapidly absorbed into the body, into inorganic mercury which is poorly absorbed and largely excreted. In contrast, most strains of yeast (candida) and *Escherichia coli* (E. coli) carry out the reverse reaction, namely, converting inorganic mercury to organic mercury.[98] Frequent antibiotic use would result in a loss of normal gut flora and an increase in yeast and E. coli populations. This would reduce and could even completely inhibit the excretion of mercury, allowing it to be absorbed into the body and brain. This may be one of the reasons why autistic children often have higher mercury levels than other children.[66]

FOOD ADDITIVES
Synthetic Dyes and Preservatives

Synthetic chemicals added to foods, like certain drugs, can affect brain function. Many parents see their children's behavior and social interaction improve when they remove artificial food colorings, flavorings, and preservatives from their diet. In fact, the Autism Research Institute's 2009 survey of more than 27,000 parents of autistic children found that 58 percent reported that their children's symptoms improved after eliminating foods containing artificial food additives.

A number of studies have shown a link between behavior and learning problems with synthetic food dyes (Yellow 5, Yellow 6, Red 3, Red 40, Blue 1, Blue 2 Green 3, and Orange B), preservatives (BHA, BHT, TBHQ, sodium benzoate), and artificial flavorings.[99-101]

Artificial food additives are commonly used in processed, packaged, convenience foods such as candy, gum, breakfast cereal, soda, flavored drinks, ice cream, popsicles, jam, chips, cookies, pies, frozen pizza, and microwave dinners. Most of these are considered "junk" foods because they provide little nutrition and are loaded with sugar and artificial ingredients.

School officials and teachers also see an improvement in students when food additives are removed from the diet. When New End Primary School in Hampstead, England banned junk foods, school officials saw a dramatic improvement in pupils' behavior. At Deganway School in Wales, additives were banned from the school menu. Packaged foods containing artificial additives were replaced with fresh fruits and vegetables. Students' behavior and concentration improved. Melrose Elementary in Tampa, Florida completely overhauled their lunch menu, removing foods high in sugar and artificial ingredients. The school principal said the effects were "amazing."

An experiment involving identical twin brothers with developmental issues provides dramatic evidence of the impact that food additives can have on a child's behavior and learning ability. Michael and Christopher Parker, age five, were put on separate diets for two weeks. Michael went on a food additives-free diet, which banned all sweets, soda, and chips. During the study period Michael became more assertive and calmer than his twin brother and outperformed him on IQ tests. Before the experiment, the twins each made the same mistakes on IQ tests and completed them in exactly the same time. After the two week experiment Michael's score improved by 25 percent. "I can't believe the changes that Michael has shown in his behavior," says his mother Lynn. In addition, she says he "has developed a sense of humor and is a lot more talkative."[102]

Excitotoxins

Many of the foods in your local grocery store contain neurotoxins. That hot dog you ate for lunch or the diet soda you drank to wash it down could damage your health and destroy precious brain cells. "Carol Hamm was a close friend," says James Bowen, MD. "We played cards together a couple of times per week and she constantly had diet drinks in her hands while she played. She, over a short period of a few weeks use, visibly deteriorated physically right in front of my eyes, and mentally. Her card playing deteriorated as well! She would defiantly look me right in the eye as she drank diet drinks to let me know that she didn't care that I had warned her of what I knew about aspartame. She was going to satisfy her addiction by damn! Come what may! What came was that, one night she didn't show for cards, and her daughter Debby called the police. When we arrived at her house she was lying dead in bed with bloody fluid running out of her mouth."

Carol was a victim of what has come to be known as *aspartame disease—* poisoning caused by consuming foods containing the artificial sweetener aspartame (AminoSweet, NutraSweet, Equal, Spoonful, and Equal-Measure). Aspartame accounts for over 75 percent of the adverse reactions to food additives reported to the FDA each year. There are over 90 different adverse effects that have been reported with aspartame consumption, among them headaches, memory loss, slurred speech, tremors, irritability, anxiety, depression, seizures, and even death. An entire weight-loss industry has been built around aspartame. It is added to thousands of diet and low-calorie desserts, snack foods, sugar-free chewing gum, and beverages.

Aspartame is made up of three chemicals: methanol (10 percent), phenylalanine (50 percent), and aspartate (40 percent). Methanol, also known as wood alcohol, is toxic. In the body, it breaks down into formic acid and formaldehyde, both of which are poisonous. The Environmental Protection Agency (EPA) recommends limiting methanol consumption to 7.8 mg/day. A single 1 liter sized beverage sweetened with aspartame contains about 56 mg of methanol—seven times the EPA limit. Heavy users of aspartame-containing products consume two or three times this amount, as much as 168 mg of methanol daily, which is 22 times the EPA limit.

Phenylalanine, the most abundant ingredient in aspartame, is an amino acid found naturally in some foods. Persons with the genetic disorder phenylketonuria (PKU) cannot metabolize phenylalanine. This leads to dangerously high or even fatal levels of phenylalanine in the brain. It has been shown that ingesting aspartame, especially along with carbohydrate (sugar and starch), can lead to excess levels of phenylalanine in the brain even in persons who do not have PKU. Excessive levels of phenylalanine in the brain can cause the levels of serotonin, a neurotransmitter, in the brain to decrease, leading to emotional disorders.

The name "aspartame" is a derivative of the third ingredient—aspartate. Aspartate is also an amino acid. It is similar to glutamate, another amino acid. Both aspartate and glutamate are found in various levels in foods. Our cells can convert aspartate into glutamate and vice versa. Aspartate and glutamate are important neurotransmitters. In fact, they are the most abundant neurotransmitters in the brain. Aspartate and glutamate in the diet, however, can become potent *excitotoxins*—substances that cause overstimulation leading to cellular death.

Glutamate and aspartate are excitatory neurotransmitters. Too many of them can overstimulate the neurons, exciting them into a feverish frenzy of electrical activity, exhausting the neurons' energy reserves, causing them to die. In the process, a large number of destructive free radicals are generated, which in turn promotes inflammation and cellular damage, compounding the problem.

The body is capable of handling a certain amount of excess neurotransmitters. Receptors and enzymes keep them under control. But if the influx of neurotransmitters is greater than the body's ability to control them, brain cells can be stimulated to death. If the situation is repeated over and over again, then more and more brain cells will be killed. In time, the accumulative loss of brain cells will manifest itself as various neurological abnormalities. A growing number of studies are linking glutamate excitotoxicity to neurodegenerative and neurodevelopmental disorders including Alzheimer's, Parkinson's, ALS, autism, epilepsy, and schizophrenia.[103-116]

The most frequent source of aspartate is from the artificial sweetener aspartame. The most common source of glutamate comes from the flavor enhancer monosodium glutamate (MSG). MSG is added to a large assortment of commercially packaged foods—soups, frozen dinners, pizza, gravies, sauces, chips, croutons, lunch meats, bouillon, canned tuna, and salad dressings. It is frequently found in restaurant foods. You can even buy MSG by itself as a flavor enhancer in the spice section of the grocery store. It is sold under the brand name Accent.

The negative effects of glutamate were first observed in 1954 by a Japanese scientist who noted that direct application of glutamate to the central nervous system caused seizure activity. This report, unfortunately, went unnoticed for several years. The toxicity of glutamate was than observed in 1957 by two ophthalmologists, D.R. Lucas and J.P. Newhouse, when the feeding of monosodium glutamate to newborn mice destroyed the neurons in the inner layers of the retina. Later, in 1969, neuropathologist John Olney repeated Lucas and Newhouse's experiment and discovered the phenomenon was not restricted to the retina but occurred throughout the brain. He coined the term "excitotoxicity" to describe the neural damage that glutamate, aspartate, phenylalanine, cysteine, homocysteine, and other excitotoxins can cause.

Animal studies have shown that MSG added to the diet can trigger seizures. The duration and intensity of the seizures are most pronounced at younger ages when the brain and immune system are still underdeveloped.[117] It is disheartening that MSG in one form or another is often added to baby foods and infant formulas.

In 1994 Russell L. Blaylock, MD, who at the time was a clinical assistant professor of neurosurgery at the University of Mississippi Medical Center, published a book titled *Excitotoxins: The Taste That Kills*. Both of his parents were afflicted with Parkinson's disease, which compelled him to research the disease in depth, seeking for the cause and an effective treatment. His research led him to an understanding of the devastating effects of excitotoxic food additives and their influence on various forms of neurodegeneration. His book summarizes the research linking excitotoxins to neurodegenerative disorders and provides details on the types of foods to avoid.

If only a few foods contained glutamate or aspartate, it wouldn't be much of a problem. Small amounts in the diet can be handled without too much worry. The problem is that the vast majority of processed, packaged and restaurant foods contain excitotoxins. It is very difficult to find a canned, frozen, packaged, or prepared food in the grocery store that does not contain excitotoxic additives in some form.

Aspartame and MSG are among the most common and the most recognizable additives. Because of the public's growing awareness of the dangers of MSG, food manufacturers often disguise this ingredient by putting it in a different form. Additives that contain MSG include hydrolyzed vegetable protein, sodium caseinate, calcium caseinate, yeast extract, autolyzed yeast, soy protein isolate, and textured protein. Of these, hydrolyzed vegetable protein is probably the worst because it also contains two other excitotoxins—aspartate and cysteine. Some food manufacturers have attempted to sell the idea that this additive is "all natural" or "safe" because it is made from vegetables, but it is not safe. Dr. Russell Blaylock says, "Experimentally, one can produce the same brain lesions using hydrolyzed vegetable protein as by using MSG or aspartate." One very ambiguous but common ingredient is "natural flavorings." Despite the word "natural," this is a general term that often includes MSG. You should get into the habit of reading the ingredient labels on everything you buy and avoiding all foods containing these additives or any additives that have similar sounding names.

Amino acids have become popular as dietary supplements. You can find individual purified excitotoxins being peddled as dietary supplements labeled as L-glutamine, L-cysteine, and L-phenylalanine. You may also see them in combination with other amino acids or with multiple vitamin and mineral supplements. Despite health claims, they are nothing more than brain-destroying drugs, and it is best to avoid them all.

Some people are more sensitive to excitotoxins than others and display allergy-like reactions. This has been called "Chinese Restaurant Syndrome" because MSG is commonly used in Asian cooking. Symptoms may include headaches, nausea, diarrhea, heart palpations, dizziness, difficulty concentrating, mood swings, heartburn, skin rashes, and asthma. Those who are allergic to MSG are lucky. They know to avoid eating foods with this additive. But the rest of us can be completely oblivious to the damage that is being done.

Those people who defend the use of MSG state that glutamate is a natural substance commonly found in many foods; if glutamate-containing foods are not harmful, then MSG is not harmful either. Our bodies can handle natural dietary sources of glutamate that are found in meats, cheeses, vegetables, and such. This is clearly seen in those who are allergic to MSG. They can eat mushrooms, tomato sauce, red meat, and other foods high in natural glutamate without a problem, but when they eat foods with added MSG they experience immediate adverse reactions. Obviously there is something very different between the glutamate that is found naturally in foods and the glutamate in food additives.

Protein is made out of amino acids. Glutamate is one of some 22 amino acids that make up the proteins in the human diet. Many of the plant and animal proteins in our foods contain glutamate. Glutamate in foods is always attached to other amino acids. The process of breaking proteins down into individual amino acids takes time, so the amino acids are released slowly. Blood levels of glutamate are kept within reasonable bounds that the body is capable of handling. Also, glutamate bound to other amino acids or proteins cannot pass through the blood-brain barrier, so it doesn't pose a problem. The glutamate in MSG, on the other hand, is in its free form and does not have to be broken off a protein, so you absorb a higher dose more quickly. MSG in this more purified form acts like a drug, passing through the blood-brain barrier with an immediate effect.

High blood levels of free glutamate in the diet tend to open up the blood-brain barrier, allowing more glutamate as well as other neurotoxins to enter the brain.[118] This extracellular glutamate, along with other neurotoxins, interferes with glutamate transporters, triggers inflammation, and stimulates free-radical production. This excitotoxicity causes the release of intracellular glutamate stored in the brain cells. The brain is flooded with glutamate, causing more inflammation and producing more free radicals, which in turn releases more glutamate. A vicious cycle continues, leading to neuron destruction.[119]

Even small concentrations of excitotoxins entering the brain can trigger this destructive cycle. Children with autism should stop eating foods with excitotoxic additives immediately. That means most processed, packaged convenience foods sold at the grocery store. Replace them with fresh, natural foods and make more meals from scratch rather than using packaged ingredients.

Nitrates, Nitrites, and Nitrosamines
Which of the following two meals supports good brain health and which can contribute to poor mental health?

1) Scrambled eggs cooked in butter, topped with cheese and sour cream

2) Tossed salad with croutons and diced lean turkey topped with low-fat Thousand Island dressing

Number 1 is the better choice. Eggs are very nutritious and actually support good brain health. However, as nutritious as the salad may sound, it can be a cause of many problems. While the vegetables are good, the toppings may not be. The croutons, turkey, and salad dressing may contain a number of additives that harm the brain, including MSG, aspartame, and, in the turkey, nitrite. Nitrite in itself is not so bad, but when eaten it can transform into one of many nitrosamine compounds, and that can spell big trouble.

Nitrosamines are potent cancer-causing chemicals formed in the stomach by a reaction between nitrite added to foods and amines (found in proteins normally present in the body). They are carcinogenic in large doses and cause liver damage, insulin resistance, and neurodegeneration at smaller doses.

Nitrite is added to many processed foods, especially processed meats such as bacon, sausage, ham, bologna, salami, pepperoni, pastrami, olive loaf, hot dogs, polish sausage, bratwurst, jerky, beef sticks, corned beef, smoked meats, preserved fish, and fish byproducts. It can be found in some processed vegetables, nonfat dry milk, and cheeses.

People often use the words nitrite and nitrate interchangeably. Although chemically similar, they are two distinct substances. We are exposed to nitrite primarily from processed foods. Nitrate, to a lesser extent, is also added to food, however, it is a greater problem in contaminated drinking water. Nitrate from fertilizers and human and animal waste may be carried by rain, irrigation, and other surface water through the soil into ground water, ultimately contaminating drinking supplies. Well water is the most susceptible. Nitrate is converted into nitrite in the digestive tract, which in turn can be converted into nitrosamine. Nitrite is ten times more toxic than nitrate.

Nitrates are also found naturally in some leafy green and root vegetables, but these sources are of little concern because they are always combined with antioxidant nutrients such as vitamins C and E, beta-carotene, and flavonoids that prevent their conversion into nitrosamines. The meat industry often tries to dispel fears about the nitrites added to their products by pointing out that nitrates (not nitrites) are found naturally in some vegetables. They fail to mention that nitrates are 10 times less dangerous than nitrites—the type most commonly used in the meat industry. Nor do they mention that nitrate toxicity is rendered impotent by other substances in the vegetables that are not found in processed meat products.

You will usually see nitrite listed on food labels as *sodium nitrite* or *potassium nitrite*. It is added to foods as a preservative. It prevents toxin production by the bacterium *Clostridium botulinum*, which is responsible for causing botulism. Because of nitrite's high carcinogenic potential, this has been an important issue within the food industry. Regulatory agencies would like to ban the chemical completely from all foods, but that would increase the risk of botulism poisoning. To limit risk of cancer, yet still provide safety against botulism, the United States government limits the addition of sodium or potassium nitrite to 120 parts per million. This is the lowest level found to be effective in controlling growth and toxin production by the bacterium.

Another source of nitrate is *thiamine mononitrate* which is often found in baked goods, baby foods, and infant formula. When whole wheat is processed into white flour, many of the vitamins and minerals are removed. One of these vitamins is thiamine (vitamin B_1). Because thiamine is an essential nutrient, the government has mandated that it and four other nutrients (riboflavin, niacin, folic acid, and iron) be added back into the white flour. This is called "enriched" white flour because it has been enriched with these missing nutrients. Manufacturers can add natural thiamine or synthetic thiamine (thiamine mononitrate). Thiamine mononitrate is found in Carnation infant formulas, some bottled baby foods, especially the junior combinations, cereals, and other infant prepared foods. If thiamine mononitrate is listed on the ingredient label, don't use it.

Nitrite and nitrosamine intake have long been linked with an increased risk of cancer of the lungs, stomach, esophagus, pancreas, bladder, colon, and liver in humans as well as diabetes and liver disease. More recently, it has been discovered that nitrosamines also promote Alzheimer's disease and other neurodegenerative disorders. A nitrosamine compound called streptozotocin is commonly used by researchers to deliberately produce diabetes in lab animals. Dr. Suzanne de la Monte and colleagues at Brown University in Providence, Rhode Island, accidently found that giving streptozotocin to her lab mice caused them to develop the equivalent to Alzheimer's.[120] Nitrosamines cause DNA damage, oxidative stress (the production of destructive free radicals), lipid peroxidation, and pro-inflammatory cytokine activation, which lead to increased cellular degeneration and death, thus promoting neurodegeneration. In young children nitrosamines promote the conditions that can lead to autism.

It would be wise to avoid all processed foods containing nitrites and nitrates. This includes most cold cuts and cured meats and products that contain them, such as pizza and canned soup. These foods also often contain MSG and sometimes aspartame as well. Avoid all baby foods containing thiamine mononitrate. Read ingredient labels. Fortunately, supermarkets are increasingly offering brands of processed meats and baked goods that are nitrite-free. You have to search for them at regular food stores, but they are readily available in most health food stores. Fresh meats are almost always free of added nitrites.

BOTTOM LINE

One of the problems with solving the mystery of autism is that until recently there has not been a theory that has been able to tie all the clues together. Vaccines in themselves do not cause autism; many vaccinated children do not become autistic. Something else is at work here. Vaccines are merely a single piece of the puzzle. Other factors such as infections, environmental toxins, food allergies, heavy metal poisoning, abnormal gastrointestinal ecology, drugs, poor nutrition, food additives, and excitotoxins can all contribute to autism. Rarely is just one of these alone the cause. This is why treatments that address one or two of these issues seem to work for some autistic children but not for others. All these factors can contribute. What ties them all together is that they all cause inflammation and excessive microglial activation. At some point, repeated insults from a combination of these factors causes the brain's immune system to lock into a perpetual state of activation that will remain activated indefinably until something happens to deactivate the microglia.

The intensity and frequency of exposure to neuroinflammatory conditions determines the age at which autism surfaces and its severity. Early infantile autism is caused by a combination of prenatal conditions and early assaults, such as initial vaccinations during the first few months of life. Late-onset or regressive autism occurs after a period of time of normal language and social development followed by a sudden regression. It is during the formative years, and especially the first 26 months, when the brain is rapidly developing that a child is most vulnerable to the events that lead to autism.

Waxing and waning of autistic symptoms is well known.[121] This probably occurs as a result of fluctuating intensity of neuroinflammation. Each new insult on the brain causing increased microglial activity and increased severity of symptoms. The opposite is also true. A reduction in microglial activity that calms inflammation is followed by an improvement in symptoms.

Since neuroinflammation is an underlying factor in autism, it has been reasoned that anti-inflammatory medications may help treat the condition. While working at Royal Free Hospital, Andrew Wakefield claimed to have had modest success in relieving some of the symptoms using anti-inflammatories. This theory, however, has been attempted on other neuroinflammatory disorders without much success. For example, when nonsteroidal anti-inflammatory drugs like Celebrex and Aleve were administered to Alzheimer's patients, it actually accelerated their mental decline, making their condition worse.[122-123] The theory was sound, but the drugs themselves caused more harm than good. Less toxic medications or methods may succeed.

In the following chapters you will learn how to calm neuroinflammation and stimulate healing and repair of the brain using harmless, natural methods involving diet, nutrition, and supplementation. You will discover how to prevent and reverse autism and other neurodevelopmental disorders.

The best time to start treating autism is when the brain is young and at its most dynamic stage of development. As the brain matures, it becomes more difficult to make significant changes in brain structure and circuitry. The sooner treatment is initiated, the greater the chances for success.

7 | The Ketone Miracle

THE BRAIN DISORDER CURED BY A "MAGIC" DIET

"On March 11, 1993, I was pushing my son, Charlie, in a swing when his head twitched and he threw his right arm in the air," recalls Jim Abrahams. "The whole event was so subtle that I didn't even think to mention it to Nancy, my wife, until a couple of days later when it recurred. She said she had seen a similar incident. That was the beginning of an agony I am without words to describe."

Charlie suddenly went from being a normal, active one-year old to a toddler racked with multiple violent seizures. He was diagnosed with Lennox-Gastaut Syndrome, a severe form of epilepsy. Charlie's attacks became so extreme that his parents padded the walls of his room and had him wear a football helmet to protect himself.

Over the next nine months Charlie experienced thousands of epileptic seizures, an incredible array of drugs, dozens of blood draws, eight hospitalizations, a mountain of EEGs, MRIs, CAT scans, and PET scans, and one fruitless brain surgery. He was treated by five pediatric neurologists in three cities, two homoeopathists, and even a faith healer. Despite all this, Charlie's seizures remained unchecked and his mental development delayed. His prognosis was that of continued seizures and progressive retardation.

At 20 months of age Charlie weighed only 19 pounds. He was taking four medications, but still suffered hundreds of seizures daily. The side effects to the drugs he was taking were nearly as bad his disease, compounding his agony.

Refusing to believe that nothing more could be done, Jim went to the library to research the disease. There, he found a book by John Freeman, MD, a professor of neurology at Johns Hopkins University, which contained references to a dietary treatment for epilepsy called the ketogenic diet. Jim learned that the ketogenic diet had been used successfully for over 70 years in treating severe cases of epilepsy.

Jim took Charlie to see Dr. Freeman at Johns Hopkins Hospital in Baltimore, Maryland, the only place in the country at the time that was prescribing the ketogenic diet. The ketogenic diet is like a low-carb diet on steroids—high in fat with adequate protein, a little carbohydrate, and no sugar. Charlie began the "magic diet" and within two days his violet seizures miraculously stopped.

90

"Charlie has been virtually seizure-free, completely drug-free, and a terrific little boy ever since," says Jim. "He has had to remain on a modified version of the ketogenic diet after being on the full diet for two years, but he goes to school and leads a normal, happy life." Charlie was successfully weaned off the diet at the age of seven. Despite worries about developmental delays and retardation, the diet corrected the problem in his brain and allowed him to develop normally, both physically and mentally.

Inspired by Charlie's success, his parents founded the Charlie Foundation to Help Cure Pediatric Epilepsy to support medical research and education about the ketogenic diet. Jim Abrahams, Charlie's father, was a successful movie producer and director in Hollywood. In 1997 Jim wrote and directed a movie based his son's experience titled ...*First Do No Harm* starring Meryl Streep and Fred Ward. The movie also included a cast of several bit players who had, in real life, been cured from epilepsy using the ketogenic diet. Millicent Kelly, a dietitian who helped run the ketogenic diet program at Johns Hopkins, played herself in the movie.

Seizures can be very dramatic involving violent, uncontrollable thrashing movements and loss of consciousness; or they may be as mild as a brief loss of awareness to one's surroundings and go essentially unnoticed by casual observers.

Depending on the sensitivity of the examination, it is estimated that at least 30 percent and as many as 82 percent of autistic children experience periodic seizures. Seizures occur as a result of the misfiring of electrical signals in the brain. In autism there already is a defect in the brain's wiring, so misfiring would be expected. One way to think of it is to imagine an electrical storm. The brain generates biochemical electrical charges, allowing brain cells to communicate to each other. A seizure happens when this electricity surges, like a lightning bolt hitting a fuse box, overloading parts of the brains' circuitry. It is known that autistic children who show a regression of mental development have a significantly higher incidence of both major and minor seizures compared to those children who do not regress.

Doctors are not completely sure why seizures occur or how to stop them. Although there are many anticonvulsive drugs available to treat the symptoms, none are completely effective or without adverse side effects, and none of them can even remotely be called a cure. The most successful treatment for epilepsy is the ketogenic diet. Not only can it reduce the occurrence of seizures, but in many cases it can bring about a complete and lasting cure. Generally, patients stay on the diet for a period of two years. In some very severe cases, a modified ketogenic diet may be continued for a longer period of time to allow the brain adequate time to heal. After that time a large percentage of patients can resume eating normally again without ever experiencing another seizure.

Thousands of children have been helped with the ketogenic diet. Bryce suffered his first seizure shortly after his fourth birthday. "I still remember the day vividly," says his mother Dr. Deborah Snyder, DO, "I was at work when the director of his preschool called to tell me. I ran to my car, leaving an office full of patients behind and barely stopping at traffic lights."

When she arrived, Bryce was in a state of mental confusion that typically follows seizures. At the hospital he had an MRI of his brain and many laboratory tests, all of which appeared to be normal. Snyder clung to the hope that this was an isolated incident and would never recur. She was wrong.

Three weeks later Bryce had another seizure at daycare and was placed on medication. He suffered many side effects from the medications, including abnormalities with his blood count and behavioral issues such as biting, kicking, and spitting. His cognitive ability began to decline. He was slow to find his words, his writing and drawing regressed, and he even fell asleep in the middle of his cousin's birthday party. To make matters worse, the seizures didn't stop.

"The first time I actually witnessed a seizure myself was one of the most horrific events I've ever experienced," says Snyder. "To see your little boy writhing on the floor, muscles contracted, eyes deviated, drooling, and unresponsive is like having someone reach into your chest and rip out your heart. As a parent, even as a doctor-parent, you are helpless."

Two months into his illness, his seizures began to spiral out of control. Five different anticonvulsive medications proved fruitless, even when he took three at once. His physicians thought he had Lennox-Gastaut Syndrome. Most children with this condition end up mentally retarded.

The Snyders received new hope after watching a Dateline NBC television special featuring Charlie Abrahams and his success with the ketogenic diet. "I had heard mention of the ketogenic diet in passing in medical school, but really knew nothing about it," says Snyder. "So I read some more. The more I learned about the diet, the more I believed it was our best option." She made an appointment for Bryce to be admitted to the hospital to start the ketogenic program, but had to wait three weeks for an opening. In the meantime, his mother began to reduce the carbohydrates in his diet and started to introduce foods that were on the diet, such as macadamia nuts, heavy whipping cream, and blueberries. His seizures improved. Bryce had up to 25 seizures daily before he started the ketogenic diet. Within three weeks, he was seizure free. He was maintained on the diet and one medication for a year, then the diet alone for another year. He was weaned completely off the diet in the summer of 2005.

"The ketogenic diet gave me my son back," says Snyder. "Bryce has been seizure free, medication free, and on no special diet for four years and counting. Rather than becoming mentally retarded as was his prognosis, he just completed third grade with straight A's. Bryce is a true modern day miracle!"

Gathering together what she learned during her two years working with what is often referred to as the "miracle diet," Dr. Snyder wrote a book to help other parents succeed with the diet, titled *The Keto Kid: Helping Your Child Succeed on the Ketogenic Diet*.

"When Matthew was 9 months old, he was having a bath when his first seizure occurred," recalls his mother Emma Williams, of Lingfield, England. "I had never seen anything so frightening, and it was happening to my son. The first one lasted for over 15 minutes." By the time Matthew was 15 months old he was having seizures daily.

He was diagnosed with uncontrolled complex epilepsy. Emma read everything she could get her hands on regarding epilepsy and contacted any organization that might help. When Matthew was two years old she learned about the ketogenic diet. When she asked her neurologist about it, he dismissed it as an unproven fringe therapy that was too difficult to manage and recommended drugs as a better option.

Matthew's seizures occurred both day and night—even when he was sleeping. He was given every antiepileptic drug available, but nothing helped. Some weeks he would lie on the couch like a zombie and other weeks, he would never sleep and spent all night shouting the house down. No one ever got a full night's sleep.

By age 6, Mathew had made no progress whatsoever. He had the mentality of a one-year-old. He could not talk and was sill in diapers. Emma was concerned because there were no drugs left for him to try and every type of brain scan had been done. He wasn't even a candidate for surgery because the doctors couldn't pinpoint which part of the brain the seizures were coming from.

Again she heard of the ketogenic diet and again she asked her doctors about it. Again she was told it was too difficult to manage and was encouraged to keep trying the drugs. However, the drugs weren't working and there was nothing else left to try, so as Matthew was approaching his eighth birthday Emma again asked about the ketogenic diet. At this time the hospital was about to conduct a clinical trial using the diet and her doctor asked if she wanted to participate. "I practically bit her hand off saying yes!" recalls Emma. "It was my last hope, there was absolutely nothing left to try and Matthew's epilepsy was worse than ever."

Matthew started the diet in the summer of 2002. It started off shakily. Matthew couldn't have his favorite foods. He was grumpy and miserable. He spent most of his time shouting with displeasure. He was still having seizures so he was either shaking or shouting. To avoid further conflict, his family didn't eat in front of him, but ate their meals secluded in the bathroom.

After the first three or four days Matthew started to calm down. Over the next few days he calmed down even more and began eating his meals without vocal protest. He soon became happier and began sleeping through the night. No longer did he wake up at 4 a.m.

Within two weeks of starting the diet, Matthew's seizures were reduced by 90 percent and within eight months he was off all medications. He began to speak his first words. "After a few months on the diet he called me 'mum' for the very first time—I didn't stop blubbing for about four days. No money in the world can buy that feeling. When he comes home on his school bus and sees me coming to get him, he says 'mum mum.' I feel like I've won the lottery every day…This Christmas for the first time ever, my son sat on my lap and opened his Christmas presents. He ripped the wrapping paper off and looked inside to see what he had got. It was the best Christmas present I've ever had."

For many years the ketogenic diet was used out of desperation, a last resort after medications had failed. The diet has proven successful with even the most severe cases of epilepsy. Because of its success, the ketogenic diet is gaining wider acceptance as a standard form of treatment rather than an alternative to drug therapy.

"Why should this diet be a last resort?" Emma questions. "I first asked about it when my son was two years old. It took me until he was nearly eight to get him on it. He now has the best quality of life he has ever had." Inspired by Matthew's success, Emma started Matthew's Friends Charity (www.matthewsfriends.org) in 2004 to share her experiences and provide support to other parents seeking help through the ketogenic diet.

THE KETOGENIC DIET

The ketogenic diet has been around since the 1920s. Its origin stems from therapeutic fasting, which in the early 20th century was a popular form of treatment for many chronic health problems. Patients would fast, consuming nothing but water, for up to 30 days and sometimes even longer. Fasting therapy was used to treat a wide variety of difficult-to-treat health problems including digestive problems, arthritis, cancer, and diabetes. In many instances prolonged fasting proved beneficial.

Some health problems responded very well to fasting therapy. One of these was epilepsy. One of the most prominent physicians of the early 1900s to promote the use of fasting therapy was Dr. Hugh Conklin. He recommended fasting for 18 to 25 days. He treated hundreds of epilepsy patients with his "water diet" and boasted of a 90 percent cure rate in children and a 50 percent cure rate in adults.

Dr. H. Rawle Geylin, a prominent New York pediatrician, witnessed Conklin's success first-hand and tested the therapy on 36 of his own patients, achieving similar results. His patients ranged in age from 3.5 to 35 years. After fasting for 20 days, 87 percent of the patients were free of seizures. Geylin presented his findings at the annual meeting of the American Medical Association in Boston in 1921, ushering in fasting therapy as a mainstream treatment for epilepsy.

In the 1920s when only phenobarbital and bromides were available as anticonvulsant medications, reports that fasting could cure epilepsy were exciting. These reports set off a flurry of clinical investigations and research activity.

As a result of fasting therapy, many epileptic patients would remain seizure free for years, if not for life. For others the cure was only temporary, lasting only a year or two. In children, long-term freedom from seizures occurred in about 18 percent of cases. Repeating the fast would stop the seizures again, but there was no guarantee for how long. Longer fasts seemed to produce better results, but for some patients the length of time required to bring a lasting cure seemed impractical. Researchers began looking at ways to mimic the metabolic and therapeutic effects of fasting while allowing patients to consume enough nourishment to sustain life for extended periods of time, and hopefully bring about a higher cure rate. The result was the development of the ketogenic diet.

Under normal conditions, our bodies burn glucose for energy. During fasting when no foods containing glucose are consumed, fat is utilized to supply the body's need for energy. Some of this fat is converted by the liver into water-soluble compounds (beta-hydroxybutyrate, acetoacetate, and acetone) collectively known as ketone bodies. Normally the brain uses glucose to satisfy its energy needs. If glucose is not available, one of the only other sources of fuel it can use is ketone bodies or ketones. Other organs and tissues in the body can utilize fat for energy, but not the brain—it must have either glucose or ketones. Ketones actually provide a more concentrated and efficient source of energy than glucose. They have been described as our body's "superfuel," producing energy more efficiently than either glucose or fat.[1] More efficient energy production also allows the brain to function better. Ketones are also neuroprotective. As a consequence, in a brain fueled by ketones, the dysfunction or short circuit caused by epilepsy is overridden and the brain is allowed to gradually rewire and heal itself.

The elevated level of ketones produced in the blood during fasting can be duplicated by simply restricting the consumption of carbohydrate (starch and sugar)—the primary source of glucose in the diet. Carbohydrate is composed of glucose molecules and other sugars that the body converts into glucose. Starch and sugar are found in all plant foods but are most abundant in grains, fruits, and starchy vegetables such as potatoes. Dietary fiber, which is also considered a carbohydrate, does not contribute glucose because our bodies do not have the enzymes to break the fiber down. So the glucose molecules in the fiber remain locked in place as it travels through and out of the digestive tract. Meat and eggs contain only a very small amount of carbohydrate. Fat contains essentially none.

The ketogenic diet consists of eating a high proportion of fat, adequate protein, little carbohydrate, and absolutely no sugar. High-fiber carbohydrate foods are preferred over those rich in starch or sugar. The diet provides just enough protein and sufficient calories to maintain growth and repair.

The classic ketogenic diet contains a 4:1 ratio (3:1 for infants and teens) by *weight* of fat to combined protein and carbohydrate. So each meal contains four times as much fat as it does a combination of both protein and carbohydrate. There are 9 calories in 1 gram of fat and 4 calories each in 1 gram of protein and 1 gram of carbohydrate. An unrestricted, ordinary diet consists of about 30 percent fat, 15 percent protein, and 55 percent carbohydrate. The 4:1 weight ratio of the ketogenic diet equates to 90 percent of calories from fat, 8 percent from protein, and 2 percent from carbohydrate. Carbohydrate consumption is restricted to 10-15 grams per day. The diet excludes most high carbohydrate grains, fruits, and vegetables, such as breads, corn, bananas, peas, and potatoes. Total calorie consumption is reduced to 80-90 percent of estimated dietary requirements because this is believed to improve ketone levels. This hasn't been too much of a problem because ketones tend to reduce hunger so patients can feel satisfied without being hungry. Initially, fluid consumption was restricted to 80 percent of normal daily needs. This was done in the belief that it increased blood levels of ketones. But the lack of fluid resulted in an increased risk of developing kidney stones. Later it was found that restricting fluid intake had no benefit and the practice was discontinued.

Since every calorie of fat, protein, and carbohydrate is precisely calculated and measured, the patient is required to eat the entire meal without receiving any extra portions. Every meal needs to have the 4:1 or 3:1 ratio. Any snacks have to be incorporated into the daily calorie allotment and must have the same ratio. Consequently, it takes a good deal of time and effort to prepare meals and snacks.

In 1921, Dr. Russel Wilder of the Mayo Clinic coined the term "ketogenic diet" to describe a diet that produced a high level of ketones in the blood through the consumption of a high-fat, low-carbohydrate diet. He was the first to use the ketogenic diet as a treatment for epilepsy. Wilder's colleague, pediatrician Mynie Peterman, later formulated the classic 4:1 ketogenic diet. Peterman documented positive effects of improved alertness, behavior, and sleep with the diet in addition to seizure control. The diet proved to be very successful, especially with children. Peterman reported in 1925 that 95 percent of patients he studied had improved seizure control on the diet and 60 percent became completely seizure-free. That is an extraordinary cure rate for a disease that otherwise had been deemed incurable.

The diet was not without its drawbacks. A number of patients found the ketogenic diet too difficult to prepare and unappetizing. Consequently, many could not keep with it long enough to achieve satisfactory results. As many as 20 percent could not tolerate the diet and failed to follow through with it. In 1938 a new anticonvulsant drug, phenytoin (Dilantin), was developed. Taking a pill was much easier than worrying about preparing and eating a specific diet. The focus of research quickly turned to discovering new drugs. The ketogenic diet was mostly ignored by researchers and was used primarily as a last resort to treat very serious cases that did not respond to drug therapy. Publicity from the Charlie Foundation in the 1990s brought the therapy out of obscurity into the limelight where it has reemerged as an important treatment for epilepsy.

IS EATING A HIGH-FAT DIET SAFE?

As much as 90 percent of the calories in the ketogenic diet come from fat. The ketogenic diet is not just a high fat diet, but an *extremely* high fat diet. The American Heart Association and other organizations have recommended for years that we limit our fat intake to no more than 30 percent of our daily calories. They make this recommendation based primarily on the now outdated lipid hypothesis of heart disease, assuming that eating much more than 30 percent fat would cause heart disease. The high-fat ketogenic diet has now been in use for 90 years. For most of that time, those on the diet ate primarily saturated fats, the kind that dietitians tell us to avoid. Yet after nearly a century of use with literally thousands of patients consuming a 60-90 percent fat diet for extended periods of time (years, in fact), no heart attacks or strokes have been reported. Indeed, just the opposite has happened. People have been healed and have overcome an otherwise incurable disease, in the process experiencing many additional health benefits.

Many people worry that blood cholesterol levels would skyrocket on such a diet. This is really not an issue to worry about. Studies on cholesterol levels in patients following the ketogenic diet do show that, on average, total blood cholesterol levels often increase. But for optimal mental health, this is actually a good thing. Lifespan as well as mental function improve with increased cholesterol levels. You would think that if the high-fat ketogenic diet was harmful, it would become clearly evident after nearly a century of clinical use!

Total cholesterol is not an accurate predictor of heart disease risk because this number includes both the so-called "good" and "bad" cholesterol. Most of the increase is due to the good cholesterol—the type that is believed to protect against heart disease. Studies have consistently shown that those people who go on ketogenic diets generally have higher HDL (good) cholesterol and lower cholesterol ratio (indicating reduced risk of heart disease).[1-3]

Despite the rise in total cholesterol, there is no evidence that the high fat diet has a harmful effect on the heart or arteries. In the biggest analytical study on the safety and efficacy of the ketogenic diet to date, investigators failed to find any harm being done over time: the effects were all positive.[4] "We have always suspected that the ketogenic diet is relatively safe long term, and we now have proof," says Eric Kossoff, MD, a neurologist at Johns Hopkins who participated in the study. "Our study should help put to rest some of the nagging doubts about the long-term safety of the ketogenic diet."

The safety of high fat diets actually extends back thousands of years. A number of populations traditionally have survived and even thrived on diets supplying 60-90 percent of calories as fat. The most notable, perhaps, is the Eskimo. The Eskimo lived near the Arctic Circle from Alaska to Greenland where edible vegetation was scarce. The traditional Eskimo diet contained virtually no carbohydrate after weaning (milk contains some carbohydrate), relying totally on meat and fat for the rest of their lives. Yet, the primitive Eskimo was described by early arctic explorers as robust and healthy, free from the diseases of civilization such as heart disease, diabetes, Alzheimer's, and cancer, and living to an age equal to that of contemporary Americans and Europeans. The same can be said of the American plains Indians before colonization by white settlers, the native Siberians (Buryat Mongols, Yakuts, Tatars, Samoyeds, Tunguses, Chukuhis, and others) of northern Russia, and the Maasai of Africa, all of whom thrived on an extraordinarily high fat diet. Their diet was not just high in fat but was high in saturated fat and cholesterol, yet heart disease was unheard of among them. Even today, those who continue their traditional high-fat diets are remarkably free from the degenerative diseases that are so common in Western society. High fat diets have withstood the test of time and have proven to be not only safe, but therapeutic.

THE MCT KETOGENIC DIET

In nature, fats and oils are composed of fat molecules known as triglycerides. Most of these are classified as long chain triglycerides (LCTs) because they are built on a long chain of carbon atoms. Smaller triglycerides are known as medium chain triglycerides (MCTs). In the 1960s, it was discovered that MCTs produce more ketones than normal dietary fats composed of LCTs. MCTs are more efficiently absorbed and are preferentially used by the liver to produce energy in comparison to the more common LCTs. As a result, a product was developed that consisted of 100 percent MCTs, appropriately named MCT oil.

The severe carbohydrate restrictions of the classic ketogenic diet made it difficult for parents to produce palatable meals for their children. In 1971, Peter Huttenlocher developed a ketogenic diet in which about 60 percent of the calories came from MCTs. This allowed more protein and up to three times as much carbohydrate as the classic ketogenic diet. Total fat consumption could be reduced from 90 percent of calories to about 70 percent (60 percent MCT, 10 percent LCT), with about 20 percent protein and 10 percent carbohydrate to round out the diet.

MCT oil is mixed with at least twice its volume of skimmed milk, chilled, and sipped during meals or incorporated into the food. Huttenlocher tested it on twelve children and adolescents with severe epilepsy and difficult-to-treat seizures. Most of the children improved in both seizure control and alertness, producing results that were similar to those of the classic ketogenic diet. The MCT ketogenic diet is considered more nutritious than the classic diet and allows patients the option to eat more protein and carbohydrate, providing a greater variety of foods and ways to prepare meals.

Despite all the positives with the MCT diet, there are some drawbacks. Consuming too much MCT oil can cause nausea, vomiting, and diarrhea. Many patients have had to abandon the MCT diet because they could not tolerate these side effects. A modified MCT diet, which is a combination of the MCT and classic ketogenic diets, is generally more tolerable and is currently being used in many hospitals.

MODIFIED ATKINS DIET

Dr. Robert Atkins is known for championing low-carb dieting for weight loss and better overall health. In his bestselling book *Dr. Atkins' New Diet Revolution,* he outlines four phases of his low-carb diet. The diet includes the induction phase, the ongoing weight loss phase, pre-maintenance phase, and the maintenance phase. The induction phase of the diet restricts total carbohydrate consumption the most, limiting it to 20 grams per day. The classic ketogenic diet restricts carbohydrates to 10-15 grams. Although Atkins induction phase allows a little more carbohydrate, it still produces ketosis (measurable levels of ketone bodies in the blood). In fact, ketosis can be produced by restricting carbohydrate to 40 to 50 grams a day in adults, depending on how carbohydrate-sensitive an individual is.

Atkins encouraged those on the diet to get into ketosis. On a moderate fat, low-carb diet, as opposed to the high-fat ketogenic diet, ketosis indicates that body fat is being dissolved and utilized to meet the body's daily energy needs. As body fat is burned for energy, weight is reduced. In this case, ketosis is a sign the body is losing its excess fat and weight.

Even though the induction phase of the Atkins diet does not produce as high a level of ketosis as the ketogenic diet, people reported that it controlled seizures. In response to these accounts, researchers at Johns Hopkins Hospital put people on the induction phase of the Atkins diet for extended periods of time, referring to it as a *modified Atkins diet*. The modified Atkins diet places no limit on calories or protein, and the lower overall ketogenic ratio (approximately 1:1) does not need to be consistently maintained in each meal of the day. Carbohydrates were initially limited to 10 grams per day in children, 15 grams per day in adults, and increased to 20-30 grams per day after a month or so, depending on the effect on seizure control. The researchers reported that the modified Atkins diet reduced seizure frequency by more than 50 percent in 43 percent of patients and by more than 90 percent in 27 percent of the patients.[5] This and other studies have shown that seizure control with the modified Atkins diet compares favorably with the classic ketogenic diet. Although a higher level of ketosis may provide slightly better protection against seizures, the lower level is still highly effective.

THE NEUROPROTECTIVE EFFECTS OF KETONES

In the treatment of epilepsy, researchers have noted that patients on the ketogenic diet not only experience reduction in the incidence and severity of seizures but also show improved cognition, alertness, attention, and social interaction.[6-8] Brain function apparently experiences improvement in many areas.

Ketones possess potent neuroprotective properties that can ease inflammation, oxidative stress, disturbed glucose metabolism, and excitotoxicity, all of which are common in many neurological disorders. Investigators have reasoned that if ketones protect against seizures and improve mental function, they may protect against other neurological disorders as well.

Case reports have shown the ketogenic diet to be of benefit in the treatment of narcolepsy (a sleep disorder characterized by sudden, uncontrollable urges to sleep), cancer, autism, depression, migraine headaches, and disturbances in glucose metabolism such as type 2 diabetes, polycystic ovary syndrome, and some rare metabolic disorders.[9-19] Animal studies suggest that ketone bodies may also be helpful in treating some forms of cardiovascular disease and male infertility.[20-21]

Ketones have been shown to have potent anti-cancer effects. Part of the reason for this is that cancer cannot live in an oxygenated environment, and ketones improve oxygen delivery to the cells throughout the body. A second reason is that cancer cells cannot use ketones to produce energy. Cancer cells burn glucose, so when ketones replace glucose in the bloodstream, cancer cells starve. Consequently, cancer cells have a difficult time surviving in an environment where ketones dominate. Studies show that in animals, ketones decrease tumor size and cancer-related muscle wasting.[22] Similar results have been reported in human cancer patients.[23-24]

The anti-cancer effects of ketones are most pronounced in the brain.[25] In the absence of glucose, cancer cells can survive on fatty acids which are released from fat storage during a fast or when calorie consumption is restricted. However, fatty acids cannot cross the blood-brain barrier. A person on a very low-carb or ketogenic diet depends on ketones to supply the vast majority of the brain's energy needs. Consequently, the brain gets very little glucose, essentially starving the cancer to death. This is exactly what has been seen in animal studies and in at least one human case study.[26-27]

Potentially the greatest benefit to ketone therapy may be in treating conditions affecting the brain. Oxygen is vital for proper brain function. The brain depends on oxygen so much that although it represents only 2 percent of the mass of the body, it consumes some 20 percent of the oxygen. Consequently, brain cells are extremely sensitive to oxygen deprivation. Without oxygen, some brain cells start dying in less than five minutes, leading to brain damage or death. Hypoxia (lack of oxygen) can be caused by asphyxiation, carbon monoxide poisoning, cardiac arrest (heart attack), choking, drowning, strangulation, stroke, very low blood pressure, and drug overdose.

Ketones block the detrimental effects of hypoxia by improving oxygen delivery. Ketones increase blood flow to the brain by 39 percent, improving circulation and oxygen availability.[28] A number of studies show that ketones protect the brain against the damage caused by the interruption of oxygen delivery to the brain.[29-31]

Hospital patients who cannot eat for one reason or another are often given nutritional formulas administered intravenously. When patients who have suffered severe head trauma are given nutritional IV solutions containing the majority of fat in the form of MCTs, recovery is significantly enhanced.[32-33] In the body, the MCTs are converted into ketones which nourish the brain and speed healing.

Evidence from animal studies and human clinical trials suggest that the ketogenic diet can provide symptomatic relief and disease-mitigating effects in a broad range of neurodegenerative disorders including Alzheimer's, Parkinson's, ALS, Huntington's, traumatic brain injury, and stroke.[34-37] Disturbance in glucose metabolism is an underlying problem common in neurodegenerative diseases. Ketones provide an alternative—and more effective—source of energy that bypasses the glucose metabolic pathways of energy production to give the neurons the life-giving energy they need to function properly and provide an environment in which healing can take place. Ketone bodies are actually the preferred substrates for the synthesis of neural lipids. In other words, ketones promote repair and reproduction of the brain cells.

In tissue cultures, ketone bodies have been shown to increase the survival of motor neurons—the neurons that control movement. This is important for those with ALS—a neuromuscular disease. In a mouse model of ALS, researchers fed a ketogenic diet to mice that were genetically modified to develop ALS. Physical strength and performance in these mice was preserved in comparison to mice that were fed a standard diet. On autopsy it was found that the ketogenic-fed mice had significantly higher numbers of surviving motor neurons than did the control mice.

Tissue cultures from dopaminergic and hippocampal cells of the brain (areas affected by Parkinson's and Alzheimer's disease) are also protected by ketones.[38] MPTP, a neurotoxic drug that causes the destruction of dopamine neurons, is administered to animals to mimic Parkinson's disease. Ketones, however, protect the dopamine neurons in these animals from the harmful effects of MPTP, maintaining energy production and function.[39]

Ketones not only prevent neurodegeneration but can restore lost function as well. This was demonstrated in a clinical study with Parkinson's patients by Dr. Theodore VanItallie and colleagues at Columbia University College of Physicians and Surgeons. "Ketones are a high-energy fuel that nourish the brain," says Dr. VanItallie. "Our study was very successful for our patients." The study involved five Parkinson's patients who were put on a ketogenic diet for 28 days. All of the participants' tremors, stiffness, balance, and ability to walk improved, on average, by 43 percent.[40]

The participants maintained a classic 4:1 ketogenic diet consisting of about 90 percent fat. Initially, seven subjects volunteered for the study, but one dropped out the first week because the diet was too difficult to maintain and the other dropped out for personal reasons. Three of the remaining five participants who completed the study adhered faithfully to the prescribed menus. The other two participants did not adhere to the diet as strictly, but still achieved and maintained ketosis throughout the study. Each participant was evaluated using the Unified Parkinson's Disease Rating Scale at the beginning and at the end of the study. The scores were compared. In each case, the subjects showed marked improvement. Interestingly, the two participants who were not as strict with the diet and had slightly lower blood ketone levels improved the most. One improved by 46 percent, while the other improved by 81 percent, indicating that a classic ketogenic diet may not be necessary, and a less restrictive diet such as the modified Atkins may be more effective.

The researchers monitored the participant's cholesterol levels closely because they were concerned about how the high fat diet might affect blood lipids. Total blood cholesterol levels in four of the subjects showed no significant difference at the end the study. The total cholesterol of one participant, however, increased by 30 percent. However, she was the one who showed the greatest (81 percent) improvement in symptoms. The increased cholesterol certainly did not do her brain any harm and was probably part of the reason she improved so much more than the others.

Ketones significantly reduce the amount of plaque that develops in the brains of mice and dogs who exhibit Alzheimer's-like dementia.[41-42] In dog models of Alzheimer's disease, ketones improve daytime activity, increase performance on visual-spatial memory tasks, increase probability of learning tasks, have superior performance on motor learning tasks, and increase performance in short-term memory.[43] A number of studies have shown that ketones protect the brain from injury and promote rapid healing after an injury occurs.[44-46]

Rett syndrome is one of the autistic spectrum disorders, affecting girls more often than boys. Over half of those with Rett syndrome suffer from epilepsy. Those with Rett syndrome are typically undersized and have difficulty controlling physical movements (caused by a defect of the motor neurons in the brain). Because of the high seizure rate among those with this condition, a study was conducted to see what effect the ketogenic diet would have in treating this condition. Seven girls aged 5 to 10 years participated in the study. All seven suffered from severe seizures that would not respond to drug therapy. The girls were put on a MCT ketogenic diet for a number of weeks. Two of subjects could not tolerate the strict diet and did not finish the study. The remaining five all showed a significant decrease in seizure activity. In addition, they demonstrated better behavior and improved motor skills.[47] This was the first study to show that the ketogenic diet could be of value in treating autistic spectrum disorders.

Another study evaluated the ketogenic diet on a group of autistic children 4 to 10 years of age that included both boys and girls. Eighteen children completed the study. The program consisted of four weeks on an MCT ketogenic diet followed by two weeks off, repeated four times. During the period of time they were off the diet they could eat anything they normally did. The study lasted six months.

At the beginning of the study each child was evaluated using the Childhood Autism Rating Scale to determine his or her severity of autism. According to this scale, scores between 30 and 36 indicate mild to moderate cases, whereas scores of 37 and over indicate severe cases. Two of the 18 children fell in the moderate range while the remaining 16 children scored in the severe range. At the end of the study each child was evaluated again using the rating scale. All 18 children showed improvement at the end of the study period. The two children who started the diet with moderate autism showed dramatic improvement with a reduction of more than 20 points on the rating scale. The improvement was so significant that they were able to enroll in regular classes at school. Their autism was essentially cured in six months. The remaining 16 children who were classed as severely autistic also improved but to a lesser degree. Eight of them experienced good improvement (8-12 points) and eight displayed modest improvement (2-8 points).[48]

The MCT ketogenic diet was highly successful for the two children with moderate autism. It was moderately successful for those with severe autism. The results would undoubtedly have been much better if the diet was not interrupted every four weeks by a two week break and had extended for a longer period of time. In treating epilepsy, children routinely stay on the diet continuously for a period of two years. If they are seizure-free after this time, they resume a normal diet. If seizures return, the diet or a modified ketogenic diet is extended until the seizures are under control.

Ketones improve the activity of *neurotrophic factors*—small proteins that exert survival-promoting and nourishing actions on neurons.[49] These factors play a crucial role in neuron survival and function. Neurotrophic factors regulate the growth of neurons, associated metabolic functions such as protein synthesis, and the ability of the neuron to make the neurotransmitters (e.g., dopamine, glutamine) that carry the chemical signals which allow neurons to communicate with each other.

Ketones also supply the lipid building blocks for neurons.[50] Thus they aid in the regrowth or repair of damaged cells and the synthesis of new brain cells. This is exciting because it means that ketones potentially provide a means to reverse much of the damage caused by neurological disorders such as autism.

One of the unfortunate consequences of converting glucose into energy is the production of destructive free radicals. It is like the exhaust expelled when a car engine burns gasoline. In the case of our cells, the exhaust is free radicals. Healthy, well-nourished cells, however, are prepared for this and carry with them a reserve of protective antioxidants that neutralize the free radicals, reducing the damage they may cause. When ketones are used to produce energy in place of glucose, much less oxygen is needed, which greatly reduces the formation of free radicals and conserves precious antioxidants. Ketones act like a high-grade, clean-burning fuel that produces little exhaust and gives more power. In people who have neurological disorders, antioxidant reserves are so depleted that free radicals generated from various sources run wild, promoting inflammation and degeneration.

Ketones can be utilized by every cell and organ in the body except the liver, where they are made. Almost every disease state, whether it is in the brain or elsewhere, involves runaway inflammation and poor oxygen and glucose utilization. Ketones improve oxygen utilization and calm inflammation, thereby potentially providing protection against a large number disease conditions.

As you see, the health benefits associated with ketones are numerous and varied. "Ketones are a superfuel for the brain," says Richard Veech, MD, a senior scientist with the United States National Institutes of Health (NIH). Dr Veech calls ketones the body's "superfuel" for good reason. Ketones increase energy production by 25 percent while reducing oxygen consumption. This boost in energy has a

Health Benefits Associated with Ketones

The following are some of the documented health benefits associated with ketones and low-carbohydrate ketogenic diets.

- Provides an alternative high-potency energy source that can be used by every organ in the body except for the liver.[51]
- Protects against brain damage caused by cerebral hypoxia (lack of oxygen) and improves survival.[52-53]
- Reduces the formation of destructive free radicals.[20, 51, 54]
- Calms inflammation in the brain and throughout the body.[20, 84]
- Protects brain cells from chemical toxins.[55]
- Protects against epileptic seizures, including difficult-to-treat drug-resistant seizures.[56]
- Protects against infantile spasms.[57]
- Protects against narcolepsy.[58]
- Mitigates symptoms of autistic spectrum disorders.[47, 59]
- Prevents migraine headaches.[60]
- Acts as an antidepressant.[61]
- Protects the brain against damage caused by physical trauma.[62]
- Protects against neurodegenerative diseases including Alzheimer's, Parkinson's, Huntington's, and ALS.[63-66]
- Protects against symptoms of hypoglycemia.[67]
- Supplies the substrate from which new neurons can be synthesized.[68]
- Protects against diabetes. Reduces the liver's output of glucose and increases insulin production, thus improving blood sugar control and carbohydrate tolerance.[69-70]
- Mitigates the effects of insulin resistance by mimicking the acute metabolic effects of insulin.[71]
- Protects against cancer, especially brain cancer.[72-73]
- Enhances heart function by improving efficiency and strength while utilizing less oxygen. Ketones increase the hydraulic efficiency of the heart by 25 percent in comparison to glucose.[20, 74]
- Protects against brain damage caused by stroke.[75]
- Increases cellular resistance to stress and improves recovery after surgery.[76-77]
- Protects against polycystic ovary syndrome.[78]
- Increases sperm vitality and motility, important for successful fertilization.[79]
- Useful aid for weight management and obesity treatment.[80]
- May be helpful in alleviating the detrimental effects of almost every disease state due to the ability to calm inflammation and increase oxygen utilization.[81-82]
- Improves overall health and increases life span.[83]

stimulating effect on the cells and the body, transforming ordinary cells into super cells. Cell metabolism is revved up. Efficiency improves. Neurotrophic factors are activated. A mild-mannered Clark Kent of a cell is transformed into a Supercell. The cells' own mechanisms of self-preservation and healing kick into high gear. The Supercell's ability to fight off harmful influences such as toxins and stress are enhanced, and the cell's ability to survive under harsh conditions increases. The cell's productivity increases too. It is no wonder that ketone bodies appear to be associated with so many health benefits.

THE COCONUT OIL MIRACLE
Homer's Story

Homer Rosales is an honor student, sings in the church choir, and speaks two languages fluently. Last year he won the "Most Behaved" award at his elementary school. In all respects Homer is a model student and a delight to his parents. He wasn't always this way, however. A few years ago he was a terror, hyperactive, uncontrollable, and noncommunicative. You see, Homer was autistic.

Homer was diagnosed with autistic spectrum disorder on March 13, 2002. He was one week away from his fourth birthday. "My primary concern at that time was his speech delay," says his mother Rosemarie. "Imagine, he was almost four years old but I had yet to hear him call me mama—the sweetest word a mother hears from her child."

His hyperactivity was a constant annoyance to his parents, other children, and the neighbors. He was so hyperactive that as soon as he stepped out of the house he would run off and get lost without any idea of how to get home. He would wander into neighbors' homes unnoticed and without their permission and destroy their property—computers, vases, TVs, stereos, etc. The owners would open the door and be shocked to find him all alone in their homes.

Homer had no fear of danger. He never indicated if or when he was hungry. He never played with other kids and usually harmed them by throwing stones or striking them with hard objects. "He was so destructive in church, restaurants, and stores that we rarely took him to public places," says Rosemarie. "Oh my, what kind of a child I have!"

Despite behavioral therapy, Homer showed little progress. "Then God guided me to PRIME Center Foundation," says Rosemarie. "Mr. Roni Romeo Ocubillo, the founder of this special school introduced me to a gluten-free and casein-free (GFCF) diet. His approach was supported by studies that demonstrated that certain foods seem to affect the developing brains of some children with autism."

Rosemarie was told that autistic children have an immune system dysfunction which causes them to have abnormal microflora populations in the intestinal tract. Candida often flourishes, damaging the intestinal wall, leading to leaky gut syndrome. Some of the symptoms of candida overgrowth in children include sugar cravings, headaches, hyperactivity, and behavior and learning problems. Many parents of children with ADHD, as well as those with autism, report that treatment for candida improves their children's behavior and concentration. Nystatin, an antifungal drug used to fight candida, is recommended to all the autistic children enrolled in the PRIME program.

At the age of six, Homer began his special school and his new diet. We eliminated all foods containing gluten and casein," says Rosemarie. "Many of my son's favorite foods such as spaghetti, oatmeal, and milk were now off limits. Nystatin was given to him to control candida and aid in building a healthy digestive tract. The program seemed to work. His hyperactivity lessened, he could focus more, and could talk a little with some sense. When I would ask, 'What are you doing Homer?' He could answer 'Safeguard, wash.'"

After following the gluten-free and casein-free diet for almost 10 months, Rosemarie felt her son was on his way to lasting improvement. His behavior improved, he became more manageable, he began to socialize with other kids, could read and write a little, and talk a little. Things were beginning to look up.

"To our dismay," says Rosemarie, "we got another blow when Homer came down with pneumonia. He was confined at the hospital and advised to rest. He was absent from his therapy for a full month. During his stay at the hospital the nurses and doctors had a hard time putting in his IV. He was very strong. It literally took hours to attach the IV. When he felt the pain, instead of calling 'Mama,' he shouted, 'Help Barney! Mickey Mouse help! Superman, Batman!' My goodness…what a child I have! He wouldn't take his medicines orally because he didn't like the taste. It was a struggle for me at the hospital taking care of him. He got his medicines, mostly antibiotics, through his IV. He didn't like to eat. He was asking for his spaghetti, wanted to drink milk and other foods prohibited on his therapy diet. He wasn't eating properly. I was worried about his ability to fight off the infection. I called PRIME and asked permission to allow Homer to eat the foods he liked for the sake of his health."

When Homer finally went back to his school, all of the staff, including Mr. Ocubillo the foundation's director, were disappointed and frustrated with his behavior. "He was back to zero," Rosemarie says. "His autism was so prevalent again! He was very hyperactive again. We had to start all over. Mr. Ocubillo told me that it was due to the antibiotics while he was hospitalized. The antibiotics not only killed the bacteria that caused his pneumonia but also the good intestinal bacteria, which help keep candida under control. I was so depressed with this development, I don't remember how many times I cried. But still, I didn't lose hope. I prayed hard to God for His guidance."

Rosemarie's prayers were answered and the answer came from an unlikely source—virgin coconut oil. "I had heard how coconut oil could be used to strengthen the immune system, prevent illness, and improve health," she says. "I began to take it daily by the spoonful as a dietary supplement. I observed that my overall health improved, including my asthma. I thought perhaps it could help Homer by building up his immune system. I tried to give it to him but he refused. It took me five months of struggle to get him to take his first spoonful. I continued to give it to him every day and sometimes three times a day. After two months, I noticed a dramatic improvement in his behavior and especially in his speech. Up until then, he had only been able to understand and speak a little in English. Now, not only was his English improving, but for the first time he was beginning to speak in Cebuano—our native dialect." (The Rosales are from the Philippines.)

Autistic children often never learn to speak and when they do, they have limited communication skills. Homer was learning to learn to speak *two* languages!

By the time Homer was seven years old his echolalia (involuntary repetition of words) and his ritualistic behavior were gone. He was beginning to read well and write clearly. He could tell stories and express his feelings and ideas, and was developing friendships with other children. His behavior improved dramatically. He would ask permission before going into the neighbors' houses and could find his way back home.

"I shared my knowledge of coconut oil with Mr. Ocubillo at PRIME," says Rosemarie. "At first, he was skeptical. So I gave him some articles to read. A coworker of mine gave him a copy of Dr. Bruce Fife's book *The Coconut Oil Miracle*. In the book Dr. Fife describes, among other things, the antifungal properties of coconut oil. That's when I realized that coconut oil killed the candida in my son's intestines. Originally, my only purpose in giving Homer the oil was to improve his immune system. I never realized that his autism would be gone with the help of coconut oil. What an amazing miracle!"

Mr. Ocubillo researched coconut oil further and now all the children at the PRIME Center Foundation are taking virgin coconut oil daily. It has replaced the antifungal drug Nystatin formerly used.

Homer's progress was so astounding that in 2006 he was enrolled in regular classes at school. "During the evaluation process the principal was impressed because Homer could read very well," says Rosemarie. "He got a score of 61 out of 65 on the written exam. Thanks to coconut oil I said goodbye to PRIME Center forever and welcome to the world of regular students."

Five years have passed since Homer was integrated into regular classes at school. In that time he has become a model student with many friends. He no longer eats a special diet, but still consumes coconut oil. His mother uses it in all her cooking. "I tell people that Homer was once autistic but they don't believe me," says Rosemarie. "What a miracle!"

Coconut Ketones

Why does coconut oil have the power to cure autism? As noted above, coconut oil can help in the treatment with autism by boosting the immune system and killing candida in the intestinal tract, but there is more to it than that, much more. The secret is in coconut ketones.

Coconut oil is ketogenic; that is, it stimulates the production of ketones. Coconut oil is composed predominately of medium chain triglycerides. In fact, the MCT oil used in the treatment of epilepsy is derived from coconut oil. Normally, a person must be fasting or on a very low-carb, high-fat ketogenic diet in order for the body to manufacture ketones. Not so with coconut oil. The body will convert the MCTs in coconut oil into ketones regardless of what other food is eaten. If you supply the body with MCTs, the body will crank out ketones even when consuming carbohydrates. However, if carbohydrate consumption is reduced, ketone production is enhanced.

When parents put their children on gluten-free and casein-free diets (GFCF diets) they no longer consume grains and dairy, both of which are usually associated with high carb foods.

Consider all the foods that must be eliminated on a GFCF diet: bread, rolls, muffins, crackers, cookies, pretzels, hot and cold breakfast cereals, toaster pastries, pie, cake, donuts, pasta, pizza, bagels, tortillas, ice cream, milk chocolate, cheese puffs, sandwiches, and many commercially prepared meals such as frozen dinners, soups, sauces, etc. If you eliminate all of these items from the diet, you must replace it with something else. Often the replacement is meat and vegetables—low-carb items. Consequently, many GFCF diets are low-carb in nature. A low-carb diet combined with ample amounts of coconut oil can work wonders for autistic children.

For years the MCT ketogenic diet has been successful in reducing seizures and even bringing about lasting cures for epilepsy. The coconut oil ketogenic diet can do the same for epilepsy as well as for autism. Coconut oil isn't just ketogenic; it provides many other benefits that protect the brain and stimulate brain cell growth.

> "Ketones are a superfuel for the brain."
> —Richard Veech, MD, National Institutes of Health

8 | The Cholesterol Factor

THE GOOD SIDE OF CHOLESTEROL

Contrary to popular belief, fat and cholesterol are not ugly beasts that lurk in our foods just to do us harm. They are valuable, even essential, nutrients. Simply put, fat and cholesterol are good for you. They nourish the body and can help protect you from disease. Our fanaticism on reducing fat and cholesterol has painted a one-sided and inaccurate picture in most people's minds about these important nutrients. Consequently, most people mistakenly believe that the less fat and cholesterol they eat, the better. This is not true. Eating too little fat and cholesterol can have serious health consequences.

Cholesterol is one of the most important substances in your body. It is vital for the proper function and regulation of all body systems. You have cholesterol in every cell in your body. It is there for an important reason.

The cells of our body are encased in a lipid (fat and cholesterol) membrane. Even the individual organelles (cell organs) inside the cell are encased in a lipid coat. Cholesterol is a vital element of the cell and organelle membranes. It is uniquely able to influence the structure, thickness, permeability, deformation, and other characteristics of cell membranes. Cholesterol is needed to regulate the entry and exit of certain hormones, fats, and proteins and typically makes up about 20 percent of the membrane. In certain areas of the membrane, cholesterol concentration increases to 30 to 40 percent. Some cells, such as the nerve cells, contain even more.

For the cells to function properly, an ample amount of cholesterol needs to be available. Cholesterol must be continually supplied to form new cells and repair damaged tissues. For example, when an injury occurs within a blood vessel, cholesterol is used in the repair process. If the injury becomes chronic, as in the case of an artery beset by chronic inflammation, cholesterol, along with protein and calcium, is laid down repeatedly. This can lead to the formation of the plaque characteristic of atherosclerosis. Promoters of the cholesterol hypothesis of heart disease claim that since cholesterol is present, it must be the cause of the clogging in the artery. But according to the newer and more widely accepted response-to-injury hypothesis, cholesterol didn't cause the plaque, but was part of the repair process that is trying to fix the problem. It is the chronic inflammation that caused the cholesterol, as well as the protein and calcium, to be deposited. The amount of plaque deposited in the artery has absolutely no relationship to the amount of cholesterol in the blood.

Cholesterol also functions as the precursor for a number of vital hormones. All of the steroid hormones, including pregnenolone, aldosterone, estrogen, progesterone, testosterone, and cortisol, start out as cholesterol. These hormones regulate sexual differentiation and behavior; mediate menstrual cycle and pregnancy; regulate the excretion of salt and water by the kidneys; affect carbohydrate, protein, and lipid metabolism; and influence a wide variety of other vital functions including inflammatory reactions and the capacity to cope with stress. It is cholesterol that makes you who you are and keeps your body running smoothly.

Bile, too, gets its start as cholesterol. Bile is secreted by the liver and stored in the gallbladder. When we eat a meal, bile is released into the digestive tract to emulsify dietary fats and fat soluble nutrients and facilitate their digestion and assimilation. Without bile we could not digest the fats which are necessary for proper health.

Vitamin D, an essential element for our bodies, is manufactured in our bodies as sunlight interacts with the cholesterol in our skin. Vitamin D has a multitude of functions including immune system support and aiding in the building of strong bones and teeth. It is also needed for healthy brain function and helps lower the risk of developing diabetes, heart and kidney disease, high blood pressure, and cancer.

Cholesterol is essential for proper immune function. When blood cholesterol is low, white blood cells, the workhorse of our immune system, are under-produced, and the body is less capable of fighting off infections, neutralizing toxins, and removing cancerous cells.[1] Cholesterol also acts as a detoxifying agent by neutralizing toxins secreted by disease-causing bacteria.[2-3]

Alcohol consumption during pregnancy is known to cause birth defects. Cholesterol helps nullify the detrimental effects of certain toxins, including alcohol. Research suggests that increasing cholesterol consumption during pregnancy may prevent at-risk mothers from conferring alcohol-related damage to their growing fetus.[4]

The toxins secreted by infectious bacteria do more harm than the organisms themselves. It is the toxins that poison the body and cause the majority of symptoms associated with the bacterial infections. Cholesterol works with the immune system to neutralize these harmful toxins. For example, *staphylococcus aureus* is a common bacterium that causes a variety of infections including skin infections, connective tissue infections (cellulitis), breast infections (mastitis), blood infections (sepsis), lung infections (pneumonia), bone infections (osteomyelitis), heart infections (endocarditis), toxic shock syndrome, and food poisoning, among others. Cholesterol helps protect against these infections by aiding the immune system in neutralizing the toxins secreted by this and other organisms.[5] For example, in one study patients with pulmonary tuberculosis were hospitalized for eight weeks and randomly assigned to receive a cholesterol-rich diet (800 mg/day) or a normal diet (250 mg/day). All the patients received the same drugs to treat the infection. Lab tests during the study demonstrated that bacteria levels of those on the cholesterol-rich diet came down much faster, which resulted in quicker recovery.[6]

Cholesterol is needed for building strong bones and protects against osteoporosis. Bone tissue is continually being dismantled and rebuilt. As we grow older, the process of dismantling bone occurs more rapidly than rebuilding. Consequently, bone density declines with age. Higher blood levels of cholesterol is associated with greater bone density and fewer fractures in the elderly.[7] Lowering cholesterol weakens the bones and increases risk of osteoporosis.

During pregnancy, low cholesterol has proven to be detrimental for baby's health and development. Over 12 percent of the births in the US are premature, meaning they are born at least three weeks early of a full 40-week term pregnancy. Preterm infants face the potential of lifelong medical problems. Women with low cholesterol are 2.5 times more likely to have a premature delivery than woman with normal cholesterol levels.[8]

Cholesterol is found as a structural component in every cell but is most prominent in the nerve cells. It constitutes a major component of the myelin sheath that coats the long axons of the neurons and forms a substantial part of the cell membrane. As a major component of nerve tissue, it is the most common molecule in the brain, making the brain the most cholesterol-rich organ in the body.

Cholesterol is absolutely essential for the transmission of nerve impulses and the communication between neurons. It is needed for storing and retrieving memories. The synapses—the highly specialized contact that sits between adjacent neurons in the brain—depend on cholesterol for their function.[9]

Cholesterol is constantly being formed to maintain, replace, and repair the cells and tissues, especially nerve tissue. Any interference with normal cholesterol synthesis can impair nerve tissue maintenance and repair, leading to neurodegeneration through neuron loss.[10] Even a small depletion of cholesterol—less than 10 percent—in the neuron endings at the synapse has been shown to be enough to inhibit the release of neurotransmitters and block nerve transmission.[11] If adequate cholesterol is not available, nerve transmission stops. If the nerve is involved in creating a memory, then the memory will not be formed. If the nerve is involved in retrieving a memory, the memory will not be found. If the nerve is involved in producing or controlling physical movement, the action will not occur as expected. If the nerve is involved in making rational decisions and thinking, then bizarre or uncharacteristic behavior may result. Cholesterol availability can affect any and all brain functions. Cholesterol is the key to our ability to learn and remember. It is the key to all mental functions. Not only must it be present, but it must be present in sufficient enough quantities to fulfill its role in normal brain function.[12]

The brain contains almost 25 percent of the body's cholesterol.[13] In fact, the brain's need for cholesterol is so great that it manufactures its own cholesterol to supplement that which is produced by the liver. The cholesterol in the brain is produced by the glial cells—the non-nervous or supporting tissue of the brain.

As cholesterol research continues, the importance of cholesterol in human health is becoming increasingly evident. Many medical professionals are questioning the sanity of prescribing cholesterol-lowering drugs. Some doctors are even beginning to prescribe cholesterol-*raising* medications to patients to take advantage of the many benefits rendered by this essential substance.

THE DANGER OF LOW CHOLESTEROL

We frequently hear warnings about high cholesterol, but we rarely hear about the dangers of low cholesterol. The overemphasis on lowering cholesterol has instilled the belief that the lower your cholesterol is, the better. Nothing could be farther from the truth. The consequences of low cholesterol can be much worse than the consequences of high cholesterol. Research over the past several years has shown that low cholesterol levels are associated with increased rates of depression, anxiety, bipolar disorder, violent behavior, suicide, Parkinson's disease, ALS, cancer, celiac disease, liver disease, malabsorption, malnutrition, and some forms of dementia. More recently, autism has been added to this list. You will notice that many of these disorders involve mental health.[14-27]

The American Heart Association suggests that adults keep their total blood cholesterol levels below 240 mg/dl and preferably below 200 mg/dl (5.2 mmol/l) to reduce risk of heart attack. However, there is no magic level at which heart attack risk suddenly becomes apparent. These numbers are arbitrarily chosen for sake of convenience in prescribing medications. Studies show that those people with total cholesterol up to 240 mg/dl (6.2 mmol/l) do not experience any more heart attacks than those who have levels at or below 200 mg/dl (5.2 mmol/l). So cholesterol lowering beyond this has no benefit in terms of heart attack risk.[28-30]

The effects on brain health from lowering cholesterol using drugs have been reported for decades. In the early studies that compared cholesterol-lowering drugs with placebos (dummy pills), an unexpected phenomenon quickly surfaced. While fatal heart attacks in some high risk middle-aged men declined slightly, deaths from suicide and violence, as well as cancer, increased. The overall results showed a total *increase* in deaths among the drug users compared to those without. Those subjects who were taking cholesterol-lowering drugs reported a significant increase in depression, irritability, and aggression that apparently led to increased incidences of suicides and violent deaths. Initially, researchers brushed these findings aside, claiming they were simply the result of chance. The studies were repeated with larger numbers of subjects. The results were the same: increased deaths due to suicide and violence.[31-32]

Dr. Matthew Muldoon and colleagues at the University of Pittsburgh found that reducing cholesterol levels *doubled* the rate of death from violence and suicide.[33] A large investigation in Sweden headed by Dr. Gunnar Lindberg measured blood cholesterol levels in more than 50,000 men and women and then kept track of them for 20 years. During the first six years, 20 men with cholesterol below 207 mg/dl (5.4 mmol/l) committed suicide. Yet only five with cholesterol above 296 mg/dl (7.7 mmol/l) had committed suicide.[34]

The Framingham Study examined the relationship between total cholesterol and cognitive performance.[35] In this study some 1,900 men and women free of dementia and stroke received biennial cholesterol checks over a 16 to 18 year period. Cognitive tests consisting of measure of learning, memory, attention, concentration, abstract reasoning, concept formation, and organizational abilities were administered four to six years after the surveillance period. The researchers found a significant association between the level of blood cholesterol and measures of verbal fluency, attention, concentration, abstract reasoning, and a composite score measuring multiple cognitive domains. Participants with cholesterol levels of less than 200 mg/dl (5.2 mmol/l) performed significantly poorer than participants with cholesterol levels higher than 240 mg/dl (6.2 mmol/l).

Several studies have found that Alzheimer's patients have lower total blood cholesterol than age matched controls with normal mental function.[36] Analyzing brain tissues from deceased Alzheimer's patients, researchers have found that the diseased portions of the brains were deficient in cholesterol.[37] This finding is consistent with the observation that the hippocampus (the memory center of the brain) of some Alzheimer's patients presents a moderate yet significant reduction in membrane cholesterol.[38] As far back as 1991, researchers suggested that increasing delivery of cholesterol to the brain may help Alzheimer's patients and recommended increasing fat consumption.[39]

The Journal of Biological Chemistry published a study showing that eating a high-cholesterol diet can protect the brain from the physiological changes that are associated with neurodegenerative disease.[40] This study showed that dietary measures can be taken to help protect the brain. It also suggests that the wrong type of diet (i.e., low-fat, low-cholesterol) can promote neurodegeneration.

CHOLESTEROL DEFICIENCY:
A COMMON FACTOR IN AUTISM

The importance of cholesterol can be seen in Smith-Lemli-Opitz syndrome (SLOS), a genetic disorder caused by a deficiency in cholesterol synthesis. In people with SLOS, an enzyme required in the production of cholesterol behaves abnormally, reducing the amount of cholesterol manufactured by the body. This leads to low cholesterol levels, often below 100 mg/dl (2.6 mmol/l).

Cholesterol is essential for every tissue and every organ in the body, so a deficiency affects the entire body, including hormone and enzyme production. During fetal development it can lead to birth defects and neurological disorders. There is a wide spectrum of severity of the effects of low cholesterol during the prenatal period, ranging from individuals who are born functionally normal to malformed fetuses that die before birth. Many affected children die in the first year from failure to thrive and from increased susceptibility to infections.

Symptoms vary from person to person depending on the amount of cholesterol they can produce. Common characteristics include developmental delays, poor growth, facial anomalies, cleft palate, webbed toes, hearing and sight defects, and malformations of the heart, brain, lungs, and genitals.

The brain, with its high cholesterol requirement, is particularly affected. Neurological symptoms include social and language impairment, repetitive behavior, repeated self-injury, self-biting, head banging, opisthokinesis (upper body movement in which there is an arched backward diving motion), and mental retardation. All of these symptoms are the direct result of a cholesterol deficiency, which shows how important normal cholesterol levels are to physical and mental health.

At least half and as many as 90 percent of those who have SLOS meet the criteria for being diagnosed with autism. Consequently, many of the symptoms characteristic of autism can result from a cholesterol deficiency. Indeed, most autistic children have low cholesterol levels (less than 160 mg/dl/4.1 mmol/l). Nearly 20 percent have extremely low cholesterol, less than 100 mg/dl (2.6 mmol/l). This finding was first revealed by researchers at Johns Hopkins University. They found that in 100 autistic children not affected by SLOS, 19 percent had total cholesterol levels lower than 100 mg/dl (2/6 mmol/l).[41] This finding was confirmed in another study involving 40 autistic children, where the majority (57.5 percent) had cholesterol levels less than 160 mg/dl (4.1 mmol/l) and 17.5 percent had levels below 100 mg/dl (2.6 mmol/l).[42]

The current treatment for SLOS is a high-fat, high-cholesterol diet. Cholesterol is supplied in natural form (e.g., egg yolk, cream, butter, liver) or as purified cholesterol in capsules. While cognitive development has not shown much improvement, treatment has been successful in reducing aggressive behavior, self injury, temper outbursts, hyperactivity, and irritability and in improving growth, speech articulation, sleep, attention span, and social interaction, including initiating hugs and showing affection.[43-49] Cholesterol therapy has been used to treat SLOS since the early 1990s. In that time, no adverse side effects have been reported from the increased cholesterol and fat consumption.[41]

The occurrence of autism in SLOS children declines with cholesterol therapy. In one study it was found that out of a group of SLOS children under the age of 5 years, 88 percent displayed autistic characteristics. However, with cholesterol supplementation, the number of those with autistic characteristics dropped to 22 percent by the time they reached their 5th birthday.[50] This study provides evidence that cholesterol supplementation can be useful in the treatment of autism. While it is not a cure, it can help reduce many of the symptoms associated with this disorder.

Cholesterol deficiency could be caused by a defect in cholesterol synthesis, reduced cholesterol absorption from gastrointestinal disturbances (a common occurrence in autism), a low-fat/low-cholesterol diet, or any combination of these. Regardless of the cause, adding more cholesterol into the diet can have beneficial results.

The therapeutic amounts of cholesterol used in studies have varied from 20 to 300 mg/kg body weight/day. For a 40 pound 5-year-old that would equate to 380 to 5,700 mg per day. A single large egg contains about 212 mg of cholesterol. For those who have moderately low cholesterol levels, eating ample amounts of eggs, meat, cream, butter, and other fats each day would probably be enough to satisfy the body's cholesterol needs. Those with very low cholesterol levels (under 130 mg/dl/3.3 mmol/l) may need to add a pharmaceutical grade cholesterol supplement. New Beginnings Nutritionals (www.sonic cholesterol.com) produces a supplement called Sonic Cholesterol which is designed to correct cholesterol deficiency. Each capsule contains 250 mg of cholesterol. It is made from raw sheep's wool. This product is only available by prescription.

For those who have low or moderately low cholesterol, there is no risk of raising cholesterol levels too high. Diet alone can only raise cholesterol levels by about 10-

---

Pilots Perform Better on High-Fat Diets

If the type of food we eat can affect our mental abilities, then the diets of people whose jobs affect the lives and safety of others must be of the best quality to assure top mental performance. This was the focus of a study commissioned by the U.S. military.

Unlike many studies financed by the food and drug industries, there was no preconceived prejudice involved in this study. The government demanded the facts, without bias from political correctness or financial influences. They simply wanted the truth; lives depended on it.

The study tracked 45 student pilots to assess how different foods affected the pilots' mental performance. Every three weeks, each pilot spent one week on one of four different diets: high-fat, high-carbohydrate, high-protein, and a control diet. The menus were similar so the type of diet wouldn't be obvious to the participants.

The study used a flight simulator that required students to navigate and descend in cloudy weather when the runway wasn't visible and using only the plane's computers. They also took tests that required memorizing and repeating numbers and comparing shapes. Although the pilots did not know the difference in the foods, they did notice the difference in their own performance. "I could tell the difference on how well I was doing on the different diets," said Jeremy Ternes, who participated in the study. "There were times I thought, "Wow, I was a lot more on today as compared to last week.'"

Based on the pilots' test scores, the researchers found that those who ate the fattiest foods, such as butter and gravy, had the quickest response times in mental tests and made the fewest mistakes when flying in challenging conditions. The pilots' mental performance was significantly better with the high-fat diet over the other diets. This was an important finding because it may help decrease the number of aviation accidents due to pilot error, which is especially important for the combat fighter.

It is also important for the non-pilot as well. It means that getting adequate fat into the diet is important for proper mental function.

Source: Dave Kolpack. Study shows high-fat diet might help pilots. Associated Press, October 7, 2009.

---

15 percent. To raise it much more than that would require extreme diet modifications or supplementation.

A normal, healthy cholesterol level is around 200 mg/dl (5.2 mmol/l). Too much below this can start affecting many aspects of health. This is especially true for children. Because children's brains are still growing and developing, they require more cholesterol than adults. Approximately 85 percent of autistic children have cholesterol levels below this level. The average cholesterol level for autistic children is about 140 and 160 mg/dl (3.6-4.1 mmol/l).

The parents of 18-year-old Paulina Shaw tried everything to treat her autism, including a GFCG diet, antifungal therapy, antibiotics for intestinal clostridia, and heavy metal chelation. The treatments helped control her severe hyperactivity, abnormal sleep patterns, and self-abusive behavior. However, she still had very little use of her hands and hadn't spoken since the age of four. Despite these handicaps, her parents report she was alert, happy, and enjoyed school.

"At the beginning of the school year, we were receiving unfavorable school reports indicating that she was losing interest in participating in school activities and was becoming increasingly withdrawn," says William, her stepfather. "She was even falling asleep in class after a full night's sleep. At home, she was becoming more and more withdrawn as well and overall, more 'autistic.'"

Something was definitely wrong. Paulina began to go to bed earlier and earlier until she was going to sleep immediately after arriving home from school at 3:00 pm. Even after sleeping 15 hours at night, she was falling asleep in school.

"I decided to review all of Paulina's test results and treatments but the only thing I could find was the egg allergy," says William.

"When did you take the eggs out of Paulina's diet?" I asked my wife.

"At the beginning of the school year," she responded.

That was the same time when the school began reporting her regression. "I realized it was the eggs!" says William. The lack of eggs was apparently affecting her cholesterol levels. At the time, Paulina's cholesterol was 142 mg/dl (3.6 mmol/l), a very low value. Her parents realized that despite her allergy, they needed to feed her eggs again.

"Within a few days of giving two eggs for breakfast every day, the smiling, happy, alert and energetic (but still autistic) Paulina had returned," says William. She stopped going to bed early and her teacher started reporting positive results. Even though the eggs upset her stomach due to the allergy, the cholesterol in the eggs had proven essential for her well-being. After six months on the egg-enriched diet, Paulina's cholesterol increased to 157 mg/dl (4.0 mmol/l), demonstrating how slowly blood cholesterol levels increase with diet. Eventually Paulina replaced the eggs with a cholesterol dietary supplement.

9 | The Facts on Fats

FAT IS GOOD FOR YOU

Dietary fat plays a very important role in mental and physical health. However, not all fats are equal. Some fats are essential while others can be harmful.

All natural fats are good. However, good fats can become bad if they are adulterated by oxidation or chemically altered. Some fats are better for us than others. Some can be consumed in larger amounts than others. Some need to be eaten in balance with others. Some fats, those that are adulterated or manmade, should not be eaten at all. The problem is that most people are confused as to which are which.

Advertising and marketing propaganda have greatly influenced and distorted our perception of dietary fats. We are told to reduce our fat intake to the bare minimum in order to lose excess weight and be healthy. In addition, some fats are portrayed as being good while others are depicted as being bad. Saturated fats get the brunt of the criticism and are blamed for contributing to just about every health problem experienced by mankind. Polyunsaturated vegetable oils, margarine, and shortening, on the other hand, are hailed as the "good" fats. The truth is that most saturated fats, and particularly coconut oil, are some of the healthiest you can eat. In contrast, many polyunsaturated fats are so far removed from their natural state as to become a serious health threat.

Natural fats which have undergone as little processing and adulteration as possible are the healthiest, regardless of whether they are saturated or unsaturated. People from all walks of life and throughout history have been eating natural fats without experiencing the health problems we commonly face today. These fats are not the troublemakers. Fats are, in fact, vital nutrients that our bodies rely upon to achieve and maintain good health. We need fat in our diet. Almost all foods in nature contain fat to one extent or another.

An adequate amount of fat is necessary for proper digestion and nutrient absorption. Fats slow down the movement of food through the stomach and digestive system. This allows more time for foods to bathe in stomach acids and digestive enzymes. As a consequence, more nutrients, especially minerals which are normally tightly bound to other compounds, are released from our foods and absorbed into the body.

116

Low-fat diets are actually detrimental because they prevent complete digestion of food and limit nutrient absorption, promoting mineral deficiencies. Calcium, for example, needs fat for proper absorption. For this reason, low-fat diets encourage osteoporosis. It is interesting that we often avoid fat as much as possible and eat low fat foods, including non-fat and low-fat milk, to get calcium, yet taking the fat out of dairy products prevents the calcium from being effectively absorbed. This may be one of the reasons why people can drink loads of milk and take calcium supplements by the handful but still suffer from osteoporosis. Likewise, many vegetables are good sources of calcium, but in order to take advantage of that calcium, you need to eat them with butter and cream or other foods that contain fat.

Fat improves the availability and absorption of almost all vitamins and minerals and is essential in order to properly absorb fat-soluble nutrients. The fat soluble vitamins include vitamins A, D, E, and K. Other fat soluble nutrients include CoQ10, lutein, zeaxanthin, lycopene, alpha-carotene, beta-carotene and other carotenoids. These nutrients are absolutely vital to good health.

Many of the fat-soluble vitamins function as antioxidants that protect against free-radical damage. By reducing the amount of fat in your diet, you limit the amount of protective antioxidant nutrients available to protect you from destructive free-radical reactions. Low-fat diets speed the process of degeneration and aging. This may be one of the reasons why those people who stay on very low-fat diets for any length of time often look pale and sickly.

Carotenoids are fat-soluble nutrients found in fruits and vegetables. The best known is beta-carotene. All of the carotenoids are known for their antioxidant capability. Many studies have shown them and other fat-soluble antioxidants such as vitamins A and E to provide protection from degenerative disease and support immune system function.

Vegetables like broccoli and carrots have beta-carotene, but if you don't eat any oil with them you won't get the full benefit of the fat-soluble vitamins they contain. You can eat fruits and vegetables loaded with antioxidants and other nutrients, but if you don't include fat with them then you will only absorb a small portion of these vital nutrients. Taking vitamin tablets won't help much because they too need fat to facilitate proper absorption. Eating a low-fat diet, therefore, can actually be detrimental to your health.

How much of an effect does fat have on nutrient absorption? Apparently a lot. In a study conducted at Ohio State University, researchers looked at absorption of three carotenoids (beta-carotene, lycopene, and lutein) in meals that had added fat. The researchers used avocado as their source of fat, which is relatively high in monounsaturated fat.

Eleven test subjects were given a meal of fat-free salsa and bread. On another day the same meal was given, but this time avocado was added to the salsa, boosting the fat content of the meal to about 37 percent of total calories consumed. Blood levels of the test subjects showed that beta-carotene increased 2.6 times and lycopene 4.4 times as compared to the meal without avocado. This showed that adding a little fat to the meal can more than double or even quadruple nutrient absorption.

A second test involved eating a salad. The first salad included romaine lettuce, baby spinach, shredded carrots, and a non-fat dressing, resulting in a fat content of about 2 percent. After avocado was added, the fat content jumped to 42 percent. The higher fat salad increased blood levels of lutein 7 times and beta-carotene an incredible 18 times!

In a similar study, subjects were fed salads using dressings with a different fat content. Salad with non-fat dressing resulted in negligible carotenoid absorption. Low-fat dressing improved nutrient absorption some, but full-fat dressing showed a significant increase. The researchers were surprised not only by how adding fat improved nutrient absorption, but also how little is absorbed in the absence of fat.

If you want to get all the nutrients you can from a tomato, green beans, spinach, or any vegetable or low-fat food, you need to add some fat. Eating vegetables without added fat is in effect the same as eating a nutritionally poor meal. Adding a good source of fat in the diet is important in order to gain the most nutrition from your foods.

Nathan Pritikin, a self-proclaimed nutritionist, became famous in the 1970s and 1980s as one of America's leading advocates for low-fat dieting as a means of achieving optimal health. He founded the Pritikin Longevity Center to promote his low-fat program. Pritikin was a fanatic about keeping fat out of the diet. He claimed there was enough fat in lettuce and other vegetables to meet our body's needs. His diet limited fat consumption to a mere 10 percent of total calories. People lost weight, but they also developed health problems as a result of fat deficiency. Charles T. McGee, MD, describes in his book *Heart Frauds* patients who tried the Pritikin low-fat diet, "Pritikin Program patients become deficient in essential fatty acids after they have been on the diet about two years. These people entered the office looking gaunt, with skin that was dry, droopy, pale, gray, and flaky. Fortunately this complication was seldom seen because most people find it difficult to keep fat intake down to the 10 percent level without cheating."

Pritikin claimed his low-fat way of eating would improve health, remove excess weight, and ward off degenerative disease. Unfortunately for Pritikin, it didn't work for him. He developed leukemia, went into a deep depression, and committed suicide. Both depression and suicide are well known side effects of low-fat dieting.[1-2] Even diets that allow 25 percent of calories as fat, over twice that recommended by Pritikin, can seriously affect mental health.[3] The diet he advocated to achieve optimal health and increase longevity and happiness was the thing that drove him out of his mind and to an early death.

Another recent low-fat advocate was Roy L. Walford, MD, a professor of medicine at UCLA medical school. Walford was considered one of the world's leading experts on calorie restriction and longevity. Since the 1930s researchers have observed that the lifespan of animals could be extended up to 50 percent by restricting the number of calories they ate. Walford believed human lifespan could be extended to 120 years on a calorie restricted diet. He wrote several books on the topic, including *The 120 Year Diet*, *Maximum Life Span*, and *The Anti-Aging Plan*. His plan was based on the concept of "calorie restriction with optimal nutrition" or what he termed "CRON." He claimed it would "retard the basic rate of aging in humans, greatly extending the period of youth and middle age; postpone the onset of such late-life disease as heart disease, diabetes, and cancer; and even lower the overall susceptibility to disease at any age."

Restricting the number of calories consumed was central to his program. Since fat contains more than twice as many calories as either carbohydrate or protein, fat was almost eliminated from his diet. Walford began eating this way when he was in his early 60s and fully expected to live to be a least 100. But things didn't work out the way he had planned. He developed a brain wasting disease called amyotrophic lateral sclerosis (ALS) and died in 2004 at the age of 79. The average lifespan for a white American male is 78 years.[4] So after nearly 20 years of following a calorie restricted, low-fat diet, he added the sum total of only one year to his life and suffered with crippling neurodegenerative disease for his last few years of it. Instead of protecting him from degenerative disease, his low-fat diet was the thing that did him in.

Calorie restriction with optimal nutrition may very well extend lifespan and forestall aging, but the problem with Walford's diet was that he did not understand the importance of fat and how it is necessary in order to achieve optimal nutrition. Studies have shown that people eating low-fat diets have a higher rate of death due to degenerative disease than those with higher fat intake.[5] High-carbohydrate, low-fat diets are known to increase risk of ALS.[6]

One of the classic symptoms of neurodegenerative disease is chronic inflammation. Chronic inflammation is destructive, and ways to reduce neuroinflammation are actively being sought. While anti-inflammatory drugs have been suggested as a possible answer, for the most part they have proven to be ineffective. In fact, some accelerate the rate of neurodegeneration. Researchers continue to search for new drugs. The answer, however, is already available, and it doesn't require any drugs. Inflammation can be lowered through diet. In a study conducted at the University of Connecticut, investigators found that a low-carb, high-fat diet does an admirable job of lowering runaway inflammation. They showed that a high-fat diet (59 percent of calories from fat) greatly *reduces* inflammation and is much more effective than a low-fat diet (24 percent fat).[7]

The amount of fat people eat varies greatly around the world. Some people eat a lot while others consume relatively little. In many traditional diets, fat historically accounted for 60 to 80 percent of their total caloric intake (and the vast majority was saturated fat). Some Pacific island communities consumed up to 60 percent of their calories as fat, 50 percent of it saturated, mostly from coconut.[8] Although these people ate large amounts of fat, diseases such as heart disease, diabetes, dementia, and autism were completely unknown to them. Relatively isolated populations that still eat natural fats do not experience the degenerative diseases common in modern society.[9-10]

A QUICK COURSE IN FATS AND OILS
Fatty Acids and Triglycerides

The terms fat and oil are often used interchangeably. There is no real difference; however, fats are generally considered solid at room temperature while oils are liquid. Lard, for example, would be referred to as a fat, while liquid corn oil would be called an oil.

Fats and oils are composed of fat molecules known as fatty acids. Fatty acids are classified into three categories depending on their degree of saturation. There are saturated, monounsaturated, and polyunsaturated fatty acids. You hear these terms used all the time, but what makes a fat unsaturated? And what are saturated fats saturated with?

Fatty acids consist almost entirely of two elements—carbon (C) and hydrogen (H). The carbon atoms are hooked together like links in a long chain. Attached to each carbon atom are two hydrogen atoms. In a saturated fatty acid, each carbon atom is attached to two hydrogen atoms (see illustration below). In other words, it is "saturated" with or holding as many hydrogen atoms as it possibly can. Hydrogen atoms are always attached in pairs. If one pair of hydrogen atoms is missing, you would have a monounsaturated fatty acid. "Mono" indicates one pair of hydrogen atoms is missing, while "unsaturated" indicates the fatty acid is not fully saturated with hydrogen atoms. If two, three, or more pairs of hydrogen atoms are missing, you have a polyunsaturated fatty acid ("poly" means "more than one").

```
H H H H H H H H H H H H H H H H H O
| | | | | | | | | | | | | | | | | ‖
H-C-C-C-C-C-C-C-C-C-C-C-C-C-C-C-C-C-C-O-H      An 18 carbon chain
| | | | | | | | | | | | | | | | | |          saturated fatty acid.
H H H H H H H H H H H H H H H H H H
```

```
H H H H H H H H         H H H H H H H H O
| | | | | | | |         | | | | | | | | ‖
H-C-C-C-C-C-C-C-C-C-C-C=C-C-C-C-C-C-C-C-O-H      An 18 carbon chain
| | | | | | | | | | | | | | | | | |            monounsaturated
H H H H H H H H H H H H H H H H H H            fatty acid.
```

```
H H H H H         H         H H H H H H H H O
| | | | |         |         | | | | | | | | ‖
H-C-C-C-C-C-C=C-C-C-C=C-C-C-C-C-C-C-C-C-O-H      An 18 carbon chain
| | | | | | | | | | | | | | | | | |            polyunsaturated fatty
H H H H H H H H H H H H H H H H H H            acid.
```

The fatty acids in the oil you pour on your salad for dinner and that is found in the meat and vegetables you eat—in fact, even the fat in your own body—come in the form of *triglycerides*. A triglyceride is nothing more than three fatty acids joined together by a glycerol molecule. So you can have saturated triglycerides, monounsaturated triglycerides, or polyunsaturated triglycerides.

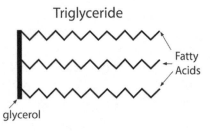

Triglyceride

Fatty Acids

glycerol

All vegetable oils and animal fats contain a mixture of saturated, monounsaturated, and polyunsaturated fatty acids. To say any particular oil is saturated or monounsaturated is a gross oversimplification. No oil is purely saturated or polyunsaturated. Olive oil is often called a "monounsaturated" oil because it is *predominantly* monounsaturated, but like all vegetable oils, it also contains some polyunsaturated and saturated fatty acids as well.

Generally, animal fats contain the highest amount of saturated fatty acids. Vegetable oils contain the highest amount of polyunsaturated fatty acids. Palm and coconut oils are exceptions; although they are vegetable oils, they contain a high amount of saturated fat.

Medium Chain Triglycerides

The different types of fatty acids can also be classified into three major categories depending on their size or, more precisely, the length of their carbon chains. There are long chain fatty acids (13 to 22 carbons), medium chain fatty acids (6 to 12 carbons), and short chain fatty acids (3 to 5 carbons). When a triglyceride is composed of three medium chain fatty acids, it is referred to as a medium chain triglyceride (MCT); likewise, long chain triglycerides (LCTs) are composed of long chain fatty acids and short chain triglycerides (SCTs) are made up of short chain fatty acids.

LCTs are by far the most plentiful in our diet, comprising 97 percent of the triglycerides we consume. MCTs make up most of the remaining 3 percent, and SCTs are very scarce. Fatty acids with chain lengths of 12 carbons or less are metabolized differently than those containing 14 or more. Consequently, many of the medium and short chain triglycerides are converted into ketone bodies, regardless of the amount of carbohydrate or glucose in the diet. LCTs are only converted into ketone bodies during severe glucose restriction, such as when fasting or eating a ketogenic diet.

Long-Chain Triglyceride

Medium-Chain Triglyceride

Most fats and oils are composed of 100 percent LCTs. There are very few dietary sources of MCTs. By far the richest natural source of MCTs comes from coconut oil, which consists of 63 percent medium triglycerides. The next largest source of MCTs comes from palm kernel oil, which consists of 53 percent. Butter is a distant third, containing only 12 percent medium and short chain fatty acids. Milk from all species of mammals, including humans, contains MCTs. Ketones produced from MCTs are essential for brain development in infants, supplying 25 percent of the brain's energy needs.

POLYUNSATURATED FATS
The Essential Fatty Acids

Polyunsaturated fats are found most abundantly in plants. Vegetable oils such as soybean oil, safflower oil, sunflower oil, cottonseed oil, corn oil, and flaxseed oil are composed predominantly of polyunsaturated fatty acids and, therefore, are commonly referred to as polyunsaturated oils.

Some fatty acids are classified as being essential. This means our bodies cannot make them from other nutrients, so we must have them in our diet in order to achieve and maintain good health. Our bodies can manufacture saturated and monounsaturated fats from other foods. However, we do not have the ability to manufacture

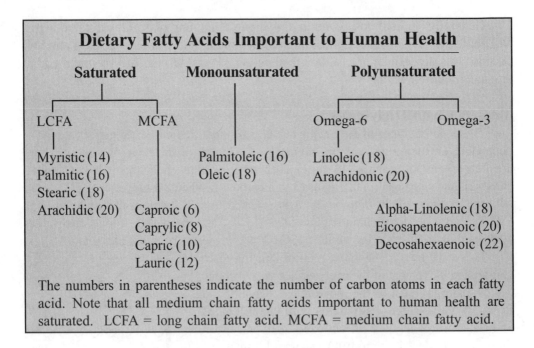

Dietary Fatty Acids Important to Human Health

Saturated   **Monounsaturated**   **Polyunsaturated**

LCFA   MCFA   Omega-6   Omega-3

Myristic (14)   Palmitoleic (16)   Linoleic (18)
Palmitic (16)   Oleic (18)   Arachidonic (20)
Stearic (18)
Arachidic (20)   Caproic (6)   Alpha-Linolenic (18)
                 Caprylic (8)   Eicosapentaenoic (20)
                 Capric (10)   Decosahexaenoic (22)
                 Lauric (12)

The numbers in parentheses indicate the number of carbon atoms in each fatty acid. Note that all medium chain fatty acids important to human health are saturated. LCFA = long chain fatty acid. MCFA = medium chain fatty acid.

polyunsaturated fats. Therefore, it is *essential* that polyunsaturated fats be included in our diet.

When we talk about saturated, monounsaturated, or polyunsaturated fats, we are not referring to just three types of fatty acids, but three families of fatty acids. There are many different types of saturated fatty acids as well as many different monounsaturated and polyunsaturated fatty acids. Two families of polyunsaturated fatty acids are important to human health: omega-6 and omega-3 polyunsaturated fatty acids. There are several omega-6 and omega-3 fatty acids. Two are considered essential because the body can use these two to make all of the rest—linoleic acid and alpha-linolenic acid. These are the essential fatty acids (EFAs) nutritionists often talk about. Linoleic acid belongs to the omega-6 family. Alpha-linolenic acid belongs to the omega-3 family.

If you eat an adequate source of linoleic acid, the body can make all the other omega-6 fatty acids it needs. Likewise, if you have an adequate source of alpha-linolenic acid, theoretically you can make all the other omega-3 fatty acids.

Nutritional studies indicate that we need about 3 percent of our total calories to come from EFAs. In a typical 2000 calorie diet, that is equivalent to about 7 grams, which isn't very much. A teaspoon holds 5 grams. So 1½ teaspoons or ½ tablespoon of EFAs will supply minimum daily needs.

Since these fatty acids are considered "essential," people often get the impression that they possess special health properties and that the more they eat the better. But this is not necessarily the case. While we must have some in our diet, too much can be detrimental. Researchers have found that the consumption of polyunsaturated oil, most notably omega-6 oils, exceeding just 10 percent of total calories can lead to blood disorders, suppressed immunity, cancer, liver damage, and vitamin deficiencies.[11]

Lipid Peroxidation

One of the reasons polyunsaturated fats have the potential to cause health problems is because they are highly vulnerable to oxidation. When polyunsaturated fats oxidize, they become toxic. Oxidized fats are rancid fats. Free radicals are a product of oxidation. Free radicals are highly reactive molecular entities that attack and damage other molecules.

When oxygen reacts normally with a compound, the compound becomes "oxidized." This process is called oxidation. Polyunsaturated fats readily oxidize in a process that biochemists call lipid peroxidation. "Lipid" is the term biochemists use to designate fat or oil, and "peroxidation" signifies an oxidation process involving unsaturated fats that produce peroxide free radicals.

When polyunsaturated oils are exposed to heat, light, or oxygen, they spontaneously oxidize and form destructive free radicals. Once they are formed, free radicals can attack unsaturated fats and proteins, causing them to become oxidized and generate more free radicals. It is a self-perpetuating process.

Liquid vegetable oils can be deceiving because they look and taste harmless even after they become rancid. The oil may not smell bad and may look as fresh as the day you bought it, yet be teaming with free radical terrorists.

When oil is extracted from seeds, the oxidation process is set in motion. The more the oil is exposed to heat, light, and oxygen, the more oxidized it becomes. By the time the oil is processed and bottled, it has already become oxidized to some extent. As it sits in the warehouse, the back of a truck, the grocery store, and your kitchen cabinet, it is continuing to oxidize. When you buy vegetable oil from the store, it has already gone rancid to some degree. In one study, various oils obtained off the shelf from local stores were tested for oxidation of the polyunsaturated fatty acids.[12] The researchers found that oxidation was already present in every sample tested. Those that had chemical preservatives added showed less oxidation than those preserved with vitamin E or other natural preservatives. When you use these oils in cooking, oxidation is greatly accelerated. This is why you should *never* cook foods using any polyunsaturated oil.

Oxidation occurs inside our bodies as well. Our only defense against free radicals is antioxidants. Antioxidants stop the chain reactions which create new free radicals. If we consume too much processed vegetable oil, the free radicals they create deplete antioxidant nutrients such as vitamins A, C, and E as well as zinc and selenium and can actually promote nutrient deficiencies.

Polyunsaturated fats are found in all of our cells to one degree or another. A polyunsaturated fatty acid in a cell membrane attacked by a free radical will oxidize and become a free radical itself, then attack a neighboring polyunsaturated molecule, likely in the same cell. The destructive chain reaction continues until the cell is severely crippled or utterly destroyed. Random free-radical reactions occurring throughout the body day after day, year after year take their toll.

Several studies have shown a relationship between processed vegetable oil consumption and damage to the central nervous system. In one study, for example, the effect of dietary oils on the mental ability of rats was determined by analyzing the animal's maze-learning abilities. Different oils were added to the rats' food. The study was initiated after rats had aged considerably, allowing enough time for the effects of the oils to become measurable. Rats were tested on the number of maze errors they made. The animals that performed the best and retained their mental capacities the longest were the ones fed saturated fats. The ones given polyunsaturated oils lost their mental abilities the most quickly.[13]

Age-related macular degeneration is the most common cause of blindness in the US, Canada, Australia, and most other affluent countries. The incidence of this condition has skyrocketed over the past 30 years. Several studies have shown that the primary culprit in causing this rise in macular degeneration is the increased consumption of unsaturated vegetable oils.[14-16]

Autistic children have been found to have higher blood levels of lipid peroxidation (oxidized polyunsaturated fats) than their non-autistic siblings. In fact, a striking correlation exists between excessive lipid peroxidation and the loss of previously acquired language skills in children with autism.[17]

Saturated fats are very resistant to oxidation. They do not form destructive free radicals. In fact, they act more like protective antioxidants because they prevent oxidation and the formation of free radicals. A diet high in protective saturated fats can help prevent lipid peroxidation that accelerates aging and promotes disease.

Polyunsaturated fatty acids are very easily oxidized. Saturated fatty acids are very resistant to oxidization. Monounsaturated fatty acids are in between. They are more stable than polyunsaturated fatty acids but less stable than saturated fatty acids.

Replacing polyunsaturated fats with saturated and monounsaturated fats in the diet can help reduce the risks associated with free radicals. Also, eating a diet rich in antioxidant nutrients such as vitamin E and beta-carotene will help protect the polyunsaturated fatty acids in the body from oxidation.

Heat Damaged Vegetable Oils

Most cooks recommend polyunsaturated vegetable oils in cooking and food preparation as a "healthy" alternative to saturated fats. Ironically, these unsaturated vegetable oils, when used in cooking, form a variety of toxic compounds that are far more damaging to health than any saturated fat could possibly be. Polyunsaturated vegetable oils are the *least* suitable for cooking.[18]

When vegetable oils are heated, these unstable polyunsaturated fatty acids are easily transformed into harmful compounds, including a particularly insidious compound known as 4-hydroxy-trans-2-nonenal (4-HNE). When you cook with polyunsaturated oils, your food is littered with these toxic substances. Cooking foods at high temperatures accelerates oxidation and harmful chemical reactions. Numerous studies, in some cases published as early as the 1930s, have reported the toxic effects of consuming heated vegetable oils.[12] However, even heating these oils at low temperatures causes damage to the delicate chemical structure of polyunsaturated fatty acids.

Over the past 20 years, an increasing number of studies have found links between 4-HNE and increased risk of heart disease, stroke, Parkinson's disease, Alzheimer's disease, Huntington's disease, liver problems, osteoarthritis, and cancer. Every time you use unsaturated vegetable oils for cooking or baking, you are creating 4-HNE.

One of the conditions linked to 4-HNE in heated vegetable oils is heart disease. This may come as a surprise to most people because polyunsaturated vegetable oils are supposed to be heart-friendly, yet recent studies show a clear link between 4-HNE and heart disease.[19-21] Studies also show that 4-HNE levels are high in the diseased regions of the brain in Alzheimer's patients.[22-23]

Studies show that diets containing heat-treated liquid vegetable oils produce more atherosclerosis (hardening of the arteries) than those containing unheated vegetable oil.[24] Any unsaturated vegetable oil can become toxic when heated. And even a small amount, especially if eaten frequently over time, will affect health. Oxidized oils have been found to induce damage to blood vessel walls and cause numerous organ lesions in animals.

The oils that are most vulnerable to the damage caused by heating are the ones that contain the highest amount of polyunsaturated fatty acids. Monounsaturated fatty acids are chemically more stable and can withstand higher temperatures, yet they too can oxidize and form toxic byproducts if heated to high temperatures. Saturated fatty acids are very heat stable and can withstand relatively high temperatures without oxidation. Therefore, saturated fats are the safest to use for day-to-day cooking and baking.

Studies show that we need some polyunsaturated fats in our diet, but if all commercial polyunsaturated vegetable oils are rancid to some degree before we even purchase them, and if they become more harmful to health when used in cooking, how are we going to get our daily requirement of essential fatty acids? The answer is simple. You can get your EFA requirement just as your ancestors did—from foods! You do not need to eat processed vegetable oils to satisfy your daily EFA requirements. You can get all your EFAs from food. This is by far the best way to get them because while they are still packaged in their original cellular containers, they are shielded from the damaging effects of oxygen and protected by naturally occurring antioxidants that keep them fresh.

Omega-6 essential polyunsaturated fatty acids are found in almost all plant and animal foods—meat, eggs, nuts, grains, legumes, and vegetables. Omega-6 fatty acids are so abundant in the diet that a deficiency isn't likely to happen. Less common are the omega-3 polyunsaturated fatty acids found in seeds, leafy green vegetables, seaweed, eggs, fish, and shellfish. You can get all the omega-3 fatty acids you need by making sure you include some fish, eggs, and leafy greens as a part of your weekly menu. Grass-fed beef and game meats also supply omega-3 fatty acids. Cattle that graze on grass, which is rich in omega-3s, incorporate these fats into their own tissues. Grain-fed beef, however, is a poor source of omega-3 fatty acids.

Hydrogenated Vegetable Oils

Many packaged foods are made using hydrogenated or partially hydrogenated vegetable oil. These are among the most health-damaging fats you can possibly eat—just as bad, if not worse, than oxidized polyunsaturated fats.

Hydrogenated oils are made by bombarding liquid vegetable oil with hydrogen atoms in the presence of a metal catalyst. In the process, polyunsaturated vegetable oils become saturated with hydrogen. This makes the liquid oil transform into a more hardened or solid fat. In the process of hydrogenation, however, a new type of fatty acid known as a *trans fatty acid* is created. Trans fatty acids are artificial manmade fats. This toxic fatty acid is foreign to our bodies and can create all sorts of trouble.

"These are probably the most toxic fats ever known," says Walter Willett, MD, professor of epidemiology and nutrition at Harvard School of Public Health.[25] Studies show that trans fatty acids can contribute to atherosclerosis (hardening of the arteries) and heart disease. Trans fatty acids increase blood LDL (bad cholesterol) and lower the HDL (good cholesterol), both regarded to be undesirable changes.[26] Researchers now believe it has a greater influence on the risk of cardiovascular disease than any other dietary fat.[27]

Trans fatty acids affect more than just our cardiovascular health. They have been linked with a variety of adverse health effects, which include cancer, multiple sclerosis, diverticulitis, diabetes, and other degenerative conditions.[28] Trans fatty acids disrupt brain communication. Studies show that the trans fatty acids we eat get incorporated into brain cell membranes, including the myelin sheath that insulates neurons. Trans fatty acids alter the electrical activity of brain cells, causing cellular degeneration and diminished mental performance.[29]

Under pressure from many health organizations and the public, the United States FDA proposed a regulation requiring food manufacturers to include the amount of trans fatty acids on the package labels. Before taking such a step, however, they waited three years for scientists at the Institute of Medicine to study the issue.

After the study was completed, the Institute of Medicine issued a statement declaring that no level of trans fatty acid consumption was safe. What surprised everyone was that the Institute of Medicine didn't give a recommendation as to what percentage of trans fats was safe to consume, as is often done with food additives, but flatly stated that *no level* of trans fats is safe. If you see a packaged food that contains hydrogenated oil, margarine, or shortening, don't touch it! If you eat out, ask the restaurant manager what type of oil they use to cook their food. If they say "vegetable oil," it almost definitely is hydrogenated vegetable oil: avoid it. The reason you can safely count on it being hydrogenated vegetable oil is because regular vegetable oil breaks down too quickly and becomes rancid. Restaurants like to reuse their oils as long as possible before they have to be tossed out. Ordinary vegetable oils have too short a life span.

Many of the foods you buy in the store and in restaurants are prepared with or cooked in hydrogenated oil. Fried foods sold in grocery stores and restaurants are usually cooked in hydrogenated oil because it makes foods crispy and is more resistant to spoilage than ordinary vegetable oils. Many frozen processed foods are cooked or prepared in hydrogenated oils. Hydrogenated oils are used in making French fries, biscuits, cookies, crackers, chips, frozen pies, pizzas, peanut butter, cake frosting, and ice cream, especially soft serve ice cream.

SATURATED FAT
Saturated Fat Is a Vital Nutrient

Probably no food component in history has been as misunderstood and maligned as saturated fat. It is labeled the cause of nearly every health problem of modern civilization. If it really is as dangerous as they say, it's truly a miracle how our ancestors survived for thousands of years eating a diet dominated by saturated fat. Animal fats, butter, palm oil, and coconut oil were the most common fats used throughout history. These fats are easy to produce using the simplest of tools. Vegetable oils from seeds such as soybeans, cottonseed, safflower seeds, and such are very difficult to extract. Consequently, polyunsaturated vegetable oils were not used much until after the invention of hydraulic oil presses near the end of the 19th century. Interestingly enough, when people ate primarily saturated fats, the so-called diseases of modern civilization—heart disease, diabetes, and the like—were uncommon. As we've replaced saturated fats with unsaturated oils, these diseases have come upon us like a plague. From a historical point of view it is easy to see that saturated fats don't cause these diseases.

The truth of the matter is that saturated fat is a vital nutrient. Yes, saturated fat is a nutrient, *not* a poison. It is necessary in order to obtain and maintain good health. Saturated fat serves as an important source of energy for the body and aids in the absorption of vitamins and minerals. As a food ingredient, fat helps us feel full and provides taste, consistency, and stability. Saturated fat is necessary for proper growth, repair, and maintenance of body tissues. It is essential for good lung function. It is the preferred source of energy for the heart muscle and also helps protect the unsaturated fats in your body against the destructive action of free radicals.

We hear a lot about the importance of the essential fatty acids. Because they are called "essential," we get the mistaken belief that they are the most important fats. However, the reason they are "essential" is because they are the *least* important of the fats. Believe it or not, saturated fat is far more important to your health than the EFAs! Let me explain why.

Saturated fat is so necessary to your health that our bodies have been programmed to make it out of other nutrients. Getting an adequate amount of saturated fat is so important to our health that it is not left to chance. The consequences of a saturated fat deficiency are so serious that the body is capable of manufacturing its own. The EFAs (polyunsaturated fats), on the other hand, are far less important to our health, so the body has not developed a means of manufacturing its own. It relies totally on what is in the diet.

The foods that we eat provide the building blocks for our cells and tissues. This is true for the fats we consume as well. The fat in our bodies consists of 45 percent saturated, 50 percent monounsaturated, and only 5 percent polyunsaturated fat. That's right. Only 5 percent of the fat in your body is polyunsaturated. Consequently, the body's need for polyunsaturated fat or EFAs is very small. Your body needs nearly 10 times as much saturated fat, as well as monounsaturated fat, as it does EFAs. So which is more essential?

While the body can manufacture saturated and monounsaturated fats, it cannot make enough on its own for optimal health. We still need them in our diet to avoid nutritional deficiencies.[30-31]

Saturated Fat Does Not Promote Heart Disease

Reducing dietary saturated fat has generally been thought to improve cardiovascular health and protect against heart attacks and strokes. This assumption is based on the belief that dietary saturated fat increases blood cholesterol, thus increasing risk of cardiovascular disease. However, even if saturated fat did raise total cholesterol, it would not increase heart disease risk. There has been debate on this issue in the medical community for decades. A recent meta-analysis study published in the *American Journal of Clinical Nutrition* now has conclusively proven that saturated fats are not harmful and do not promote heart disease.[32]

Over the years, many studies have sought to prove the lipid hypothesis of heart disease—that diets high in saturated fat and cholesterol promote heart disease. Results have been mixed. Some seemed to support it, while others did not. However, the majority of the medical community, along with the pharmaceutical industry (which profits greatly from the saturated fat-heart disease idea) supports the theory. Those studies that support the theory receive national press and are used as justification to establish government policies on health, while those that do not support the theory are generally ignored.

The evidence in favor of the lipid hypothesis is no greater than the evidence that contradicts it. In fact, there is a substantial amount of evidence that challenges the hypothesis. The number of studies for or against is not the major issue; some of the studies have used relatively few participants, while others have used much larger numbers. Obviously, the results of a study involving 50,000 test subjects carries more weight than one involving only 1,000. One large study using 50,000 participants produces more reliable results than 10 small studies with a total combined number of 10,000 participants. So the total number of studies is not as important as the number of people *in* the studies. If *all* the subjects in these many different studies were combined and evaluated equally, what would the final outcome be? Would it prove the lipid hypothesis or disprove it?

Researchers at the Children's Hospital Oakland Research Institute in California and Harvard School of Public Health got together to find out. They analyzed all the previous studies with data for dietary saturated fat intakes and risk of cardiovascular disease. The studies also had to be reliable and of high quality. The investigators identified twenty-one studies that fit their criteria. This meta-analysis included data on nearly 350,000 subjects. With such a large subject database, the results would be far more reliable than a study consisting of only 10,000 or even 100,000 subjects. The focus of the research was to determine if there was sufficient evidence linking saturated fat consumption to cardiovascular disease. Their results said "no." Intake of saturated fat was not associated with any increased risk of cardiovascular disease. Those people who ate the greatest amount of saturated fat where no more likely to suffer a heart attack or stroke than those who ate the least. It didn't matter how much saturated fat one ate, the incidence of heart disease was not affected. This study demonstrates that the combined data from all available studies in the medical literature disprove the lipid hypothesis.

This recent study is not likely to change policies and recommendations about eating saturated fat any time soon. Doctors have been warning us about the dangers of eating saturated fat for so many years that it is thoroughly ingrained into their minds, and they are likely to continue giving this outdated advice despite facts to the contrary. In other words, many health professionals will continue to ignore these studies and try to convince you to accept their opinions based on nothing more than a longstanding prejudice against saturated fat. The bottom line here is that you do not need to fear eating saturated fat or cholesterol even when you hear criticism about it in the media or from your own doctor.

A Word of Caution

In the world of scientific investigation there is often a difference of opinion. Consequently, studies are frequently published that contradict one another. We see this in the newspaper and on the Internet all the time. The media is constantly reporting new studies that show results contrary to previous studies.

The outcome of many studies is influenced by personal bias of the investigators or by the corporation funding the study. This is plainly evident in the investigation of fats and oils. Numerous researchers and their funding institutions (pharmaceutical, supplement, and weight loss industries, as well as others) have a bias against fat and especially saturated fat. Their studies often reflect this bias and perpetuate common myths. One of these myths is that saturated fat and cholesterol promote heart disease.

There have been a number of animal studies published that implicate saturated fat as a contributing factor in heart disease. When one of these studies is published, news reporters and anti-fat proponents immediately jump on it, writing blaring articles about the dangers of eating saturated fat and cholesterol, reinforcing the fat-heart disease myth. What most people do not understand, and for that matter neither do the reporters or anti-fat proponents, is that these studies are scientifically meaningless. The studies are purposely designed to give these results.

In many of these studies, the researchers combine relatively high amounts of saturated fat with cholesterol and mix it in the rats' food. After a period of time, these rats are compared to a group of rats that were fed normal rat chow. What they find is that within weeks the fat/cholesterol fed rats start developing arterial lesions that are commonly associated with heart disease. Such studies appear to suggest that saturated fat is the cause of heart disease.

However, that is not the case. When people eat the most heart-damaging foods around, they do not develop clogged arteries in just a few weeks like the animals in these experiments do. Atherosclerosis is a lifelong process that takes decades to develop. This should tell you that something is wrong with the diet that is fed to the rats and that it does not match what happens in real life.

What is wrong in these studies is the cholesterol. The cholesterol used in these studies comes in powder form. The cholesterol powder is dissolved in fat and then added to the rat chow. The problem here is that powdered cholesterol is not ordinary cholesterol. It is not the same as the cholesterol in most of your foods or in your body. When the cholesterol is "dried," it becomes fully oxidized. Oxidized cholesterol is highly toxic, just like oxidized polyunsaturated fats are. Oxidized cholesterol damages artery walls, promoting atherosclerosis; normal cholesterol does not.

It is the oxidized cholesterol that is used in these studies that causes the damage to the rats' arteries. When oxidized cholesterol is added to *any* type of fat, be it saturated or unsaturated, it causes arterial lesions. If the investigators combined oxidized cholesterol with soybean oil or corn oil the outcome would be the same: the rats would all develop lesions. However, the conclusions the authors of these types of studies come to is that it is the saturated fat that is the culprit.

In other studies, saturated fat is combined with high amounts of sugar and then added to the rat chow. When the rats develop insulin resistance or some other problem they blame it on the saturated fat and conveniently ignore the added sugar!

A little common sense will tell you these studies are deceptive. Ketogenic diets that consist of 90 percent fat, mostly saturated fat, have been used successfully for nearly a century without causing heart attacks or strokes. In fact, contrary to the rat studies, they improve health. Likewise, many populations around the world who eat traditional diets consisting of 60-80 percent fat, again mostly saturated fat, do not experience increased rates of heart disease.

In contrast, the rats in these studies are given only about 20 percent fat, nothing near the 90 percent of the ketogenic diet, yet in a few weeks they were developing atherosclerotic lesions and memory impairment. Obviously, something is wrong with the fat they fed the rats, and that something is the oxidized cholesterol. So when you see studies reported in the news or when people tell you of some study that shows that high-fat diets or saturated fat promotes heart disease, don't believe it!

Now that you are aware of the trouble oxidized cholesterol causes, you might be wondering if there are sources of this type of cholesterol in our diet. The answer is yes! Cholesterol is not found in plants, so you don't have to worry about getting any from plant-based foods. Cholesterol comes only in animal foods like meat, dairy and eggs. When animal products are dehydrated or powdered, the cholesterol in them becomes oxidized. Examples of these types of products include powdered whole milk, powdered infant formula, dried grated cheese, and powdered eggs and butter. Right now you may be saying to yourself, "Well, I don't eat powdered foods." Well, think again. Powdered products are used in the ingredients of many processed foods sold at your local grocery store, the most obvious being prepared cake, pancake, and muffin mixes. They may also be found in some salad dressing, gravy, and sauce mixes. If the ingredient label lists eggs, milk, buttermilk, sour cream, or butter, you know for sure it means *powdered* eggs, milk, buttermilk, sour cream, or butter, otherwise the product wouldn't be in a *dry* mix. Even non-fat powered milk contains oxidized cholesterol. When fat is removed from non-fat and reduced-fat milks they become relatively tasteless and watery. To improve their taste and color, powdered milk is added back into them. Most soft ice cream served in restaurants, particularly fast food restaurants, is made from a powdered mix. Sometimes the label on foods will identify a powdered ingredient, but not always. Products such as frozen pizza, TV dinners, cookies, bread, and the like could include powdered ingredients without specifying it on the label. This is a good reason to make your own meals at home rather than rely on prepared packaged foods.

Although vegetable oils do not contain cholesterol, if they are oxidized they become toxic. If an oil is powdered or dehydrated, it is oxidized and should never be eaten. This includes powdered shortening, powdered fish oil, powdered coconut oil, and powdered MCT oil. Powdered oils are often found in dietary supplements and protein shake mixes.

10 | The Ultimate Brain Food

COCONUT OIL: THE ULTIMATE BRAIN FOOD

If any food could be labeled as "Brain Food," it would have to be coconut oil. The MCTs in coconut oil are converted into ketones, which act as high-potency fuel for the brain. This superfuel bypasses the glucose metabolic pathway to overcome defects in glucose metabolism. In doing so, it boosts energy output, normalizes brain function, stops erratic signal transmission that leads to seizures, improves cognition and memory, improves motor function, and supplies building blocks for the repair, maintenance, and growth of new brain tissue. Ketones reduce the brain's need for oxygen, protecting it from injury caused by physical trauma, asphyxiation, or other causes. Ketones have proven useful in stopping the progression of neurodegenerative diseases and even reversing the symptoms.

Coconut MCTs are also converted into MCFAs, which provide additional brain support. Unlike long chain fatty acids, MCFAs can pass through the blood-brain barrier. They provide the brain with a third source of energy. Although not as potent as ketones, MCFAs still provide more energy than glucose and are preferred over glucose by brain cells as a fuel. The energy-producing, antioxidant, anti-inflammatory, antimicrobial, and antitoxic properties of MCFAs protect the brain from a variety of insults.

MCTs are absolutely *essential* for the growth and development of the fetal and newborn brain. From what researchers have been discovering in recent years, they are also of great value in maintaining healthy brain function and protecting against neurological disorders.

THE IMPORTANCE OF KETONES
FOR BRAIN GROWTH AND DEVELOPMENT
Building Blocks for the Brain

In adults, ketones are used mostly to fuel brain cells along with maintenance and repair. In young children they are essential for growing new brain tissue. The lipids that make up the majority of brain tissues are constructed from ketones. During pregnancy, a woman's ketone production increases sharply in order to supply the energy and building blocks required for her developing child's brain.[1] Even when her blood glucose levels are normal, ketone production is elevated. The fetus doesn't rely solely on its mother's ketones but produces them itself as well. After birth, the infant's blood ketone levels remain elevated as the brain continues to grow and develop.

Ketones are most critical during the third trimester of pregnancy and for the first several months of life.[2] This is the time of most rapid brain growth. An infant's brain increases in weight from 350 g (about 12 oz) at birth, to about 800 g (just over 28 oz) during the first year of life. By age two, another 400 g is added, giving it a total weight of 1,200 g. That's almost two pounds of brain in as many years! From this point on the brain increases in weight by only 200 g, so that by adulthood the brain weighs about 1,400 g. During this period of rapid growth ketones are essential for building brain mass.

After birth, the infant no longer receives ketones directly from its mother. The mother's milk, however, is enriched with medium chain triglycerides, which are readily converted into ketones by the infant's liver. In the first few weeks of life, ketones provide about 25 percent of the energy newborn babies need to survive. As long as the child is nursing and receiving MCTs, ketones are continually produced. When nursing is discontinued, there usually is no other natural source of MCTs in the baby's diet so ketone production declines dramatically. This can have a significant impact on brain growth and development. This is one of the reasons why mothers are encouraged to continue nursing for at least 12 months and up to two years. This is also one of the reasons why coconut oil, a natural source of MCTs, is added to infant formulas.

Ketones Are Neuroprotective

Ketones not only provide the brain with energy and building materials, but also protect it from harm to assure proper development. When glucose is used for fuel, it produces free radicals as a byproduct of energy production. When ketones are used for fuel, not only is energy production enhanced but free-radical production is greatly reduced, thus significantly reducing the oxidative stress in the brain and preserving protective antioxidants.[3]

The brain requires more oxygen than any other organ in the body. The adult human brain uses approximately 20 percent of all the oxygen the body consumes. Since a child's brain in comparison to its body is proportionately much larger than an adult's, the child's brain uses up to 40 to 50 percent of the available oxygen. Because of the brain's high demand for oxygen, any interruption in its delivery can have dire consequences. Without oxygen, brain cells begin to die within minutes. Such a situation is often encountered at the time of birth, before the newborn takes its first breath.

Interfering with the normal blood flow and delivery of oxygen to the brain is one of the most prominent causes of brain damage. Asphyxiation during birth is one cause of cerebral palsy. Ketones reduce the brain's need for oxygen, providing some degree of protection in incidences where oxygen delivery is interrupted.

Ketosis can alleviate much of the damage caused by virtually any condition where oxygen supply to cells may be diminished. This list would encompass almost every disease state.[4] Strokes are caused by the blockage of oxygen-carrying blood to the brain. They can cause movement, speech, and memory defects, paralysis, and death. These symptoms are all the result of brain cell death caused by a lack of oxygen. Studies show that ketones can alleviate these effects and speed recovery.[5]

Many toxic chemicals interfere with oxygen utilization. Ketones have been shown to preserve brain cell viability when exposed to certain neurotoxins. For example, Parkinson's disease is a neuromuscular disorder caused by the destruction of dopamine-producing cells in the brain. Researchers can induce Parkinson's in lab animals by giving them neurotoxic drugs. Ketones, however, completely block the damaging effects of these drugs while maintaining normal metabolism.[6]

The effect of ketone bodies in limiting the damage caused by oxygen deficiency has been extensively reported in animal studies.[7] For example, neonatal rats subjected to severe oxygen deprivation for three hours experienced severe brain damage. However, when ketosis was induced in neonatal rats subjected to the same conditions, their brains suffered little or no harm.[8] Even the heart, lungs, and other organs are protected when the fetus is in a state of ketosis.

Ketones also activate special protective proteins known as brain derived neurotrophic factors (BDNFs). BDNFs exert survival-promoting and nourishing actions on brain cells and play a crucial role in brain cell function and survival. They regulate protein synthesis and neuron growth as well as influencing neurons' ability to make the neurotransmitters which allow the cells to communicate with each other. BDNFs also have a calming effect on inflammation and can help reduce chronic inflammation which is a common feature in autism and other neurological disorders.

Protection Against Environmental Toxins
Environmental toxins can have a profound effect on the initiation and progression of neurological disorders. Everyone is exposed to chemical toxins to some degree. According to a study by the US Centers for Disease Control and Prevention (CDC), Americans carry in their bodies dozens of pesticides and toxic compounds used in consumer products, many of which are linked to potential health threats. These chemicals include pyrethroids that are ingredients of virtually every household pesticide and phthalates found in nail polish and other beauty products as well as in soft plastics.

The CDC study looked for 148 toxic compounds in the urine and blood of about 2,400 people. The discovery of more than 100 chemicals in human bodies is of great concern because we don't know what effect they can have on health. Evidence suggests that the rise in autism, Alzheimer's, cancer, and other health conditions over the past several decades may be due, in part, to the accumulation of these chemicals in our bodies.

However, removing pesticides, drain cleaners, plastic bottles, and other items isn't going to happen anytime soon. The best solution to the problem is to remove the toxins from our bodies. Certain foods have detoxifying effects that can absorb or neutralize the effects of environmental chemicals in our bodies. Simply adding these detoxifying foods to the diet can help eliminate many of the toxins we are exposed to each day. Coconut oil is of particular interest because it has been shown to be highly effective in nullifying the toxic effects a variety of chemicals, many of which are dangerous neurotoxins.

An interesting case report published in the journal *Human and Experimental Toxicology* revealed the effectiveness of coconut oil in neutralizing aluminum phosphide, a poison used in rodent control. The article recounted an incident involving a 28-year-old man who ingested a lethal amount of the chemical in an attempt to commit suicide. There is no known antidote for aluminum phosphide poisoning. Doctors had little hope of saving him. He was given the standard treatment for acute poisoning with no hope of recovery. Seeing the futility of their efforts, one of the attending physicians decided to add coconut oil the patient's treatment. To the surprise of the medical staff, the patient survived. As a result of the success, the authors recommend that coconut oil be added to the standard treatment protocol of all cases of acute aluminum phosphide poisoning.[9]

Using coconut oil to help nullify the effects of a poison is not as strange as it may sound. Researchers have known for some time about the detoxifying properties of coconut oil. Numerous animal studies have shown that coconut oil blocks the deleterious action of a number of chemical toxins. While the exact mechanisms involved are not fully understood, part of the reason for coconut oil's protective effects can be attributed to its antioxidant, anti-inflammatory, and immune-boosting properties, as well as its ability to improve oxygen circulation and utilization.

Many toxins, especially neurotoxins that attack nerve and brain tissues, are dangerous because they interfere with or block oxygen transport to the cells. Nerve cells are especially sensitive to oxygen deprivation. Without oxygen the cells suffocate and die. Much of the protection provided by coconut oil is no doubt derived from the ketones produced from the MCTs. Ketones increase blood flow to the brain by 39 percent, improving circulation and oxygen delivery. Ketones also make it possible for nerve, brain, and other cells to maintain normal energy production and function while consuming 25 percent less oxygen. Thus brain cells and other tissues are able to survive in an oxygen-starved environment long enough to allow the body time to detoxify and remove the poisons.

In addition, MCTs themselves improve oxygen circulation and delivery by stimulating the production of red blood cells in the bone marrow. Red blood cells carry oxygen throughout the body. With more red blood cells in circulation, more oxygen is delivered to the tissues. Toxins that interfere with oxygen utilization and transport are, therefore, rendered impotent or at least less harmful because of the increased oxygen availability. For these reasons, MCTs are being investigated as a means to aid cancer patients and to block the detrimental side effects of chemotherapy drugs.[10-11] MCTs don't necessarily interfere with the therapeutic action of the drug, but can reduce or eliminate the toxic side effects.

Studies show that coconut oil or MCTs can protect animals from a variety of carcinogenic chemicals.[12-14] Dr. C. Lim-Sylianco and colleagues demonstrated coconut oil's antimutagenic effects against six potent mutacarcinogens—benzpyrene, azaserine, dimethylhydrazine, dimethynitrosamine, methylmethanesulfonate, and tetracycline. Administration of coconut oil either in bolus form or as part of the diet protected the animals from the toxic effect of all six mutagens. Fertility tests were also performed and coconut oil was shown to protect fertilized female mice against the sterilizing and abortifacient effects of the carcinogens. Dr. Lim-Sylianco reported that coconut oil was "strongly protective" against all six chemicals.[15-16]

Aflatoxin is a very potent carcinogen that comes from a fungus that often infests grains, especially corn. In Asia and Africa, aflatoxin is a serious problem. Corn has been found to be the most aflatoxin-contaminated food eaten in the Philippines. In certain areas of that country corn consumption is high, and a correlation exists between the incidence of liver cancer caused by aflatoxin and the amount of corn consumed. Those people who eat the most corn also have the highest rates of liver cancer. Coconut oil consumption appears to protect the liver from the cancer-causing effect of aflatoxin. The population of Bicol, in the Philippines, has an unusually high intake of aflatoxin-infested corn, yet they have a low incidence of liver cancer. The reason for the low cancer rate is believed to be due to the high coconut consumption in the area.[17]

Studies have shown that the harmful effects of exotoxins and endotoxins—the poisons produced by bacteria that cause illness—can also be neutralized or reduced by the use of coconut oil and its monoglycerides. Monoglycerides of coconut oil are individual MCFAs that are attached to a glycerol molecule. They function much like MCFAs and possess the same antimicrobial and antitoxic properties. Monoglycerides are commonly used in the food and cosmetic industry to inhibit the production of exotoxins produced by streptococci and staphylococci.[18-19]

Both monoglycerides and MCFAs mitigate the effects of these poisons inside the body. For example, in one study guinea pigs were separated into two groups. One group was given a mixture of MCTs and fish oil in their diet. The other group received safflower oil. After 6 weeks on this diet the animals were injected with an endotoxin. The group fed safflower oil developed severe metabolic and respiratory shock. The group that received MCTs showed only mild symptoms.[20]

In another study, the protective effect of coconut oil was tested on E. coli endotoxin shock in rats.[21] A total of 180 rats were used in the study. The animals were separated into three equal groups. The first group was given coconut oil at 5 percent of daily calories in their diet, the second group 20 percent, and the third received no coconut oil and served as the control. After one month on the diet the mice were given a dose of E. coli endotoxin via oral tube. The number of survivors was monitored at intervals of up to 96 hours. The results showed that rats in the control group had only a 48 percent survival rate. Those given coconut oil at 5 percent and 20 percent of total calories had survival rates of 77 percent and 72 percent, respectively. Both coconut oil fed groups had about the same level of survival. This indicated that even a small amount of coconut oil (5 percent of calories) offered the same amount of protection against E coli endotoxin as a larger amount (20 percent of calories). In humans consuming a typical 2,000-calorie diet, 5 percent of calories would equate to about 1 tablespoon of coconut oil.

Glutamic acid, a potential neurotoxin that affects the function of the brain and nerves, is tempered by monoglycerides from coconut oil.[40] Glutamic acid is the primary component of monosodium glutamate (MSG), a common food additive. In animals, glutamic acid causes brain lesions and neuroendocrine disorders. It can do

Toxins Mitigated by Coconut Oil or MCFAs/Ketones

Coconut oil or MCFAs/ketones can prevent or reduce the toxic effects of many chemicals including the following:

Acrylamide	Aflatoxin (mycotoxin)
Aluminum phosphide (rodent poison)	Arsenic
Azaserine	Azoxymethane
Azo dyes	Benzpyrene
Botulinum toxin (endotoxin)	Carbon disulfide
Carbon monoxide (air pollutant)	Chemotherapy drugs
Dimethylbenzanthracene	Dimethylhydrazine
Dimethynitrosamine	E. coli endotoxin
Ethanol	Ethylene glycol (antifreeze)
Fluoroacetate (rodent poison)	Glutamic acid/MSG
Hydrogen cyanide	Hydrogen sulfide
Methanol	Methylmethanesulfonate
N-nitrosomethylurea	Organophosphate insecticides
Paracetamol	Streptococci endotoxin/exotoxin
Sodium nitrate (food preservative)	Staphylococci endotoxin/exotoxin
Tetracycline (antibiotic)	Trimethyltin

2,4,6-trinitrobenzenesulphonic acid (TNBS)
1-methyl-4-phenyl-1,2,3,6-tetrahydropyridine (a synthetic opioid neurotoxic drug)

the same in humans. Some of the symptoms associated with it include seizures, stroke, and heart irregularities.

Many environmental toxins can adversely affect the brain. The antitoxic effects of coconut oil provide another reason for adding it into the diet.

We come into contact with brain-damaging neurotoxins all the time. When exposure is frequent or intense, it can cause brain damage. Exposure is usually subtle and unnoticeable, like pesticides blowing in from nearby farms or preservatives and flavor enhancers added to foods. Their effects are usually not immediately noticeable but that doesn't mean they are harmless. During pregnancy the unborn baby is much more vulnerable than the mother. The mother may have no symptoms from neurotoxin exposure, yet the baby may be harmed. Young children are also much more sensitive to toxins than are adults.

Exposure to these chemicals can cause an immune reaction that triggers microglia activation. Repeated exposure, along with other assaults from vaccines, infections, and such, can keep microglia chronically activated, seriously interfering with normal brain development. Coconut oil offers a means by which these brain-destroying toxins can be nullified. If the mother consumes coconut oil regularly when pregnant and nursing, she is providing her child a degree of protection against unseen environmental and industrial toxins that could otherwise interfere with normal brain development and perhaps cause autism.

MEDIUM CHAIN TRIGLYCERIDES:
ESSENTIAL FOR INFANTS AND YOUNG CHILDREN
Digestion and Nutrient Absorption

Not only do our bodies need good nutrition to be healthy, but our brains do too. Studies show that poor nutrition in the first few years of life leads to lower IQ as well as antisocial and aggressive behaviors.[22] Intellectual performance declines with the severity of malnutrition. Even moderate malnutrition affects memory, verbal reasoning, comprehension, visual perception, and visual motor integration.[23] Malnutrition can occur due to a lack of food (total calories) or to a deficiency in essential nutrients—protein, fat (including MCTs), minerals, and vitamins. A diet of poor quality foods can provide ample calories but still be nutritionally deficient. Such a diet can be deceiving because a child can be normal weight or even overweight, yet still suffer from malnutrition due to a vitamin or mineral deficiency.

For a child's brain to reach its full genetic potential it needs good nutrition. Some children have difficulty absorbing the nutrients in their foods due to various malabsorption problems. For example, most premature infants have difficulty digesting foods because their digestive tract is still immature, while other infants may have trouble digesting particular types of foods such as fats or proteins. Often parents are unaware that such problems exist and don't understand why their children are undersized, fail to thrive, or display developmental delays. If the problem is severe it is likely to be diagnosed early on. If the problem is less pronounced, it may never be identified. If the child is autistic, malnutrition can compound the problem. Coconut oil can help.

MCTs from coconut oil provide many other benefits beyond their ability to produce ketones. MCTs are included in hospital infant formulas to serve as a primary source of energy for premature infants. They are used in feeding formulas given to patients recovering from surgery and those with malnutrition and absorption problems.[24] They are even used by athletes to improve performance and endurance and by dieters to control appetite and stimulate fat burning.

One of the advantages of MCTs over the more common LCTs is their speed and efficiency in digestion. LCTs require pancreatic digestive enzymes and bile in order to break down into individual fatty acids. MCTs, on the other hand, break down so quickly that they do not need pancreatic digestive enzymes or bile, thus reducing stress and conserving the body's enzymes. The digestive systems of young infants are still maturing and LCTs put a great deal of strain on their bodies. LCTs are often incompletely digested and, therefore, do not provide their full nutritional potential. Not so with MCTs. Consequently, MCTs provide a superior source of energy and nutrition to infants than do LCTs.

The difference in the way MCTs are digested is of great interest in medicine because it provides a means by which a number of medical conditions can be successfully treated. Replacing a portion of the LCTs normally found in the diet with MCTs has allowed doctors to successfully treat a variety of malabsorption syndromes in children including defects in fat digestion and absorption, pancreatic insufficiency, liver and gallbladder disorders, defects in protein metabolism, cystic fibrosis, and celiac disease.[25-31] MCTs can even speed recovery after intestinal surgery.[32]

Because MCTs are digested so efficiently, they also improve the absorption of other nutrients. As far back as the 1930s researchers noticed that adding coconut oil to foods enhanced the food's nutritional value. While all fats can increase the bioavailability of the nutrients in foods, coconut oil appears to be the most efficient in this respect. For example, researchers at Auburn University studied the effects of vitamin B_1 deficiency in animals given different types of fats. Vitamin B_1 deficiency leads to a fatal disease called beriberi. The fats and oils evaluated included coconut oil, olive oil, butter, beef fat, linseed (flaxseed) oil, cottonseed oil, and several others. When rats were given a vitamin B deficient diet, coconut oil was by far the most efficient in preventing the disease and extending lifespan. In fact, those receiving coconut oil actually gained weight, indicating continued growth even though the diet was nutritionally poor.[33] None of the oils tested, including coconut oil, contained vitamin B_1. So how did coconut oil prevent a vitamin B_1 deficiency? Coconut oil made what little of the vitamin that was in the diet more biologically available, thus preventing the deficiency disease.

A number of studies have found similar effects. Coconut oil improves the absorption of not only the B vitamins but also vitamins A, D, E, K, beta-carotene, lycopene, CoQ10, and other fat soluble nutrients, minerals such as calcium, magnesium, and some amino acids—the building blocks for protein.[31]

What this means is that if you add coconut oil to a meal, you will get significantly more vitamins, minerals, and other nutrients out of the food than if you used any other oil or no oil at all. Simply adding coconut oil to a meal greatly enhances the food's nutritional value.

This fact has led researchers to investigate its use in the treatment of malnutrition. For example, coconut oil, mixed with a little corn oil, was compared with soybean oil for the treatment of malnourished preschool-aged children in the Philippines. The study involved 95 children from a slum area in Manila aged 10-44 months who were 1st to 3rd degree malnourished. The children were given one full midday meal and one afternoon snack daily except Sundays for 16 weeks. The food fed to the children was identical in every respect except for the oil. Approximately two-thirds of the oil in their diet came from either the coconut oil/corn oil mix or soybean oil. The children were allocated to one of the two diets at random: 47 children received the coconut oil diet and 48 children the soybean oil diet. The children were weighed every two weeks and examined by a

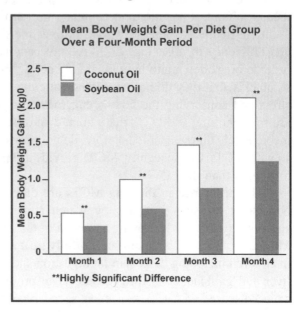

pediatrician once a week. At the start of the study the ages, initial weight, and degree of malnutrition of the two groups as a whole were essentially identical.

After 16 weeks, results showed that the coconut oil diet produced significantly faster weight gain and improvement in nutritional status compared to the soybean oil diet. The weight gain was not due to simply fat accumulation, but to growth.

The graph on the preceding page illustrates the weight gain of the children at monthly intervals on the two experimental diets. As can be seen, there was a significantly faster weight gain in the children consuming coconut oil over those eating soybean oil. A mean gain of 2.08 kg (5.57 lb) after four months was recorded for the coconut oil group, almost twice as much as the weight gain of the soybean oil groups of 1.22 kg (3.27 lb).[34]

Premature and underweight infants are particularly vulnerable to nutritional deficiencies. Their digestive systems cannot assimilate nutrients, especially LCTs, as effectively as normal weight babies. Adding coconut oil or MCTs to hospital infant formulas has greatly improved these children's nutritional status and their chances for survival.[35-37]

Since the 1970s coconut oil or MCTs have been added to hospital infant formulas. In fact, they are also included in the feeding formulas given to hospital patients of all ages. If you have ever been in a hospital and needed to be fed through a tube or an IV, then you have probably received MCTs as part of your treatment. Studies have shown that when MCTs are added to nutritional formulas, patients recovering from surgery or illness get better faster.[38-41]

Premature infants and older hospital patients are not the only ones who benefit from coconut oil. All commercial infant formulas now contain coconut oil. Adding coconut oil to infant formula makes a lot of sense because it gives the formula characteristics similar to natural mother's milk that would not be available otherwise.

A Natural Defense Against Infection

One of the most remarkable characteristics about MCFAs is their potential to combat infections. MCFAs possess potent antimicrobial properties that can kill disease-causing bacteria, viruses, fungi, and parasites.[42] This is apparently another reason why nature puts MCFAs in mother's milk. A young infant's immune system is still developing and not yet capable of effectively fighting off many infectious organisms. In fact, the MCFAs in mother's milk provide the primary protection from infection in newborns for the first few months of their lives. [43]

MCFAs not only protect the body from infection, but the brain as well. Since MCFAs can cross over the blood-brain barrier, they can support the brain's immune system by aiding in the fight against invading microorganisms. This is important because most drugs, including antibiotics, cannot pass through the blood-brain barrier. MCFAs are among the only aids available to fight off brain infections, especially viral infections for which antibiotics are useless. Prenatal and postnatal brain infections are a known cause of autism. MCFAs are one of the only defenses against these infections.

The MCTs in coconut oil are identical to those found in mother's milk and possess the same antimicrobial potential. For this reason, food manufacturers have been putting coconut oil, or MCTs derived from coconut oil, into baby formula for years in order to give the formula disease-fighting capability similar to natural breast milk.[44] The advantage of coconut oil is that it contains a much higher concentration of MCTs than human milk, so a little can go a long way.

MCFAs derived from coconut oil have been studied extensively as potential antimicrobial agents that can be used in foods, cosmetics, and drugs. Studies show that these MCFAs are effective in killing bacteria that cause health problems such as ear infections, gastric ulcers, sinus infections, bladder infections, gum disease and cavities, acne, pneumonia, gonorrhea, and many other illnesses.[45-50] They kill fungi and yeasts that cause ringworm, athlete's foot, jock itch, thrush, diaper rash, and vaginal yeast infections.[51-53] They kill viruses that cause influenza, measles, herpes, mononucleosis, and hepatitis C.[54-58] They are so potent that they can even kill HIV—the AIDS virus.[59-61] There are numerous published studies and even entire books describing the antimicrobial effects of MCFAs derived from coconut oil.[62]

Because of the published studies that have shown MCFAs to be effective in killing HIV, many HIV-infected individuals have added coconut in one form or another to their treatment programs with success. For example, Tony V. was diagnosed with full-blown AIDS but was able to overcome the disease using coconut oil therapy. HIV attacks the immune system of its victims, thus increasing their vulnerability to other infections. In fact, AIDS patients usually die from secondary infections rather than from the virus itself. Before beginning his coconut oil regimen, Tony was in terrible shape. His immune system was so weakened that he was riddled with secondary infections. He had lost a substantial amount of weight, suffered from chronic pneumonia, struggled with chronic fatigue, experienced repeated bouts of nausea and diarrhea, had oral candidiasis, and was covered from head to foot with skin infections. His flesh was an angry red, cracking, flaking, and weeping. His skin was so bad that the hair on his head was falling out in clumps. He wore a wig to hide the bald spots and oozing sores. He was so far gone that his doctors told him he had only a matter of months to live.

Unable to work because of his illness, he had little money and could not afford to continue buying medication. He asked the government for help. He was referred to a doctor who had just published a study on the therapeutic effects of coconut oil in treating AIDS. He told Tony to consume 6 tablespoons of coconut oil daily, along with rubbing more oil on the lesions all over his body. Tony began doing as he was instructed. Nine months later, to the surprise of his other doctors, Tony was not only alive, but thriving. The coconut oil healed him from all of his secondary infections and brought the HIV under control. He regained his lost weight, his hair grew back, and his skin was clear and healthy with no sign of infection.[63] While Tony may never be completely free of HIV, coconut oil has given him a better life.

Studies by Gilda Erguiza, MD, and colleagues have shown that coconut oil added to standard antibiotic therapy improves recovery from community-acquired pneumonia. Community-acquired pneumonia is an infection of the lungs that is contracted outside a hospital setting. It is a serious infection in children. In a presentation delivered to the American College of Chest Physicians in Philadelphia, Dr. Erguiza described her findings.[64] The study included 40 children between the ages of three months to five years, all suffering from community-acquired pneumonia and treated intravenously with the antibiotic ampicillin. Half of the group was also given a daily dose of coconut oil at 2 ml per kilogram of body weight. The oil was given for three days in a row. The researchers found that the respiratory rate normalized in 32.6 hours for the coconut oil group versus 48.2 hours for the control group. After three days, patients in the control group were more likely than those in the coconut oil group to still have wheezing in the lungs—60 percent of the controls still had wheezing compared to only 25 percent of the coconut oil group. Those in the coconut oil group also recovered from their fevers quicker, had normal oxygen saturation faster, and had shorter hospital stays.

MCFAs are used in a variety of medications and dietary supplements. Caprylic acid, one of the MCFAs in coconut oil, is a popular ingredient in some anti-candida formulations. Monolaurin, another coconut oil-derived supplement, is used as a general-purpose antibiotic. Fractionated coconut oil, also known as MCT oil, is a common ingredient in many health and fitness products. Coconut oil has even been put into gel capsules as a dietary supplement. Of course, you can also find pure coconut oil in just about any health food store.

All dietary fats and oils consist of various combinations of different fatty acids. Coconut oil has 10 different fatty acids. Volume-wise, about 85 percent of the fatty acids in coconut oil possess antimicrobial activity. The most important germ-fighting fatty acids in coconut oil are lauric acid, myristic acid, caprylic acid, and capric acid. All of these are saturated fats and all except myristic acid are MCFAs. These fatty acids are generally absent from other oils.

While each of these fatty acids demonstrates antimicrobial properties, lauric acid has the greatest overall antibacterial, antiviral, and antifungal effect. It is also the most abundant fatty acid in coconut oil, constituting about 50 percent of the oil. Each of these fatty acids, however, exerts a different effect on various microorganisms. For example, one may be more effective at killing *Chlamydia pneumonia* than another, but less effective against herpes. All of them work together synergistically to provide the widest and strongest germ-killing effect.

The fact that coconut oil can be used to fight infection has important implications to those with autism. Unlike most drugs, MCFAs can cross over the blood-brain barrier and actively kill infections. Herpes, *Chlamydia pneumonia*, *Helicobacter pylori*, cytomegalovirus, and other microorganisms that frequently invade the brain, as well as vaccine-related viruses such as measles, rubella, and chicken pox are all killed by MCFAs. In addition, MCFAs also kill many other microorganisms such as candida, streptococcus, and staphylococcus which can cause systemic infections that can trigger neuroinflammation.

While MCFAs are effective in killing many different types of microorganisms, they do not kill all of them. Rhinovirus, which causes the common cold, and the hepatitis A virus are two such organisms. So consuming MCFAs is no absolute guarantee against infections. This is actually a good thing. If MCFAs did kill all microorganisms they would destroy every living thing in the gut, including the friendly bacteria that are so important for good digestive health. However, MCFAs kill troublesome organisms like H. Pylori, clostridia (tetanus), candida, and the measles virus, but leave the good bacteria alone.

How can MCFAs distinguish between the good and the bad bacteria? The difference, in part, involves the type of skin (fatty membrane) surrounding the organism. Some membranes are highly vulnerable to MCFAs. When MCFAs come into contact with these microbes, they are readily absorbed into the microbe's fat-rich membrane, weakening it to the point that it ruptures, killing the organism. It's like popping a water-filled balloon. White blood cells then come in and clean up the mess by eating the debris. Some microorganisms are sensitive to MCFAs and some are not. Most friendly bacteria are not affected by the MCFAs, while many potentially harmful gut organisms are. This is part of nature's design. This is why MCFAs from mother's milk can kill disease-causing microorganisms and at the same time bypass bifidobacteria and other friendly bacteria.

"The medium chain fatty acids and monoglycerides found primarily in these two tropical oils (coconut oil and palm kernel oil) and mother's milk have miraculous healing powers," says Jon Kabara, PhD, emeritus professor of pharmacology at Michigan State University. "It is rare in the history of medicine to find substances that have such useful properties and still be without toxicity or even harmful side effects."

Theoretically, coconut oil has the potential to assist in combating almost any type of infection. Although MCFAs may not have a direct killing affect on all disease-causing microorganisms, they can boost the overall efficiency of the immune system. MCFAs stimulate white blood cell production in the bone marrow, thus increasing the number of protective white blood cells in circulation that can attack foreign invaders and neutralize chemical toxins. Currently researchers are developing a new "drug" consisting of MCTs for the purpose of stimulating white blood cell production to prevent infections in cancer patients whose immune systems are severely compromised.[65]

Gastrointestinal Health, Coconut Oil, and the Brain

Inflammation anywhere in the body causes inflammatory proteins to be released into the bloodstream. When these proteins are carried to the brain they trigger an inflammatory response in the brain. The digestive tract is a primary location for inflammation in the body. In this manner colitis—inflammation in the colon (large intestine)—can cause inflammation in the brain.

About half of those with autism have gastrointestinal abnormalities, whether symptoms are evident or not.[66] Those with autism often have an imbalance in the type of microflora living in their digestive tracts. Too many troublemakers can lead to digestive problems including Crohn's disease and colitis. The result is chronic inflammation that instigates and fans the flame of microglia hyperactivity in the brain. Coconut oil can be an excellent aid in rebalancing the environment in the digestive tract, calming inflammation.

When coconut oil is eaten, the MCTs are broken down into MCFAs. The majority of these MCFAs will go to the liver were they will be used to produce energy and ketone bodies. A portion, however, will travel down the digestive tract to destroy troublesome bacteria, viruses and yeasts. Populations of unfriendly microflora are reduced, allowing good bacteria a better chance to grow and establish dominance.

MCFAs can also calm inflammation and accelerate tissue repair. When applied on the skin, coconut oil has a soothing and healing effect. Wounds and ulcers heal faster. This effect appears to be evident in the digestive tract as well. MCFAs have been shown to calm inflammation associated with Crohn's disease and ulcerative colitis and to reduce their severity and frequency of occurrence.[67] One of the reasons for its soothing and healing effect is due to their nourishing properties on epithelial cells—the cells that make up our skin and line our gastrointestinal tract.

Short chain fatty acids (SCFAs) are the main energy source for the tissues lining the small intestine and colon. They are avidly absorbed by the tissues lining the intestinal wall. SCFAs are produced by friendly gut bacteria as they break down and digest the fiber in the foods we eat. This is one of the reasons why it is important to have a healthy digestive environment with ample good bacteria. These bacteria provide the SCFAs necessary for good intestinal health. Without SCFAs, the tissues along the intestinal wall would become malnourished and sickly. The risk of disease (e.g., Crohn's, etc.) and infection would increase. Tissues would degenerate and become porous or leaky, allowing food particles to pass through the intestinal wall and be absorbed into the bloodstream. These food proteins would be interpreted by the immune system as invading foreign bodies, triggering allergic reactions and systemic inflammation. In this way, ordinarily harmless protein molecules, like casein from milk and gluten from grains, could initiate an allergic reaction. This is one reason why dietary fiber is so important to health.

In addition to low levels of SCFAs, inflammation, food intolerances (celiac disease), infection, candida overgrowth, parasites, toxins, and drugs (such as aspirin) can also damage the intestinal wall and contribute to a leaky gut. In fact, when SCFAs are deficient, the intestinal wall is weakened so that these other factors have a greater impact.

Fortunately, there is another source of nutrition for the intestines—MCFAs. In fact, MCFAs are absorbed by the intestinal cells better than SCFAs, providing an excellent alternative source of nutrition for the digestive tract.[68] MCFAs are absorbed 2-13 times faster than SCFAs. MCFAs provide the energy the intestinal tissues need to function normally and to promote healing, especially in an environment where SCFAs may be lacking. For this reason, coconut oil/MCTs have been used for the treatment of patients with various diseases of the lower intestine and colon.

It's of interest to point out that during infancy when milk or formula are the only foods babies consume, they do not eat any dietary fiber. Therefore, no SCFAs are produced in their digestive tract. However, MCTs from breast milk or MCT/coconut oil-enriched formula provide MCFAs which supply all the energy needed to nourish the infant's intestinal tract. As the infant begins to eat more solid foods and milk consumption declines, SCFAs become the primary source of energy for the intestinal epithelial cells.

Since MCFAs are better utilized as a source of energy than SCFAs, they can have a revitalizing and healing effect on the intestinal walls. Studies have shown that MCFAs ease inflammation in the digestive tract caused by unfriendly bacteria and harsh chemicals.[69-70] For example, researchers chemically induced colitis in rats by injecting into their colons a caustic chemical to inflame and irritate the intestinal walls.

The rats were then fed a liquid diet that contained either MCTs or corn oil (as the control). The MCT diet was highly effective in reducing inflammation and preventing further damage to the colon wall. As a result of this and other studies, MCTs have been recommended for the treatment of inflammatory bowel diseases and as anti-inflammatory aids.[71]

WHAT PEOPLE ARE SAYING ABOUT COCONUT OIL

Thousands of people are currently using coconut oil as a home-remedy for infections and other health concerns with good success. Some people prefer to use *virgin* coconut oil over ordinary coconut oil. The term "virgin" indicates that the oil has undergone minimal processing so it retains all of its natural nutrients and flavor. Both forms of coconut oil have been used successfully.

"I've had chronic bladder infections for twenty years," says Cindy D. "I've been to numerous doctors with no positive results and most of the time I was worse. After the last doctor I swore I would not go to another doctor unless I was dying and had no choice. I began to research natural remedies. I tried so many things it would be hard to list. They helped to some extent but didn't cure my infections. I found your website and tried coconut oil. In one month's time I have not had one bladder infection. I'm taking one tablespoon 3 times a day with meals. I've put the oil on cuts and healed so quickly I couldn't believe it. My husband eats popcorn every night and I started using coconut oil instead of canola oil. He loves the flavor of the popcorn."

"Thursday night I had a bad ear infection," says Kevin K. "I hurt so bad I could not even touch my ear and it hurt down to my jaw and midway between the ear and cheek. I know that this is caused by bacteria or fungi so I thought what kills these better than coconut oil? I took a Q-Tip and dipped it into the coconut oil and carefully dabbed it in my ear where I felt the most pain. The next morning I woke up with no ear infection, and I could touch the opening of the ear without any pain. There was just a hint of soreness that I could feel inside the ear, but this was gone by Friday evening."

"I started using virgin coconut oil to de-frizz my hair," says Amber. "Over the holidays, my aunt complimented my long shiny hair, and I told her my secret. I found out she is an avid virgin coconut oil user too. She went on and on about the many health benefits I hadn't heard of. She mentioned that it cured her athlete's foot. I had tried everything on my athlete's foot and nothing ever worked. I gave it a shot, and it worked! The nail fungus is completely gone! It is now the only product I use on my skin head to toe, it even got rid of my acne! I wish I had known how dramatic the change would be, I would have taken before and after photos. My skin is naturally oily, but coconut oil is so light, it soaks in in a few seconds….Apparently, this stuff does much more than de-frizz hair!"

Diaper rash can occur when candida, a yeast that normally inhabits the bowels, infects the skin. It can be very painful. "I witnessed a miracle of coconut oil when my two-month-old baby developed this horrible diaper rash," says Dee. The rash was a swollen, angry red and even started to bleed. "Diaper rash creams, which I applied faithfully, were not working at all. I decided to apply the virgin coconut oil to the affected area with each changing and stopped using wipes, and it was healed in less than 48 hours."

"I am not scratching for the first time in a month," says Elizabeth. "What a relief. I first noticed it as persistent itchiness at the top of my thigh. After a week or so, a small rash appeared. It quickly spread across my hip. Then the rash appeared on my other hip. Before long, I was itchy on the back of my knees, the inside of my elbows, and the back of my hands, as well as across both hips. I went to a conventional doctor who couldn't diagnose the source but prescribed antihistamines and a prednisone 'burst.' After a week on prednisone, the rash was as itchy as ever, and my skin was even more red and swollen. I tried every topical remedy I could think of with little relief. I saw a naturopathic doctor who was also unable to diagnose my problem but suggested treating it through a process of elimination, trying an antifungal first, and going to an antibacterial if the antifungal didn't work. After several days on the antifungal with no relief—in fact, the rash was now spreading to my back, my belly, and my forearms—it flashed through the back of my mind that I had once read that coconut oil had antifungal, antibacterial, and antiviral properties. Feeling fairly desperate—and with nothing to lose—I pulled my bottle of virgin coconut oil out of the kitchen cupboard and applied it topically to all my itchy places. The results were miraculous. Almost instantly, the itching stopped. Within hours, my skin began to soothe, and the redness faded. This absence of itching is such a wonderful feeling that I'm truly grateful. I am now a coconut oil convert."

"I was desperate to find something to help my son Jayden's severe atopic eczema, which is often infected with yeast or bacteria," says Heidi Carolan. "After months of trying the creams given to me by doctors, nothing worked. Many of the creams seemed to make the condition even worse! Apparently, he is sensitive to some of the chemicals in the creams. Every week the doctor would give him another cream, followed by an angry reaction of weeping and inflammation that would eventually scab over. The following week the doctor would prescribe yet another cream and the cycle would happen all over again! Since the medicines didn't work, I began searching for something natural, without harmful chemicals, to treat his skin condition. I found information about organic virgin coconut oil and decided to give it a try. To my amazement, after using it for only a short time, his skin showed a huge improvement! After months of failure, virgin coconut oil is the only thing that has worked for him. I have been using it on him every day since and am pleased with the results. His skin is now normal again." (See before and after photos of Jayden on the following page.)

In some cases, like those noted above, coconut oil can be more effective than drugs and medicated creams and lotions. The epithelial cells of the skin are similar to those that line the digestive tract, so they often show a similar response to coconut oil treatment. Colitis, Crohn's disease, and other inflammatory gastrointestinal disorders are notoriously difficult to treat. They are usually considered lifelong afflictions that gradually get worse over time. Yet, in many cases coconut oil can bring about significant improvement, if not a complete recovery.

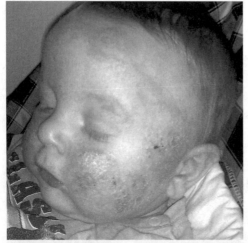

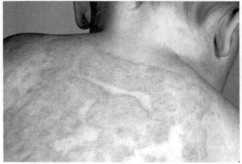

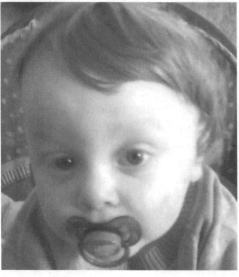

Jayden's chronic skin condition showed no improvement despite the use of numerous medicated creams and lotions (top two photos). After using coconut oil Jayden's skin cleared up nicely (bottom photo).

"I am 29 years old and have been suffering with ulcerative colitis for 14 years," says Mike. "My father had ulcerative colitis that went untreated and led to cancer and his death at the age of 46, so I have always been aware of the seriousness. I never experienced coconut oil until my wife found your cookbooks! I visited your website and ordered your *Coconut Cures* book and was blown away page after page. In addition to colitis, I have several other medical problems that were treated with coconut oil so how can I not give it a shot. I built up to a maintenance level of 1-2 tablespoons in my coffee every morning and started feeling better after about one month. Nine months later I had my yearly colonoscopy check up (required for colitis patients of any age) and my doctor was shocked! Not only has the disease reversed itself, none of the biopsies revealed any indication of colitis and I essentially have a normal person's colon! I told him about coconut oil and, of course, my doctor thought that the medication was cause for improvement but said to definitely keep doing whatever I'm doing. If only my father had this knowledge when my father was young, he could have seen his kids grow up."

"Last year I was diagnosed with celiac disease," say Lindsey Avery, a college student majoring in exercise physiology. "After not yet having developed a regular coconut oil regime I changed my diet to eliminate gluten but incorporated coconut oil instead of prescription anti-inflammatories to heal the walls of my intestinal tract. As an experiment, I had intestinal biopsies taken at the time of the diagnoses and five months following the incorporation

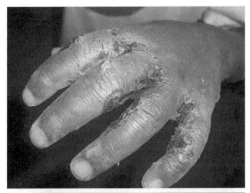

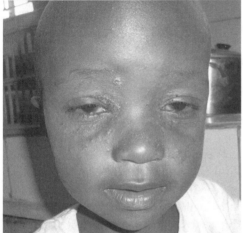

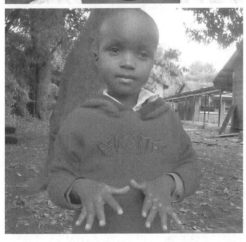

Four-year-old boy with a severe skin infection covering his hands, face, and head (top two photos). A poultice made with coconut oil was applied to the infected areas. Within two weeks the infection was completely gone (bottom photo).

of coconut oil into my diet. The results were dumbfounding. I was able to reverse the damage to my GI tract in five months, to the opposition of my GI specialist who told me this health process would take at least a year with necessary prescriptions."

"Six months ago, I was diagnosed with endometriosis, irritable bowel syndrome, and irritable bladder syndrome, with a significant yeast overgrowth," says Amanda H. Surgery was offered as a possible treatment option. Amanda, knowing her diet had to play a significant role in her diagnosis, turned down the surgery, and started looking for another solution. She found some resources on the web and decided to follow a radical diet that eliminated wheat, dairy, soy, sugar, and other potentially problematic foods. "After three months there was a noticeable improvement, however, not as much as I expected or would have liked," she said. "Remembering a visit to Sri Lanka some years previously and feeling utterly marvelous after spending three weeks consuming coconuts in abundance, I wondered if perhaps there was a significant ingredient that I was missing that the coconut contained." Convinced that coconut oil was the missing ingredient, she began taking it daily. "Well what a miracle indeed," Amanda exclaims. "All symptoms of disease disappeared within a month and I now have an excess of energy I haven't had for years."

"I am a mother of an 8-year-old with epilepsy," says Debbie H. "At least once a month she would have a bad week where she would experience multiple seizures and lose control of her left arm and drool terribly. Her mouth would seize a lot and her speech would be unclear. She always jokes and says her mouth and arm 'dances'…I have found introducing coconut and coconut cream or coconut yogurt to be very successful. Dried coconut flakes are yummy. My daughter loves them and so do I. I am finding that I am using coconut more and more. Over the last three months she has had only one seizure and I am hoping the seizures will disappear completely."

"My son (Charlie) has grand mal and petit mal seizures and status epilepticus (severe continuous unremitting seizures lasting longer than 5 minutes)," says Sharon. "He is considered medically fragile. He's also had some strokes and about 30 neurosurgical procedures. We first evaluated the ketogenic diet for him in the mid 1970s shortly after we adopted him and decided it was too hard. Now, nearly 30 years later, as his body is not tolerating antiepileptic drugs very well, I looked at the ketogenic diet again and noticed the inclusion of medium chain triglycerides from coconut oil. Charlie's been on virgin coconut oil for several months…he's not had a life threatening seizure since last December (seven months ago), a very pleasant respite for both of us as his seizures do not stop by themselves…We are doing a modification of the ketogenic diet. But Charlie is an adult. I would strongly suggest that the ketogenic diet be given careful thoughtful consideration. Seizures are no fun, they cause brain damage and long term use of antiepileptic medications can cause its own set of problems."

Holistic-minded medical doctors, nurses, and nutritionists are also using coconut oil and recommending it to their patients. "Virgin coconut oil is immunoprotective in children, superior to vitamin C," says Arturo C. Ludan, MD, pediatrician/gastroenterologist. "Clinical studies show virgin coconut oil's significant role in pediatrics as a source of energy, an immune system booster, a local antiseptic, and an anti-inflammatory."

Dr. Eliza Perez Francisco, MD, says, "In my clinical practice at St. Luke's Medical Center, I use virgin coconut oil for the elderly in relation to physiologic changes that occur with aging. Virgin coconut oil can address sensory losses, tooth and gum problems, changes in the intestinal tract, changes in the immune system, changes in body composition, and changes that come with menopause and andropause…A combination of old age and malnutrition makes older people vulnerable to pneumonia, UTI, and bedsores. Virgin coconut oil can help fight infection in the early stages. Take the case of a 76-year-old who developed painful herpes zoster on his trunk. The antibiotic cream given to him only lasted for one application because the area affected was so wide. But when virgin coconut oil was applied all over the skin for a week, the patient reported relief from itch and the lesions dried up."

Dr. S. Kumar, MD, states, "I am a primary care practitioner or general practitioner with priority in nutritional medicine as the healing component. I have read Dr. Fife's, Dr. Dayrit's, and Prof Mary G. Enig's books and am using only virgin coconut oil (VCO) for cooking and also orally when down with the flu, etc. I strongly advise my patients to consume more VCO when sick and advocate to all ages from newborns to the old and sick, including those with diabetic, hypertensive, heart, and skin ailments and even those stricken with cancer. Over the last two years I've seen patients get better. It is difficult sometimes for some patients initially to accept VCO. They think I am going 'nuts'! The truth is being revealed and allopathic medicine has to admit all this while they have been wrong and it is still not too late to rectify this mistake. I still get criticisms from many but I believe in due time the critics will be silenced."

"I grew up in Puerto Rico, where coconut was widely available and consumed for a myriad of remedies," says Carlos Diaz. "I remember my mother using the coconut milk to feed us in lieu of regular milk. I come from a big family and none of my brothers and sisters had any serious health problems when they were young. This is amazing, when you consider we had no running water at that time, and access to healthcare was very scarce. Coconut oil was used as a remedy for any stomach problem (i.e., constipation, diarrhea, ulcers, etc). It was also used as a purging agent and as an ointment to prevent wound or insect bite infections…It's interesting that when a Puerto Rican wants to say he is in superb good health, he says 'estoy como coco' which literally means 'I'm as good as a coconut.'"

ADDING COCONUT OIL INTO YOUR DAILY LIFE

As you have learned about some of the many benefits of coconut oil, it should be obvious that this extraordinary brain food can play a central role in the fight against autism and other neurological disorders. Therefore, understanding how to incorporate it into your daily life is important. The simplest way to do this is to prepare your foods with it. Coconut oil is very heat stable, so it is excellent for use in the kitchen. You can use it for any baking or frying purpose. In recipes that call for margarine, butter, shortening, or vegetable oil, use coconut oil instead. Use the same amount or more to make sure you get the recommended amount in your diet (see Chapter 14 for details on dosage).

Not all foods are prepared using oil, but you can still incorporate the oil into the diet. You can add coconut oil to foods that aren't normally prepared with oil. For example, add a spoonful of coconut oil to hot beverages, hot cereals, soups, sauces, and casseroles, or use it as a topping on cooked vegetables.

Although I recommend that you consume coconut oil with foods, you don't have to prepare your food with it or add it to the food. You can take it by the spoonful like a dietary supplement. Many people prefer to get their daily dose of coconut oil this way. If you use a good quality coconut oil, it tastes good. Many people don't like the thought of putting a spoonful of oil, any oil, into their mouths. It may take some people a little time to get used to it.

There are two primary types of coconut oil you will find sold in stores. One is called *virgin* coconut oil; the other is refined, bleached, and deodorized (RBD) coconut oil. Virgin coconut oil is made from fresh coconuts with very minimal processing. The oil basically comes straight from the coconut. Since it has gone through little processing, it retains a delicate coconut taste and aroma. It is delicious. RBD coconut oil is made from copra (air dried coconut) and has gone through more extensive processing. During the processing all the flavor and aroma has been removed. For people who don't like the taste of coconut in their foods, this is a good option. RBD oil is processed using mechanical means and high temperatures. Chemicals are not generally used. When you go to the store, you can tell the difference between virgin and RBD coconut oils by the label. All virgin coconut oils will state that they are "virgin." RBD oils will not have this statement. They also usually do not say "RBD." Sometimes they will be advertised as "Expeller Pressed," which means that the initial pressing of the oil from the coconut meat was done mechanically, without the use of added heat. However, heat is usually used at some later stage in the refining process.

Many people prefer the virgin coconut oil because it has undergone less processing and retains more of the vitamins and phytonutrients that nature put into it. This is why it maintains its coconut flavor. Because more care is taken to produce virgin coconut oil, it is more expensive than RBD oil.

Most brands of RBD coconut oil are generally tasteless and odorless and differ little from each other. The quality of the different brands of virgin coconut oil, however, can vary greatly. There are many different processing methods used to produce virgin coconut oil. Some are better than others. Plus, the care taken also affects the quality. Some companies produce excellent quality coconut oil that tastes so good you can easily eat it off the spoon. Other brands have a strong flavor and may be nearly unpalatable. You generally cannot tell the difference just by looking at the jar. You have to taste it. If the oil has a mild coconut flavor with a mild coconut smell and tastes good to you, then that is a brand you should use. If the flavor is overpowering or smells smoky, you might want to try another brand.

Coconut oil is available at all health food stores and many grocery stores, as well as on the Internet. There are many different brands to choose from. Generally the more expensive brands are the best quality, but not always. All brands, however, have basically the same culinary and therapeutic effects and are useful.

If you purchase coconut oil from the store, it may have the appearance of shortening, being firm and snow white in color. When you take it home and put it on your kitchen shelf, after a few days it may transform into a colorless liquid. Don't be alarmed. This is natural. One of the distinctive characteristics of coconut oil is its high melting point. At temperatures of 76 degrees F (24 C) and above the oil is liquid like any other vegetable oil. At temperatures below this, it solidifies. It is much like butter. If stored in the refrigerator, a stick of butter is solid, but let it sit on the countertop on a hot day and it melts into a puddle. A jar of coconut oil may be liquid or solid depending on the temperature where it is stored. You can use it in either form.

Coconut oil is very stable, so it does not need to be refrigerated. You can store it on a cupboard shelf. Shelf life for a good quality coconut oil is 1 to 3 years. Hopefully, you will use it long before then.

MCT Oil

Most of the health benefits associated with coconut oil comes from its medium chain triglycerides. If MCTs are good, then it might be reasoned that a source that contains more than coconut oil may be even better. Coconut oil is the richest "natural" source of MCTs, but there is another source that contains more: MCT oil. Coconut oil consists of 63 percent MCTs, while MCT oil is 100 percent. MCT oil, which is sometimes referred to as "fractionated coconut oil," is produced from coconut oil. The 10 fatty acids that make up coconut oil are separated out and two of the medium chain fatty acids (caprylic and capric acids) are recombined to form MCT oil.

The advantage of MCT oil is that it provides more MCTs per unit volume than coconut oil. It is tasteless and, being liquid at room temperature, can be used in cooking or as a salad dressing. The disadvantage of MCT oil is that it has more of a tendency to cause nausea and diarrhea than coconut oil, so there is a limited amount that can be used without experiencing this side effect. It also contains no lauric acid—the most important of the medium chain fatty acids.

In contrast, about 50 percent of coconut oil consists of lauric acid. Lauric acid possesses the most potent antimicrobial power. When combined with the other fatty acids in the oil, its antimicrobial potential is enhanced. Consequently, coconut oil has a far greater germ-fighting ability than MCT oil.

Another difference between MCT oil and coconut oil lies in the rate of ketone production. The MCFAs in MCT oil are quickly converted into ketones. Blood ketone levels peak 1½ hours after consumption and are gone after 3 hours. However, the conversion of lauric acid in coconut oil into ketones is slower. Ketone levels peak at 3 hours after consumption of coconut oil, but remain in the blood for about 8 hours. MCT oil may give a quicker and higher peak in ketosis, but fizzles out much sooner.

MCT oil would need to be administered every 2 hours or so day and night to maintain blood ketone levels. During sleep, brain function remains fully active and needs energy just as it does when awake. An autistic child taking this product would need to be awakened constantly throughout the night to receive doses of MCT oil. This amount of MCT oil is unrealistic not only because it is impractical and not advisable to wake a child every two hours each night, but also because of the undesirable digestive disturbances it would cause.

Coconut oil only needs to be taken three or four times a day to maintain blood ketone levels and can last throughout the night. MCT oil can, however, be added to coconut oil which may produce a quicker rise in ketosis, but it really isn't necessary. Coconut oil lasts longer, has fewer side effects, and is more effective in treating chronic infections.

SUMMARY

Looking at all that coconut oil can do, it can definitely be called the ultimate brain food. The MCTs in coconut oil are converted into MCFAs during digestion. A large portion of these MCFAs provide immediate energy or are converted into ketones. Ketones are produced specifically to feed the brain. They provide an alternative source of high-potency fuel for the brain, activate certain proteins in the brain that calm inflammation, stimulate healing and repair, and provide the basic building blocks for new brain tissues. Ketones improve oxygen delivery protecting against conditions that promote hypoxia. Ketones also help protect the brain and body from a variety of environmental, industrial, and dietary toxins.

MCFAs improve digestion and nutrient absorption, supplying the brain and body with the nutrients its needs for good health. They also provide protection against troublesome bacteria, viruses, and fungi that can infect the brain, digestive tract, and other organs. Infection anywhere in the body will stimulate the release of proinflammatory proteins that can travel to the brain and trigger an inflammatory response. The digestive tract is a common location for low-grade chronic infections that can keep brain inflammation continually active. MCFAs can eliminate harmful microorganisms in the gut, reestablish proper flora populations, soothe and heal inflamed tissues, and nourish the intestinal wall, thereby improving digestive health and eliminating chronic inflammation.

Mother's milk is one of nature's primary sources of MCTs. Their presence in milk serves a multitude of purposes that are essential in the proper growth and development of infants and therefore, are absolutely essential during this period of time. For this reason, MCFAs are considered to be *conditionally essential fatty acids*. We must have them during this critical phase of life in order to develop properly. This is why hospital and commercial infant formulas all include coconut oil or MCTs.

MCTs used for medical and commercial purposes come from either coconut or palm kernel oils—the highest natural sources for these unique fats. Coconut oil contains about 10 times more MCTs than breast milk, making it a super rich source of this special group of fats and a useful tool in the fight against autism.

11 | Prenatal and Postnatal Nutrition

PRENATAL CARE

Environmental factors play a significant role in the development of autism. While some factors can and do occur after birth, many are encountered during pregnancy. Researchers at Stanford University studying autism rates among siblings and twins have recently learned that conditions in the womb can have a profound effect on autism rates. They found that autism occurred in 77 percent of male identical twins and 50 percent of female identical twins. Among fraternal twins the rates were lower: 31 percent for males and 36 percent for females. The rate of autism occurring in two siblings who are not twins was much lower, suggesting that the conditions the twins shared in the womb contributed to the development of autism.[1] The researchers estimated that 58 percent of autism cases are caused or at least initiated by conditions in the womb.

A woman's nutrition prior to and throughout pregnancy is crucial to both her health and the health of her baby. Sound nutrition during pregnancy and nursing promotes proper growth, development, and health so that the infant can achieve its full genetic potential. Pregnancy has such a major impact on an infant's development that women should enter pregnancy well informed and prepared. What a mother does during pregnancy can have a huge impact on the baby's physical and mental health. The fetus draws its nutrients from the mother's body, so if the mother is deficient in any nutrient, her baby will be also.

The mother's nutritional needs during pregnancy and lactation are higher than at any other time in her adult life and are greater for certain nutrients than for others. Pregnant women must select foods high in nutrient density—foods that build health, not destroy it. Junk foods should be avoided. The worst foods to eat are those filled with empty calories—foods that supply calories but little nutrition. Processed convenience foods loaded with sugar and chemical additives should be limited. Generally, the more processing a food has undergone, the less nutritious it is and the more chemical additives it contains. The best foods are whole natural foods such as whole grains, fresh vegetables and fruits, and fresh meats, dairy, and eggs, preferably organic.

Women who don't eat properly increase their risks of giving birth to a premature or low birth weight child. Low birth weight is defined as 5.5 pounds (2,500 g) or less. The birth weight of an infant isn't just about size; it has a significant impact on the baby's health. An infant's birth weight is the most potent single indicator of the infant's current and future health. A low birth weight baby has a statistically greater chance than a normal weight baby of developing diseases (e.g., diabetes, ear infections, etc.), experiencing developmental disorders, including autism, and of dying early in life. Studies show that low birth weight children are more likely to experience multiple cognitive and behavioral problems and are less likely to complete high school.[2] About one in every 13 infants born in the US is a low birth weight infant, and about one-fourth of those die within the first month of life.

Some low birth weight infants are premature—they are born early although they are the right size for their gestational age. Others have suffered growth failure in the womb and may or may not be born early, but they are small for gestational age.

Every single week in the womb is important, even the last few weeks. A full term pregnancy takes about 40 weeks. Pregnancies lasting at least 37 weeks are regarded as full-term, but new research finds that babies born in the 37th or 38th week of pregnancy have a higher risk of dying before their first birthdays than those born after 39 weeks of gestation. Research has revealed that infants born at 37 weeks are twice as likely to die in the first year of life as those born at 40 weeks.[3]

Good eating habits should start *before* pregnancy. A strong correlation exists between pre-pregnancy nutrition and infant birth weight. A major reason why the mother's pre-pregnancy nutrition is so crucial is that it determines whether she will be able to grow a healthy placenta during the first month of gestation. The only way nutrients can reach the developing fetus is through the placenta. In the placenta the mother's and baby's blood vessels intertwine and exchange materials. The fetus receives nutrients and oxygen and the mother's blood picks up carbon dioxide and other waste materials for disposal. If the mother's nutrient stores are inadequate during placental development, then no matter how well she eats later on, the fetus will not receive optimum nourishment. The infant will be a low birth weight baby, with all of the accompanying health consequences.

Certain critical organs develop early. At eight weeks gestation, the embryo is called a fetus and has a complete central nervous system, a beating heart, a fully formed digestive system, and the beginning of facial features. Over the next seven months of pregnancy the fetus increases rapidly in size. The amniotic sac fills with fluid to cushion the infant. The mother's uterus and its supporting muscles increase greatly in size, her breasts change and grow in preparation for lactation, and her blood volume increases by half to accommodate the added load of materials it must carry. Fat stores increase to provide nutrients for milk production.

Weight gain during pregnancy directly influences infant birth weight. For a normal sized woman (about 120 lb/54 kg), total weight gain should be about 22-28 pounds (10-13 kg). If the mother does not gain the full amount of weight recommended, she may give birth to a low birth weight baby.

POTENTIAL HAZARDS DURING PREGNANCY
Infections

Poor lifestyle and eating habits, especially consuming excessive amounts of sugar-laden foods, seriously depresses immune function, making the mother more vulnerable to infection. Infections during pregnancy are more than just an inconvenience to the mother: they can be disastrous for the fetus. It is well known that if a mother-to-be is stricken with rubella, it can lead to birth defects. *Any* infection during pregnancy is potentially dangerous.

There are critical windows of time during pregnancy in which the fetus is most vulnerable to infection.[4] Studies show that babies born to mothers who experience a viral infection during the first trimester or a bacterial infection during the second trimester have an increased risk of developing autism.[5]

It is also known that women who are infected with the flu during pregnancy are significantly more likely to give birth to a child with neurological disorders. At first, researchers assumed this was due to the virus being passed to the fetus, but subsequent studies found that it was not necessarily the virus, but the mother's immune reaction to the virus that caused the problem by triggering an immune response in the brain of the unborn child.[6]

Mothers who experience infections during pregnancy produce inflammatory cytokines that affect and interfere with normal fetal brain development. For example, women who have infections during the second trimester have an increased risk of their children developing schizophrenia and other psychotic disorders.[7-9]

Pregnant women are often encouraged to get the flu vaccination. This is not a good idea. These vaccines contain live viruses as well as mercury-laden thimerosal, neither one good for the developing fetus. The mother will likely experience some type of immune reaction, as this is the purpose for the vaccination. In the process, inflammatory cytokines will be released into her bloodstream that will trigger a like reaction in the fetus, activating microglia in the unborn child's brain, which will interfere with normal brain development.

Drugs and Toxins

Certain substances can harm the growing fetus: alcohol, caffeine, tobacco, drugs, hydrogenated vegetable oils, artificial sweeteners, nitrates, chemical food dyes, and other food additives. Most of these products act as drugs and serve no useful purpose for the developing infant or the mother during pregnancy.

Drugs taken during pregnancy can cause serious birth defects and developmental delays. We live in a society in which the use of drugs is routine for many people. The side effects of these drugs, particularly on unborn children, aren't always well understood. Many drugs are on the market for years before it is discovered that they cause birth defects or other harm. It is wise to avoid all drugs, even common over-the-counter ones.

Antidepressant medications like Prozac, Zoloft, Celexa, or Lexapro taken before or during pregnancy have been found to substantially increase the risk of autism.

When mothers took antidepressants the year before delivery their children were twice as likely to be born with autism. The risk increased another 30 percent if the mothers used these drugs during the first trimester of pregnancy.[10]

One of the most common drugs that can adversely affect fetal development is caffeine. Like many other substances, caffeine is rapidly absorbed across the placenta. The developing fetus has a very limited ability to metabolize caffeine, making it much more harmful to an unborn infant than to an adult. Caffeine can kill. In one study the daily use of just two cups of coffee (equivalent to four 12-ounce cola drinks) was linked to an increased risk of spontaneous abortion.[11] If the caffeine in two cups of coffee can increase the risk of death, then a lesser amount can have serious effects on growth and development.

Smoking restricts the blood supply to the growing fetus, limiting the delivery of oxygen and nutrients and the removal of wastes. It stunts growth, thus increasing the risk of low birth weight, delayed development, and complications at birth. The brain has an especially high demand for oxygen. If oxygen is restricted, it will have a pronounced effect on brain development and function. Smoking is a well known cancer risk. It is not only a high risk for pregnant users but also for their unborn children. One study found that the incidence of cancer and leukemia in children of women who smoke while pregnant is twice as high as in nonsmokers.[12] The surgeon general of the United States has issued a warning that smoking can be a direct cause of fetal death.[13]

You can assume that whatever drug, food, or product you consume, your fetus will consume as well. If something affects the mother's brain, it will certainly affect the unborn child's brain and will do so to a much greater extent. A prime example of this is alcohol.

Alcohol consumption during pregnancy can cause irreversible brain damage and mental and physical retardation in the fetus. Alcohol crosses the placenta freely and enters the fetal brain, causing both glucose and oxygen deficiency, to which developing nerve tissue is extremely vulnerable. The results can lead to fetal alcohol syndrome (FAS), comprising a combination of growth retardation, mental retardation, and physical defects. About 1 in every 750 children in the US is born with FAS. For every baby with this condition, ten more are born with less pronounced symptoms. This is known as subclinical FAS. The mothers of these children drank, but not enough to cause obvious, visible defects. The subtle abnormalities associated with subclinical FAS often show up later as learning disabilities, behavioral abnormalities, motor impairments, and other problems.

When alcohol crosses the placenta, fetal blood-alcohol concentrations increase until they equal that of the mother's blood-alcohol level. This may seem to be of little concern if the mother is not drunk and is functioning normally. However, while blood levels are the same for the mother and fetus, the fetus' body is significantly smaller and its detoxification system is less developed. Also, blood-alcohol concentrations remain in the fetus longer than in the mother. Even when alcohol can no longer be detected in the mother's blood, it can be detected in the unborn child's blood for hours afterward. Consequently, a pregnant woman need not be an alcoholic in order to give birth to a baby with FAS or subclinical FAS. Social drinking can be all it takes.

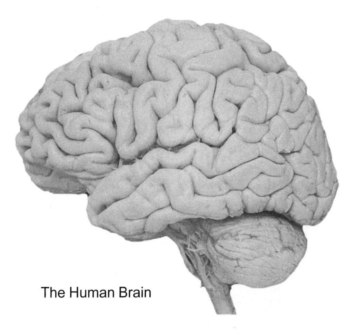

The Human Brain

She only needs to consume enough to exceed the capacity of her unborn child's liver to detoxify the alcohol.

How much is too much? The surgeon general of the United States has issued a statement that women should drink absolutely no alcohol during pregnancy. The American Medical Association advises women to stop drinking as soon as they *plan* to become pregnant.[14] The responsibility of caring for another life requires that women abstain from alcohol during pregnancy. So far, no safe level of alcohol consumption during pregnancy has been established. Women who choose to drink during pregnancy, even moderately, are putting their children at greater risk than those who abstain completely. Why take the risk?

Any drug or harmful substance can cause havoc on the growing, developing brain. Whether it is alcohol, nicotine, caffeine, or whatever, the effects on the fetus are prolonged and disruptive. The mechanisms of brain growth are disturbed, often giving rise to abnormal development.

In the 1960s Dr. Peter Witt performed a series of experiments to see how various drugs affect brain function. To do this he used spiders and tested their ability to build their webs while under the influence of various drugs. A normal spider would build an intricate and functional web. However, if the spider was fed a fly that had been injected with a drug, the spider's web became seriously flawed. We can make a visual analogy between fetal brain development and Dr. Witt's spider webs.

Think of a spider web as the multitude of intricate circuits in the human brain. When the brain building processes work unencumbered as they should, the result is an orderly and functional brain. But when the processes are influenced by drugs, the result is an altered abnormal and dysfunctional structure, like the irregular spider webs shown in the illustratiosn on the following page. Obviously, if the brain's circuitry is as messed up as these spider webs, there will be major developmental problems with the child.

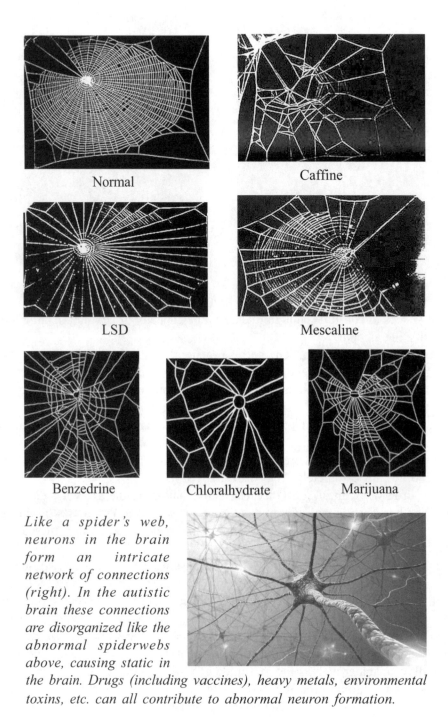

Normal

Caffine

LSD

Mescaline

Benzedrine

Chloralhydrate

Marijuana

Like a spider's web, neurons in the brain form an intricate network of connections (right). In the autistic brain these connections are disorganized like the abnormal spiderwebs above, causing static in the brain. Drugs (including vaccines), heavy metals, environmental toxins, etc. can all contribute to abnormal neuron formation.

Eating healthfully and avoiding all unnecessary drugs and drug-like substances provides the growing fetus the best opportunity to develop optimally.

YOU CAN HAVE A HEALTHY BABY

If you were offered a simple, natural, no-risk, low-cost method that would greatly increase your chances of giving birth to a full term, normal weight, healthy baby with normal or better brain development, and almost no risk of any neurodevelopmental problems, including autism, would you take it? Believe it or not, you do have this choice.

Eating a healthy, toxin-free diet is the first step in helping your unborn child develop to its full genetic potential. This includes eating a diet with ample protein and fat. Often, mothers-to-be avoid high-protein and high-fat foods, thinking they are unhealthy. Many needlessly worry about their cholesterol levels. The last thing an expectant mother needs to worry about is high cholesterol. If anything, she should worry about low cholesterol (see Chapter 8).

The mother's cholesterol level can affect her unborn baby. If her cholesterol is low, so is her unborn baby's. This can seriously affect fetal brain development, possibly setting the stage for autism later on. Cholesterol is necessary for normal embryonic and fetal development. Pregnant women with low cholesterol (below 160 mg/dl) are twice as likely to have premature babies or babies with microcephaly (underdeveloped heads).

Researchers from the US National Institutes of Health found that infants born to women who used drugs to lower their cholesterol during pregnancy experienced an increased incidence of severe central nervous system defects and limb deformities.[15] The study showed that nearly 40 percent of babies exposed to cholesterol-lowering drugs in the womb were born with serious malformations. "Birth defect studies suggest that these are the kinds of problems that occur if the embryo does not get enough cholesterol in early pregnancy to develop normally," said one of the study's authors, Dr. Maximilian Muenke, a senior investigator and chief of the medical genetics branch at the National Human Genome Research Institute. The mother's cholesterol levels can be affected by drugs or by low-fat dieting—a common occurrence in our modern anti-fat society.

Eating good sources of fat is important for the health of the baby. In many traditional cultures around the world pregnant women are encouraged to increase their fat intake to assure a healthy pregnancy. In Southeast Asian and the Pacific island communities it is the custom for pregnant women to add more coconut or coconut oil into their diets, especially during the last few months before delivery. It is their belief that coconut helps to make deliveries easier and the babies stronger and healthier. Over numerous generations they have witnessed how coconut oil protects both the mother and developing child.

In Malaysia where coconuts grow in abundance, coconut oil is used in late pregnancy for this purpose. For generations Malaysian women have been encouraged to eat coconut oil while pregnant. Researchers at the Universiti Sains Malaysia medical school wanted to find out if this practice was just an old wives' tale or if it really offered some benefit. To answer this question they set out to find out if coconut oil consumption had an effect on infant mortality just prior to or soon after birth. They examined dietary and birth information from 316 mothers. They discovered that infants whose mothers had consumed coconut oil during pregnancy had a significantly higher survival rate, thus validating the age old practice.[16]

Adding coconut oil during pregnancy not only increases the infant's chances for survival but can affect its health throughout life. Evidence suggests that children whose mothers eat coconut oil during pregnancy are less likely to become obese as adults.[17] This effect is likely due to improved health of the mother which results in better fetal development. Defects in fetal development can affect the child's health for life.

Coconut oil supplies an ample source of dietary MCTs that can be converted into ketones in the mother's body. We always have some level of ketones in our bodies. Ketone production increases during pregnancy. Besides the brain, the fetus itself is a major consumer of ketones. Adding a source of MCTs to the diet increases ketone levels. Ketones, being high-potency sources of energy, are readily utilized by almost every organ in the growing infant's body. For this reason, MCTs have been suggested as a means to supply ketones to support better growth of the fetus, especially when intrauterine growth is slow.[18]

MCTs have the potential to help with a number of pregnancy issues. The following incident recounted by Rosemarie Rosales illustrates this point. I'll let her tell the story.

My sister in faith (we both belong to the Church of Christ) Mechelle Mandal Tirol, 33 years of age, who at seven months pregnant had a problem with her pregnancy. She underwent an ultrasound to know the gender of her baby. She was shocked to learn that her amniotic fluid had decreased to 9.8 cm. The normal count should be 10 cm or more. She was advised to have another ultrasound a week later. By this time it had decreased to 8.6 cm. She was admitted to the hospital. She was given medications and advised to drink lots of water. After three days in the hospital her AFI (Amniotic Fluid Index) decreased to 6.2 cm.

Her doctor told her that if she reaches the critical level of 4.0 cm, she would have to deliver the baby immediately by caesarian section. Mechelle was extremely worried because her baby was two months premature.

In addition, she was experiencing some other problems. Fetal movement had dramatically slowed down, she had a urinary tract infection (UTI), and her lips were cracked and very dry.

She convinced her doctor to let her go home so that she could attend church the following day, Sunday, and to ask her minister to pray for her and her unborn child. Another thing, she really wanted to see me and asked my advice regarding virgin coconut oil. Her doctor was very worried with her condition and was very hesitant to let her go home. She made her promise to return on Monday and have another ultrasound. If the result was still negative, for sure she would have the operation.

Sunday afternoon right after church service, she consulted me about virgin coconut oil and told me about her condition. She asked me these questions: "Can virgin coconut oil help me with my condition? How many tablespoons shall I drink?" I remembered what I read in your book that if ever you're not feeling well, double the dose. I told her to drink 30ml (2 tbsp) right away when she arrived home, another 30ml before bedtime and 30ml the following day after breakfast. Pray hard, be positive and hope for the best. Her ultrasound was scheduled for 10:00 am the following day.

Monday afternoon she called me and was very ecstatic with the result of the ultrasound. Her AFI had increased from 6.2 cm to 7.3 cm. She felt better now. Her UTI has gone and no more drying of her lips. And that from only 90ml (6 tbsp) of virgin coconut oil. What an amazing miracle!

Five days later her AFI measured 8.0 cm. Fetal movement which had slowed down during this ordeal also improved. The doctors were surprised with the results and kept asking what had she done. Mechelle wouldn't tell them. No caesarian necessary. As of this writing the child and mother are doing well.

I still could hardly believe that the oil can really make a difference, can save people's lives and unburden them with anxieties as to whatever health condition they are in. God is really soooooo good for giving us the coconut—the Tree of Life.

How much coconut oil should a pregnant woman be taking? Anywhere from 2-4 tablespoons a day beginning with the first indication that she is pregnant or as soon as she begins to plan to become pregnant. Of course, coconut oil offers so many health benefits that it is a good idea to be taking some every day whether you plan to become pregnant or not.

Add the oil slowly into your diet, especially if you are already pregnant. If you are not accustomed to eating much fat, the added fat may cause a bit of nausea or diarrhea. If you consume the oil with food, these symptoms are less likely to happen. You may want to start by adding only 1 tablespoon of coconut oil daily; if you experience no problems, then increase the dose to 2 tablespoons. If you do experience a problem, cut back on the dose for a while and allow the body to adjust to the added fat intake. After a couple of weeks try increasing the dosage again. In time, you will be able to take 3 or more tablespoons of coconut oil daily without any problems.

BREASTFEEDING

After their baby daughter Louise became listless, Sergine and Joel Le Moaligou frantically called an ambulance to their home 90 miles north of Paris. By the time paramedics arrived, baby Louise was dead.

Medical examiners noticed the baby was pale and thin. The 11-month-old child weighed only 12.5 pounds (5.7 kg); she should have weighed around 20 pounds (9 kg). She was obviously malnourished. On closer examination they found she was suffering from severe vitamin A and B_{12} deficiencies, which had apparently left her susceptible to infection. She died of a pneumonia-related illness.

The parents were shocked to learn of their daughter's nutritional deficiencies because she had been exclusively breastfed. Believing that breast milk provided the best nutrition for their daughter, they couldn't understand why she failed to thrive.

The problem wasn't the breastfeeding itself but an issue with the milk. The child's parents were both vegans and avoided consuming any animal products, including dairy and eggs. As a consequence, the mother's milk was deficient in fat as well as several important nutrients, including vitamins A and B_{12}. The mother's strict vegan diet is what ultimately led to her daughter's death.

Breast milk holds a place in the infant's diet that no other food can fulfill. If the mother is healthy, it contains a perfect blend of vitamins, minerals, proteins, and fats for optimal growth and development. It provides all the nutrients needed for the first year or so of an infant's life. Although breast milk is a perfect food for an infant, it can become less than perfect if the mother isn't careful with her diet. What she eats can have a profound effect on the quality of her milk.

For breast milk to provide all the nutrition the baby needs, the mother must continue eating a good, nutrient dense diet, free from drugs and food additives. Trans fatty acids, rancid fats, alcohol, caffeine, MSG, and other potentially harmful substances consumed by the mother can contaminate breast milk. Even vaccines given to the mother can do harm. For instance, five days after receiving a vaccine for yellow fever a mother reported two days of headache, malaise, and low fever. Her 23-day old infant who was exclusively breast-fed also become sick and was hospitalized with seizures, requiring continuous infusion of intravenous anticonvulsants. The infant received antimicrobial and antiviral treatment for meningoencephalitis. After 24 days of intensive care in the hospital the baby eventually recovered.[19]

During the first few months of life, an infant grows at an amazing rate, so good nutrition is very important. Birth weight doubles around four months of age and triples by the end of the first year. To put this in perspective, if the same rate of growth happened to a 120 pound (54 kg) woman she would weigh 360 pounds (163 kg) after one year. By the end of the infant's first year, the growth rate slows significantly, so that between the first and second birthdays, the weight gained amounts to less than 10 pounds.

Due to their small size, infants need a smaller total quantity of nutrients than adults, but because of their rapid growth rate, infants need over twice the nutrients for their size than do adults. For this reason, mothers should eat ample amounts of healthy fats and protein. Fat is a major component of mother's milk. It supplies about 50-60 percent of the calories in breast milk. Breast milk is rich in cholesterol and supplies about six times the amount adults ordinarily consume.[20] In many parts of the world nursing mothers are encouraged to add extra fat into their diets to enrich their milk. In China, for instance, new mothers are encouraged to eat 6-10 eggs (a good source of cholesterol) a day along with about 10 ounces of chicken or pork.

Eggs, fish, shellfish, and grass-fed beef are particularly important because they supply docosahexaenoic acid (DHA), an omega-3 essential fatty acid, and cholesterol, both of which are needed for proper brain development. Interestingly, even though coconut oil does not contain DHA, coconut oil consumption increases brain levels of DHA.[21] It does this by improving the brain's absorption of DHA from other foods.

Breast milk generally contains between 2-20 percent MCTs depending on the mother's diet. Adding coconut oil to her diet can increase the milk's MCT content to around 20 percent or more. This would be to the advantage of the baby.

Vitamin D is of particular concern. Vitamin D has long been known to be important for proper bone development. It also plays a role in protecting against cancer, arthritis, inflammatory bowel disease, diabetes, cardiovascular disease, macular degeneration, hypertension, multiple sclerosis, depression, and infections.

Defense against infections and the speed at which the body can overcome infection are directly related to vitamin D levels. Activation of white blood cells to fight infection requires vitamin D. Without adequate vitamin D, the immune system is sluggish. Infections can be more frequent, last longer, and even linger indefinitely when the immune system is crippled by a lack of vitamin D. This holds true for infections in the brain, the gut, and elsewhere.

Neurons in the brain contain vitamin D receptors, suggesting that the vitamin may play a role in brain development and protection. Vitamin D acts as a molecular switch, activating more than 200 genes. This may be one of the reasons why it can have such great influence on health.

Vitamin D is known as the "sunshine vitamin" because it is produced by exposure to sunlight. The ultraviolet (UV) rays from the sun penetrate the skin and initiate chemical reactions that convert cholesterol into vitamin D.

John J. Cannell, MD executive director of the Vitamin D Council believes that vitamin D deficiency in women during pregnancy increases the child's risk of developing autism. Studies have repeatedly shown that severe vitamin D deficiency during pregnancy deregulates dozens of proteins involved in brain development.[22] Cannell has noted that the months of birth of autistic children are not evenly distributed throughout the year as would typically be expected. More autistic children are born in the winter than in summer, with peaks in March and November. There also appears to be a strong association between latitude and autism. The farther away from the equator you live, the less sunlight you are exposed to during the year. Those people who live in Canada get less sun exposure than those who live in Florida. Recent CDC prevalence data for 14 states showed that New Jersey, with the highest prevalence of autism, was also the second most northern, while Alabama with the lowest prevalence of autism, was the most southern. In addition, the incidence of autism in Goteborg, Sweden, in children born to dark-skinned women from Uganda is 15 percent—200 times higher than in the general population. Vitamin D supplementation has shown to be of benefit in treating autism. For example, treatment of one autistic boy with 3,000 IU per day of vitamin D_3 (cholecalciferol) for three months resulted in great improvement in behavior and learning, with better scores on IQ tests.[23]

There are few foods that are good sources of this vitamin. We get most of it from the action of sunlight on our skin. Newborns generally have limited exposure to sunlight, so they depend on the vitamin D in their mother's milk. Unfortunately, breast milk is often deficient in vitamin D. This is not a defect in the milk but a result of a vitamin D deficiency in the mother.

Most children are vitamin D deficient, especially during the winter. A study by researchers at the Shriver National Institute of Child Health and Human Development in Rockville, Maryland found that in the US during the winter 78 percent of breastfed infants who did not receive supplementation were severely vitamin D deficient.[24]

Dr. Cannell says that the risk of autism could be lowered significantly by women using vitamin D supplements before conception, during pregnancy, and after birth. He recommends that pregnant and nursing women get 6,000 IU (150 mcg) per day of vitamin D.

The best way to get vitamin D is from sunlight. However, most people living in temperate climates are vitamin D deficient. It is estimated that 85 percent of the population in North America has sub-optimal levels of vitamin D. People living in Europe and other temperate climates are similarly deficient. Vitamin D deficiency is the result of too little sun exposure. In ages past, people spent much of their time outdoors working in the fields and doing other chores. They received ample sunlight to produce the vitamin D they needed. Today we spend most of our time indoors, in vehicles, and in the shade. When we do go into the sun we've become so paranoid about skin cancer that we block the sun's rays with sunscreen lotion. Mothers need to take special efforts to get adequate sun exposure without overdoing it.

Mother's milk is not just a source of nutrition but also provides protection against disease. Breast milk contains the mother's antibodies, protecting the infant from infections to which she has developed immunity. These diseases are the ones in her environment and precisely those which the infant needs the greatest protection. This is one reason why it is beneficial for mothers to have encountered all the childhood infections while she was young so that she can pass that protection to her children, at least while they are nursing. Vaccines given to young girls often short circuit this maternal protection because the effects may wear off by the time they are of childbearing age. Further, antimicrobial enzymes, proteins, and medium chain fatty acids in breast milk provide protection against a broad spectrum of infectious organisms for which there is no antibody immunity. For example, when E. coli (the nasty bacteria that dwells in toilets) is added to human breast milk, 80 percent of it is killed off within two hours.[25]

The gastrointestinal tract of a normal newborn is sterile. During birth and rapidly thereafter, bacteria (microflora) from the mother's vaginal canal and the surrounding environment colonize the infant's gut. It takes about a month for a vaginally born infant to fully establish its intestinal microflora. Infants born by caesarean section are also exposed to their mother's microflora through nursing, kissing, and the surrounding environment, but their gut flora may be disturbed for several months after birth. This may set the stage for abnormal gut flora in the years to come, especially if the infant is formula fed.

Mother's milk contains bifidus factors that encourage the growth of the "friendly" bifidobacteria in the infant's digestive tract. Bifidobacteria are the most abundant type of bacteria found in the digestive system of breastfeeding babies. They are important because they inhibit the growth of harmful microorganisms, boost immune function, prevent diarrhea, synthesize vitamins and other nutrients, protect against cancer, and help digest complex starches and dietary fiber. Bifidobacteria are used in probiotic dietary supplements to reestablish normal gut microflora after antibiotic use and to treat certain bowel diseases like ulcerative colitis and yeast infections (candidiasis).

Be aware that skin creams and lotions are absorbed into the body. You shouldn't put anything on your body that you wouldn't put inside of it. The chemicals in skin

The Colicky Baby

Colic is characterized by agonizing outbursts of inconsolable crying that persist for hours in an otherwise healthy baby. Colicky babies aren't simply fussy babies, they are in pain. They scream and squirm, because they hurt. Fussy babies respond to holding and coddling, colicky babies usually do not. They cry for hours despite all attempts to placate them, making parents feel helpless and frustrated.

Between 20 to 40 percent of all infants suffer from colic. Diagnosis involves the rule of threes: begins within the first three weeks of life, lasts at last three hours a day, occurs at least three days a week, continues for at least three consecutive weeks, and seldom lasts longer than three months. Colic is usually worst at around 6 to 8 weeks of age.

Colic has long been an enigma to medical science. Doctors aren't sure what causes it or how to ease the agony. Both bottle fed and breastfed babies get colic. Dietary changes by nursing mothers sometimes helps; for example, avoiding caffeine, alcohol, or too many cruciferous vegetables (cabbage, turnips, broccoli, etc.). Scientists have investigated a number of possible culprits—allergies, hormones in milk, even stress in the womb, without much success.

Colic has long been believed to be caused by a digestive disturbance of some type. In fact, the term "colic" comes from the Greek *kolikos*, meaning "suffering in the colon." Research suggests this is the most likely cause. Researchers have recently found that colicky babies have abnormal intestinal flora along with active inflammation, which could be the source of the discomfort.[43]

Rebalancing the infant's intestinal environment offers the most promising solution. In a 2007 study researchers examined 83 colicky babies. Over 28 days, some of the infants were given simethicone, a medication that reduces gas; the others were given a probiotic supplement containing *Lactobacillus reuteri*, one of the beneficial gut bacteria found in yogurt. At the end of the study, the babies who received the anti-gas medication continued to cry on average for two and a half hours daily. Those who received the probiotic, however, reduced their crying to 51 minutes a day.[44]

Another study published in 2010 with 48 colicky babies showed similar results.[45] In this study, stool samples from the infants taking the probiotic supplement showed an increase in good bacteria and a reduction in bad bacteria, such as E. coli.

The microflora living in the infants digestive tract is influenced by many factors including the type of birth (vaginal or caesarean), health of mother's digestive tract, bottle fed or breastfed, and if breastfed, the quality of the milk and of the mother's diet. The above studies show probiotic supplementation can also have an influence.

Colic usually subsides after the baby is three or four months old. The relief of symptoms, however, is no guarantee the problem has been corrected, especially if no action has been taken to correct it. The problem just moves to an asymptomatic phase for a time, only to possibly resurface later in the form of indigestion, constipation, bloating, colitis, and such. Colic can be viewed as a warning sign that there is something wrong in the infant's digestive tract. With the use of probiotic supplementation and a proper diet, steps can be taken early to prevent possible digestive problems in the future.

lotions, especially when applied on the breast, can be absorbed into and contaminate mother's milk. Many common skin lotions and sunscreens contain mineral oil, a petroleum product similar to the oil used in your car. You certainly would not want to put motor oil in your baby's milk. Ironically, baby oil which is sold for use on infants is made from 100 percent mineral oil. Mineral oil has been linked to dozens of health problems, including autoimmune diseases and cancer.

Coconut oil makes the best natural skin lotion. It softens the skin, promotes healing, acts as a natural sunscreen, and is completely safe for you and your baby. It is a much better choice over commercial products.

INFANT FORMULA

Formula manufacturers market their products as "scientifically formulated" and would have us believe that infant formula is nearly identical to breast milk. Some go so far as to claim that formula is better than breast milk because of the added ingredients that are otherwise lacking in breast milk. One of these is iron. While iron is an essential nutrient, it is also a potent oxidizer (free-radical generator) and encourages the growth of unfriendly bacteria. For some reason not clearly understood by scientists, breast milk is low in iron. You would think that if the perfect infant food was low in a certain ingredient, there is a reason for it. But scientists believe they know better than nature and fortify infant formula with extra iron because a growing body needs it, or so they believe. However too much iron can be detrimental and for a small infant, just a little can be too much.

One of the protective features of breast milk is its ability to inhibit the growth of disease-causing bacteria such as E. coli, staphylococcus, and streptococcus, which are common causes of illness in newborns. However, when supplemental iron is added to breast milk, the antibacterial properties of the milk are destroyed.[26] Iron acts like a fertilizer for bacteria stimulating their growth. Doctors recommend that mothers of premature infants add a powdered supplement known as *human milk fortifier* to their breast milk to enhance its nutritional content. Of course, iron is included in these fortifiers. Yet adding iron-fortified products to the milk renders the mother's milk ineffective in protecting the baby from infection. This may be one of the reasons why infants who receive either iron-fortified formula or fortified human milk formula are more susceptible to infections than those who are breast fed.[27-28]

Studies also show that babies that consume iron-fortified formulas are more likely to experience neurodevelopmental delays as they grow older. For example, researchers at the University of Michigan showed that children fed iron-fortified formula as infants scored an average of 11 points lower on IQ tests at 10 years of age than similar children fed low-iron formula.[29] If an infant has a diagnosed iron deficiency then iron fortification is warranted; otherwise, it is not necessary or desirable.

Another "improvement" scientists have made is adding soy protein and soybean oil to formula. This has proven to be a big mistake. Soy blocks thyroid function, which can lead to a number of adverse effects later on. In addition, soy protein mimics the female hormone estrogen, which can lead to significant hormone imbalances in the infant that can seriously affect sexual development.

Formulas also contain incidental contaminants that can play havoc on the mind and body of a growing infant. Perchlorate, a chemical used in rocket fuel, has been found in numerous brands of baby formula. The Environmental Protection Agency has stated that the amounts of this chemical present in the infant formula are considered safe, but the Centers for Disease Control and Prevention say that there is still some concern, especially in areas with high levels of perchlorate contamination in the water used to make the formulas.

Liquid infant formulas are sold in cans that are lined with plastic. Chemicals in this plastic can leach into the formula. Trace amounts of melamine and bisphenol-A, both toxic chemicals used to make plastics, have been found in baby formulas. Melamine has been known to cause death as a result of high concentrations in some formulas. Bisphenol-A can adversely affect the infant's brain and reproductive organs.

Powdered infant formula has been suggested as a safer alternative, but this isn't so. Powdered formula may be even worse because it contains oxidized fats that promote inflammation and free-radical generation. When fats are "powdered" they become oxidized. In other words, they become rancid and very unhealthy. In addition, powdered infant formulas are not sterile and may contain bacteria that could cause illness or adversely influence gut flora.[30] Don't use them.

Formula fed infants don't receive all the antimicrobial protection available from breast milk or the bifidus factors to promote healthy gut bacteria. For these reasons, formula fed infants have a much wider variety of gut bacteria, including larger quantities of troublesome ones such as clostridium, which is commonly elevated in autistic children. These bacteria can promote inflammation that can trigger an inappropriate immune response in the brain.

Studies have found that infants who consume formula in place of breast milk are at increased risk of allergies, ear infections, gastrointestinal disorders, respiratory tract infections, atopic dermatitis, eczema, asthma, obesity, diabetes, sudden infant death syndrome, and autism.[31-33] Some research suggests that breastfed children may even develop higher intelligence compared to bottle-fed children.[34]

Because of the MCT content in breast milk, newborns develop ketosis at the onset of breastfeeding. Recognizing the importance of MCTs, food manufacturers add them to all infant formulas. Even when infant formula has the equivalent amount of MCTs as mother's milk, the same degree of ketosis doesn't occur. Most likely the MCTs have been adulterated, probably through oxidation. This would be expected with a powdered formula. Oxidized fats, including oxidized MCTs, are useless in terms of their nutritional value and cause significant distress to living tissue.

In a survey of mothers with autistic children it was discovered that most had not breast fed their infants, thus denying their children the full protection and benefits offered by MCTs.

Despite the marketing propaganda of the food industry, infant formulas are not and will never completely imitate human breast milk. In fact, creating an infant formula equal to human milk would be impossible. "Infant formula can never duplicate human milk," writes John D. Benson, PhD, and Mark L. Masor, PhD, in the March 1994 issue of *Endocrine Regulations*. "Human milk contains living cells, hormones, active enzymes, immunoglobulins, and compounds with unique structures that cannot be replicated in infant formula."

Some mothers prefer to use formula rather than breast milk for fear that their exposure to environmental toxins or drugs has tainted their milk, making it unhealthful. While the milk may be less than ideal, it may not be any worse than the alternative. Formula is usually combined with cow's milk. Dairy cows are exposed to higher levels of pesticides in their feed and to hormones and antibiotics which they are given routinely. Plus the milk has been processed and pasteurized, making it a nutritionally inferior food in comparison to breast milk. In most cases, breast milk is superior to cow's milk or formula. Of course, if the mother is addicted to drugs or alcohol that is another matter.

What about those mothers who cannot nurse for one reason or another? What options do they have? Better alternatives to commercial formulas are the homemade infant formulas developed by nutritionists at the Weston A. Price Foundation. These recipes contain whole, natural foods, including coconut oil. Recipes for homemade infant formulas can be found on their website at www.westonaprice.org.

BREAST MILK ENHANCEMENT

When mothers adopt a healthy diet and lifestyle their breast milk can provide their newborns with the best source of nutrition. However, you can enhance the nutritional value and strengthen the antimicrobial properties of the milk by adding coconut oil to your diet. MCT-enriched milk will also encourage a healthy intestinal environment.

Human milk fat has a unique fatty acid composition. The primary fat is saturated, comprising about 45-50 percent of the total fat content. The next most abundant fat is monounsaturated, which makes up about 35 percent of the milk fat. Polyunsaturated fat comprises only 15-20 percent of the total. A significant portion of the saturated fat in human breast milk can be in the form of MCTs. Sadly, many mothers produce very little. This can have dramatic consequences on the health of their children.

It is important that mother's milk contain as high a percentage of MCTs as possible. This can be done with diet. Given an ample supply of food containing MCTs, a nursing mother will produce milk rich in these health-promoting nutrients. While cow's milk and other dairy products contain small amounts, the foods richest in medium chain fatty acids are tropical oils, principally coconut oil.

The three most common MCFAs in both coconut oil and mother's milk are lauric acid, caprylic acid, and capric acid. The levels of these antimicrobial fatty acids can be as low as 3 to 4 percent, but when nursing mothers eat coconut products (shredded coconut, coconut milk, coconut oil, etc.) the levels in their milk increase significantly. For instance, eating 40 grams (almost 3 tablespoons) of coconut oil in one meal can triple the amount of MCTs in the mother's milk after 14 hours.[35] If the mother consumes coconut oil daily while nursing, the MCT content can increase even more.

Preparation by the mother should start before the baby is born. Pregnant women store fat to be used later in making their milk. After the baby is born the fatty acids stored in the mother's body and supplied by her daily diet are used in the production of her milk. If she has eaten and continues to eat foods that supply ample amounts of MCFAs, her milk will provide maximum benefit to her baby. These mothers can have as much as 30 percent of the saturated fatty acids in their milk in the form of MCTs. If the mother does not eat foods containing MCTs and does not eat them while nursing, her mammary glands will only be capable of producing about 3 to 4 percent.

Eating 2 to 4 tablespoons of coconut oil a day is one of the best things a nursing mother can do for her child. The child will eat better, sleep better, and feel better. Common health problems such as colic and thrush are dramatically reduced. Mothers often report how their baby's health or growth improves with the addition of coconut oil to their own diet. Many nursing mothers are adding coconut oil to their diet with good results.

"A few months ago I recommended virgin coconut oil to a young mother who was still nursing at the time," says Helen R. "This will of course increase the [MCT] content of the mother's milk. The baby became so fond of the milk that she almost choked and could not get enough and she grew 5 centimeters (2 inches) in two weeks when the virgin coconut oil supplementation (of the mother) was started." At present, the young mother no longer nurses, but she adds one teaspoon of virgin coconut oil to the jar of baby food she feeds her daughter.

Coconut oil can work wonders in helping underweight or premature infants grow. "I have personal experience with this," says Jan. "In fact, this is why I started taking virgin coconut oil in the first place. My baby was very low weight and I just knew that something wasn't right. Our pediatrician was no help, he said because she hadn't lost weight she was fine. I finally went to a naturopathic doctor and explained my situation (besides the baby gaining only a few ounces, I had postpartum depression). My baby was nine pounds and I'd nursed the last six months. He said that I probably didn't have enough good fats in my system. That would account for my milk not being rich enough in fat to help her grow and it also probably had a great deal to do with my hormones being out of whack and me struggling with postpartum depression. I started taking virgin coconut oil when the baby was five months old. By the time she was seven months old she'd gained three whole pounds! My postpartum depression had disappeared also."

Jan goes on to say, "We went back for a weight check when the baby was nine months old and she had gained another two pounds and was not only back on the weight chart, but on the correct curve for her age, etc. I had also noticed that she was developing new skills all at once, that maybe she'd not been able to before. My pediatrician was so impressed he asked me what I'd done. I was a little nervous about telling him, but truthfully, the only thing I'd done differently was to take the virgin coconut oil! So I told him and he never rolled his eyes or treated me like I'd lost my mind. He even wrote it in his chart."

The best way for a nursing baby to get additional MCTs is through the mother's breast milk. Consuming 2 to 4 tablespoons of coconut oil daily will accomplish this. If bottle feeding, 1 teaspoon of coconut oil can be added to 8 ounces of warm milk or formula.

Some women may be concerned that if they start adding coconut oil into their diet they might gain unwanted weight. Weight gain, however, is not an issue with coconut oil. The MCTs in coconut oil are converted into ketones and MCFAs that

Maternal Uses for Coconut Oil

Nipple Cream. Sooths and heals tender, cracked skin due to nursing.

Baby Lotion. Moisturizes and softens baby's skin. Also good for mother's skin.

Thrush Treatment. Taken orally can help fight thrush—an oral yeast infection.

Diaper Rash Solution. Applied topically on baby's bottom can prevent and heal rash.

Prevent Colic. Colic is caused by an excess of unhealthy bacteria in the gut. Consuming a source of milk rich in MCTs will improve the microbial environment in the infant's digestive tract.

Stretch Mark Remover. Applied to the abdomen during and after pregnancy prevents and heals stretch marks.

Remove Cradle Cap. Apply to infant's scalp, allow to soak in for 10-15 minutes and wash out with shampoo and water. Repeat daily as needed.

Fight Urinary Tract Infections. Taken orally, can help fight UTIs.

Fight Yeast Infections. Taken orally and applied vaginally can help ease yeast infections.

Breast Milk Enhancer. Consumed orally by mother enriches breast milk with medium chain fatty acids.

Enrich Infant Formula. Add to baby formula to enrich medium chain fatty acid content.

Energy Booster. Add to diet to boost mother's energy.

Immune Enhancer. Taken orally helps strengthen immune system and ward off infections.

Gestational Diabetes Prevention. Taken orally with each meal helps prevent gestational diabetes and maintain blood sugar balance.

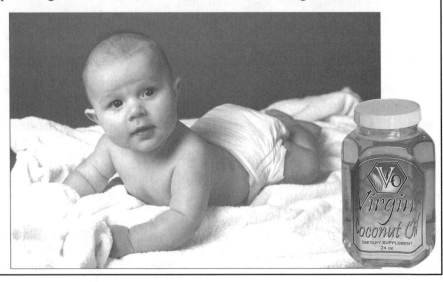

are utilized for energy production and not stored to any great extent as body fat.[36] The body prefers to use them for energy, not storage. In fact, replacing all the fats and oils in the diet with coconut oil can help a person lose excess weight. MCTs are now being studied as a means to manage weight and even as a treatment for obesity.[37-38]

Also, consider the fact that a nursing mother produces approximately 23 ounces of milk a day. At 23 calories per ounce, this milk output amounts to about 530 calories per day. In addition, her body requires extra energy to produce this milk. Therefore, the amount of energy needed for a lactating woman just to produce milk is a generous 640 calories a day above her ordinary needs. She needs these extra calories during the entire time she is nursing. This is far more calories than what she would get from eating 4 tablespoons of coconut oil every day.

SOLID FOODS

Some parents are anxious to start giving their babies solid foods, partially in the belief that it will keep them satisfied longer, so they don't need to feed as frequently and can sleep longer at night. However, studies indicate that introducing solid foods does not significantly affect sleep patterns. The mother's primary concern should not be longer periods of uninterrupted sleep, but the baby's health.

There are a number of reasons why solid foods should not be introduced too soon. The infant's digestive system and capacity to handle foods other than mother's milk gradually develops over a period of time. The ability to even swallow solid food doesn't develop until four to six months of age. We often take little thought in what foods we eat, knowing that we can digest most common foods. An infant's digestive system isn't as adaptable, and even simple carbohydrates (sugars and starches) can pose a problem. The immature stomach and intestine can digest milk sugar (lactose) just fine, but doesn't develop the ability to digest the starch found in grains and vegetables for several months. Introducing foods too early also increases the risk of developing food allergies that will plague the child for the rest of its life.

Mother's milk is the best food for infants for the first year or so of life. Solid foods should not be introduced until the baby is at least six months old and then only gradually, one at a time. When solid foods are introduced, they should not replace breastfeeding, but merely complement breast milk, the infant's main source of food.

After the first year, as the variety and volume of solid foods gradually increase, breast milk remains an ideal addition to the child's diet. The American Academy of Pediatrics (AAP) recommends that breastfeeding continue for at least 12 months, and thereafter for as long as mother and baby desire. The World Health Organization recommends continued breastfeeding up to two years of age or beyond.

By introducing foods one at a time, if your infant has an allergic reaction (irritability, skin rash, digestive discomfort, or respiratory problems) you can identify it. Suspect foods should be discontinued before going on to the next food. Foods should be simple and pure, with no added ingredients. Baby food does not need to be spiked with salt, sugar, seasonings, flavor enhancers, or other additives. The infant should be allowed to experience the goodness and flavor of whole, natural foods and enjoy them as they are.

Cooked egg yolk should be the baby's first solid food. Preferably, the eggs should be from cage-free hens produced under organic certification standards as opposed to conventional factory farmed eggs. Egg yolks from cage-free hens contain the omega-3 fatty acid DHA, which is important for optimal brain and eye development. The egg white may cause an allergic reaction and should not be given until the baby reaches its first year.

Rice cereal is often recommended as a baby's first food because it is one of the least likely to cause an allergic reaction. Oats, wheat, and other cereals are then gradually introduced. Fruits are also some of the first foods an infant receives, probably because parents like them and they are sweet. There is no place in a baby's life for baby food "desserts." Feeding infants desserts and sweets only sets the stage for diabetes, obesity, and all the accompanying health problems later in life.

The foods you feed your baby affect later development and start eating habits that will influence his or her nutritional status for a lifetime. We develop our eating likes and dislikes early in life. If a young child is raised on sugary fruit juices, sweet foods, and refined cereal products, he or she will grow up preferring sweet, high-carbohydrate foods, most of which provide little real nutrition. The child will become a fussy eater, wanting only highly sweetened foods, and will refuse more nutritious foods like vegetables. Often parents will give their children sugary breakfast cereal as a snack. These cereals are little more than candy. Fruit juice, likewise, is essentially liquid candy. The idea that a "fruit" juice comes from fruit gives the false impression it is nutritious. Most fruit juices contain relatively little nutrition and are loaded with just as much sugar as colas.

A better choice for the baby's first year is pureed vegetables without additives. Coconut oil or butter can be added to improve nutrition. As explained in a previous chapter, adding a good source of fat to vegetables and other foods greatly increases their nutritional value. Coconut oil makes a good addition to solid foods because of all the benefits it provides to the growing baby. Coconut oil is hypoallergenic; that is, it is safe for young children because it rarely causes allergic reactions. In fact, true coconut allergies are so rare that only a handful of cases have ever been reported.[39-40] Even when children are allergic to peanuts (a legume) and tree nuts, they are almost never also allergic to coconut.[41-42] So there is little threat of coconut allergy.

Infant's tastes are much more acute than ours. They can taste and enjoy the natural sweetness and flavors of ordinary foods without the need for added sugar or flavorings. Pureed meat in addition to some fruit (without added sugar) can gradually be added to the baby's diet. Cereals and breads should be the last items introduced and then given in moderation. Junk foods, especially those containing sugar (in all its various forms), nitrates, hydrogenated vegetable oils, MSG, and other additives should be completely avoided.

All infants require additional water once they start receiving solid foods. Our kidneys filter out and concentrate waste from the bloodstream. Infants are unable to concentrate this waste material as efficiently, so an infant must pass relatively more

Liquid Candy

Most parents are aware that sodas are not the best drinks for their children and believe that fruit drinks are a healthier option. After all, fruit drinks do supply a source of vitamins and minerals and are definitely better than many other beverages. However, most fruit drinks are no better than sodas. On average fruit drinks contain only 10 percent juice. Actual ingredients are water, high fructose corn syrup, artificial colorings and flavorings, and preservatives.

To be labeled as a "fruit juice," the Food and Drug Administration (FDA) requires that a product be 100 percent fruit juice. Any beverage that is less than 100 percent fruit juice must list the percentage of juice and include a descriptive term, such as "drink," "beverage," or "cocktail."

Even pure fruit juice is not the best for your children. Although they do contain some vitamins and minerals, they generally are not significant sources of these nutrients and are poor sources of other nutrients such as dietary fiber and amino acids. The biggest concern, however, is their high sugar content. On average, 8 ounces (1 cup) of fruit juice contains the equivalent of about 7 teaspoons of sugar. That's the same amount of sugar found in an 11-ounce serving of Coke, 1 cup (2 scoops) of vanilla ice cream, or three medium sugar-glazed donuts. This is why fruit juice is really nothing more than liquid candy. Do you really want to be feeding your children this much sugar?

Americans consume more than 2 billion gallons of juice a year. Children are the single largest group of juice consumers: children younger than 12 years of age comprise only about 18 percent of the total population, but consume 28 percent of all juice. By one year of age, almost 90 percent of infants consume juice. On average, infants consume approximately 2 ounces per day, but 2 percent consume more than 16 ounces daily, and 1 percent of infants consume more than 21 ounces. Toddlers consume approximately 6 ounces a day. Ten percent of children two to three years old and 8 percent of children four to five years old drink on average more than 12 ounces a day. Twelve ounces of juice contains 11 teaspoons of sugar. Sixteen and 21 ounces of juice contain 14 and 18 teaspoons of sugar respectively. That's a lot of sugar for a young child to be eating on a daily basis. In addition, sugar in other foods increases their total daily sugar intake.

Studies show that excess sugar in children's diets can increase the risk of many health problems such as malnutrition, tooth decay, attention deficit hyperactivity disorder (ADHD), and obesity and increases susceptibly to infectious disease.

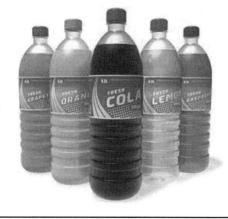

water than an adult to carry off a comparable amount of waste. This means that once solid foods are introduced, there is a risk of dehydration.

Next to milk, water is the preferred choice of liquid for an infant. Parents often give their babies sugary fruit juices to supplement their milk. Plain water is a far better choice. Children don't need liquid candy to quench their thirst. Feeding them a sugary drink every time they are thirsty only trains them to crave sweetened beverages. As they grow older, this habit will turn to a preference for sodas and other sugary beverages. At some point cow or goat milk or even formula may be given to the child. This milk can be fortified with added coconut oil to improve its MCT content.

To maintain all the benefits of MCTs after weaning, you can add coconut oil to your child's food. As a general guideline, normally developing children weighing between 12-25 pounds (5-11 kg) can be given 1½ to 3 teaspoons of coconut oil daily. Children weighing between 25-50 pounds (11-23 kg) can be given 3 to 4½ teaspoons and 50-75 pounds (23-34 kg) 4½ to 6 teaspoons. Don't give the total daily amount all at one meal. Divide it into equal portions and mix it into the food given throughout the day (note: 1 teaspoon equals 5 ml, 3 teaspoons equals 1 tablespoon). You can give your children a little more or less without worry. Keep in mind that coconut oil is a food and, therefore, is not toxic even in large doses; however, too much at any one time can produce runny stools.

12 | Nutrition and Brain Health

SUGAR AND STARCHES
Sugar, Sugar Everywhere

Throughout human history, sugar has never been a very significant part of the diet. Two hundred years ago people ate, on average, only about 15 pounds (6.8 kg) of sugar a year. During the latter half of the 1800s, as sugar refining technology improved and more of it became available, sugar consumption dramatically increased. By 1900 annual sugar consumption in the United States had risen to 85 pounds (38.5 kg). Today we consume an average of about 160 pounds (72.6 kg) of sugar per year. This is over ten times the amount consumed in 1815.

On average, we consume about 200 grams (nearly half a pound) of sugar every day. Total carbohydrate consumption from all foods (fruits, vegetables, grains, beverages, etc.) for an average size adult amounts to about 300 grams a day. If 200 grams of that is in the form of sugar, then two-thirds of our total daily carbohydrate intake comes from empty calories with no nutritional value whatsoever.

Just because you don't add sugar to your foods or eat candy doesn't mean you are not consuming massive amounts of this sweet poison. Sugar is found as an ingredient in thousands of products from bread to nuts to soda and fruit drinks. Today sugars come in a variety of forms: sucrose (white table sugar), fructose, high fructose corn syrup, dextrose—the list goes on and on. Ingredient labels list the contents, starting with the most predominant one followed in order to the least at the end. By using many names for sugar, such labels can be misleading about the proportion of sugar in the product. In many packaged products, although sugar may not be listed first, if you combined all the many forms of sugar under the name "sugar," it would be the first ingredient on the list.

We get additional sugar that comes naturally in foods. Fruits and especially fruit juices are loaded with sugar. If you include these sources, our total daily sugar intake is even higher than 200 grams.

Modern processed foods are loaded with sugar. As sugar has increased in the diet over the years, more nutritious foods have been displaced. Despite the variety of foods available to us nowadays, the nutritional value of these foods are so poor that we can eat and eat and even overeat, yet still be malnourished. We can easily get way too many calories without getting the nutrients needed for optimal health. Our foods, in effect, are slowly killing us.

Sugar Affects Brain Function

Sugar has become a major component of the modern human diet. Studies show that excess consumption of sweet foods, particularly sugar-sweetened beverages, plays an important role in the epidemic of obesity and diabetes.[1] Evidence is now emerging that shows a relationship between high sugar consumption and mental deterioration, learning difficulties, and memory loss.[2]

Researchers at the University of Alabama in Birmingham have shown that mice fed diets high in sugar develop defects in memory and learning. Over a period of 25 weeks, one group of mice received a diet consisting of mouse chow and regular water. The other group ate the same chow, but drank a sugar water solution. The sugar-fed mice performed worse on tests designed to measure learning and memory retention.[3]

The amount of sugar water consumed by the mice was equivalent to a human drinking five 12-ounce cans of regular soda a day. Five cans of soda contain about 210 grams of sugar. While most people don't drink five cans of soda every day, they do get sugar from other sources—fruit juice, candy, donuts, pancakes, cocoa, pastry, ice cream, and even everyday foods like spaghetti sauce, catsup, barbeque sauce, bread, and fruit. It is interesting that the mental defects in the sugar-fed mice occurred after only 25 weeks. What happens to our children's brains after months or years of consuming sugary fruit juices and other sweetened foods?

Advanced Glycation End Products (AGEs)

Oxygen is a very reactive molecule and readily causes oxidation and free-radical generation. Likewise, glucose can react in a similar manner to cause *glycation*. Sugar in the blood tends to glycate or "stick" to proteins and fats, causing permanent damage to tissues and generating destructive free radicals. The glycation of proteins and fats forms what are called advanced glycation end products (AGEs).

AGEs are involved in a vicious cycle of inflammation and generation of free radicals, which amplifies production of AGEs, which causes more inflammation, and so on. They are known to contribute to inflammation and microglia activation in the brain that promotes neurodegenerative disorders.[4-6]

Most of the AGEs in our bodies come from eating sugar and refined carbohydrates. Sugar and refined carbohydrates (i.e. white flour products) raise blood sugar, which in turn increases the rate at which AGEs are formed. While we most often think of glucose when we talk about glycation, another sugar, fructose, undergoes glycation at about 10 times the rate of glucose.

In recent years fructose, in the form of high-fructose corn syrup, has overtaken sucrose (table sugar) as the primary sweetener in commercially prepared products. The reason for this is that fructose is nearly twice as sweet as sucrose so less of it is needed to impart the same amount of sweetness. In other words, it's cheaper and reduces manufacturing costs. High-fructose corn syrup is used in the majority of packaged foods in place of sucrose or other sugars. Look at the ingredient labels of ice cream, candy, cookies, breads, and other prepared foods. If sugar is added, it most likely is in the form of high-fructose corn syrup.

Fructose is often recommended to diabetics and those with insulin resistance because it raises blood sugar less than table sugar. Ironically, while fructose does not affect blood sugar as dramatically as sucrose, it has a much greater overall damaging effect because it increases AGE generation and intensifies insulin resistance, making diabetic conditions worse.

All sources of fructose have the same effect on the body. It does not matter if the fructose is from high-fructose corn syrup or a natural source such as agave syrup (a popular sweetener used in the health food industry). The effects are all the same.

Depressed Immune Function

We are not completely defenseless against AGEs; the white blood cells of our immune system can remove some of these little troublemakers. They do this by eating them in a process biologists call *phagocytosis.* AGEs are engulfed by the white blood cells, broken down or digested and made harmless. The same process is used on invading bacteria.

The ability of white blood cells to phagocytize toxic particles and bacteria, however, is strongly influenced by sugar consumption. Sugar depresses the white blood cells' ability to phagocytize these harmful substances. Studies have shown that after a single dose of sugar, phagocytosis drops by nearly 50 percent and remains depressed for at least five hours.[7] If you eat a sugary meal, your immune system will be severely depressed and remain that way at least until your next meal. So if you eat pancakes or sugary breakfast cereal in the morning, drink a sugary soda with your lunch, and end your dinner with a bowl of ice cream, your immune system will be severely depressed all day long. You will be less able to remove AGEs and more susceptible to infection and inflammation, all of which can adversely affect the brain.

Sugar comes in a variety of forms. Sucrose, commonly known as white table sugar, is the most common. Others include brown sugar, honey, corn syrup, maple syrup, sucanat (unrefined dehydrated sugarcane juice), molasses, date sugar, fruit juice concentrate, barley malt, agave nectar, and brown rice syrup. In addition to these sugars, you may find others included on ingredient labels such as dextrin, dextrose, fructose, high fructose corn syrup, glucose, and maltodextrin. So-called "natural" sugars such as fruit juice concentrate or agave nectar are no better than refined sucrose. The end results are the same. Whether you eat table sugar, honey, or molasses makes little difference. Sugar by any other name is still sugar.

Starch Is Just Another Form of Sugar

Refined sugar isn't the only problem. Starch can be nearly as bad. Starch is the carbohydrate found in grains, potatoes, beans, and other starchy vegetables. Starch is sugar. It is composed of pure glucose. The only difference is that in starch, the glucose molecules are all linked together in a long chain. Once we eat it, however, digestive enzymes break the links into individual sugar molecules. Like any other source of sugar, starch causes blood sugar levels to rise rapidly, increases AGE formation, depresses immune function, and has all the other detrimental effects associated with sugar. Eating a slice of white bread is essentially equivalent to eating 3 teaspoons of sugar. White bread begins to turn into sugar in our mouths as soon as we start chewing. Saliva contains digestive enzymes that immediately begin to transform the starch into sugar.

People who do not eat many sweets or use sugar often may think they are immune to sugar's detrimental effects. Yet if they eat white bread, white rice, white potatoes, and products made with white flour, they are getting just as much sugar as anyone else and maybe even more.

White flour is made by refining whole wheat flour. During the refining process, many nutrients are removed, along with most of the fiber. Manufacturers add back a few of the nutrients but not the fiber. Fiber plays an essential role in the digestion of starch by slowing down the release of glucose into the bloodstream, making the sugar more manageable for the body.

Starch in and of itself is not necessarily bad. After all, the glucose in starch is used as a source of fuel for our cells. The problem is the *overconsumption* of starch or the disproportion of starch in the diet in comparison to fat, protein, and fiber. A moderate amount of starch and even sugar can be handled as long as adequate amounts of fat, protein, and fiber are also consumed.

Artificial Sweeteners

If real sugar wasn't bad enough, we now can "enjoy" artificial sugar—aspartame, saccharin, and Splenda. These man-made products have the sweetness of sugar with fewer calories. Like sugar, these crystalline powders are addictive, but they are even more detrimental to health than ordinary sugar. Yes, they contain fewer calories than sugar, but like any drug, they have undesirable side effects that range from headaches to death.

Sugar, even as refined as it is, is still a product the body recognizes and can process, even though the processing causes the body a great deal of stress and drains nutrients. Artificial sweeteners, on the other hand, are strange new creatures the human body has never seen before and isn't programmed to handle safely or efficiently. This creates problems. While the materials that scientists use to make artificial sweeteners may come from "natural" sources, they are combined in such a way as to form unique chemicals that are unnatural and cause all types of mischief.

One of the most widely used artificial sweeteners is aspartame. Aspartame is sold under the brand names AminoSweet, NutraSweet, Equal, Spoonful, and Equal-Measure. Discovered in 1965, it was approved for use as a food additive in the US in the early 1980s. The US Food and Drug Administration allowed its use even under the heavy criticism by several scientists who warned of its dangers. Despite objections, approval was granted based on research funded by aspartame's manufacturer (Monsanto and its subsidiary, The NutraSweet Company).

Since its approval, aspartame has accounted for over 75 percent of the adverse reactions to food additives reported to the FDA. Many of these reactions have been serious enough to cause seizures and death. At least 90 different symptoms have been documented as being caused by aspartame. Some of these include headaches/migraines, dizziness, seizures, nausea, numbness, muscle spasms, rashes, depression, fatigue, irritability, tachycardia, insomnia, vision problems, hearing loss, heart palpitations, breathing difficulties, anxiety attacks, slurred speech, loss of taste, tinnitus, vertigo, memory loss, joint pain, and, believe it or not, weight gain. In addition, aspartame has triggered or worsened brain tumors, multiple sclerosis, epilepsy, chronic fatigue syndrome, Parkinson's disease, Alzheimer's disease, birth defects, fibromyalgia, and diabetes. Would any sane person knowingly eat a substance that caused or even contributed to these types of problems?

Saccharin, discovered in 1879, was the first of the artificial sweeteners. In 1937, cyclamate came on the scene. This was followed by aspartame in the 1960s and then acesulfame K, and now sucralose. These artificial sweeteners are many times sweeter than sugar. Saccharin has a sweetening power 300 times that of table sugar, cyclamate is about 30 times as sweet as sugar, and aspartame is 200 times sweeter. Gram for gram, these sweeteners contain about the same number of calories as sugar, but since they are so much sweeter, only a fraction of the amount is needed for the same effect.

Saccharin and cyclamate have fallen in stature since the late 1960s when it was discovered that they caused tumorous growths in laboratory animals. Cyclamate was banned in the US in 1970, although it has remained in limited use in the United Kingdom and Canada. In Canada it is only allowed as a tabletop sweetener on the advice of a physician and as an additive in medicines.

In 1977, a ban was also proposed for saccharin. Since it was the only remaining artificial sweetener in use at the time many people opposed the ban, claiming the action was unfair to diabetics and the overweight. In response to the public outcry the ban was put on hold. Instead of the ban, products containing saccharin are required to carry a warning which reads "Use of this product may be hazardous to your health. This product contains saccharin, which has been determined to cause cancer in laboratory animals." Saccharin, however, is banned completely in Canada.

Acesulfame K is of the same general chemical family as saccharin. It has the same potential drawbacks as saccharin in regards to cancer. Like saccharin, it also stimulates insulin secretion, which makes it less desirable for diabetes.

The newest kid on the block is sucralose, better known by the trade name Splenda. It is 600 times sweeter than sugar. This chemical sweetener is so alien to our bodies that the digestive system doesn't know what to do with it. It travels through the digestive tract without being absorbed. Thus it provides no calories and does not affect insulin or blood sugar levels and, therefore, is considered safe for diabetics. Sound too good to be true? Judging from the number of complaints filed with the FDA, it is. Among the major complaints are nausea, diarrhea, abdominal pain, and other digestive disturbances. It appears that Splenda irritates the lining of the digestive tract causing inflammation and ulceration—problems that are already common among many autistic children. Such problems need not be exasperated.

If you're not convinced that artificial sweeteners are harmful, I recommend that you read *Excitotoxins: The Taste That Kills* by Dr. Russell L. Blaylock. This book provides details on the medical research documenting the dangers of aspartame and other food additives.

SUBCLINICAL MALNUTRITION

Most of the foods we eat nowadays are nutrient deficient. Processing and refining remove and destroy many nutrients. Sugar, for example, has a total of zero vitamins and minerals but contains fattening calories. White flour, likewise, has been stripped of its vitamin- and mineral-rich bran and germ, leaving almost pure starch. When you eat products made with white flour, you are eating primarily sugar. White rice is the same; the vitamin-rich bran is removed, leaving the white starchy portion behind. Potatoes are almost all starch. The skins contain most of the nutrients, but how many people eat the skins with their potatoes?

Most of the foods we typically eat are made from sugar, white flour, white rice, and skinless potatoes. These foods supply roughly 60 percent of the daily calories of most people. Another 20 to 30 percent comes from fats and oils. The most popular oils are margarine, shortening, and processed vegetable oils like soybean and corn oils. Oils are often hidden in our foods. All packaged, convenience, and restaurant foods contain loads of fats, including a high percentage of hydrogenated fats. Like sugar, processed oils contain little or no vitamins or minerals, only calories.

For the most part our typical diet consists of foods which are mostly empty calories—starch, sugar, and processed oils. Few of us eat fruits and vegetables. When we do, it's generally as condiments—pickles and lettuce on a sandwich, tomato sauce and onions on a pizza. Our food is loaded with calories but nutritionally deficient. We consume lots of calories but few nutrients. The consequence is that you can eat and eat and eat even to the point of becoming overweight, yet still be malnourished.

The US Department of Agriculture states that most of us don't get enough (100 percent RDA) of at least 10 essential nutrients. Only 12 percent of the population obtains 100 percent of seven essential nutrients. Less than 10 percent of us get the recommended daily servings of fruit and vegetables. Forty percent of us eat no fruit and 20 percent no vegetables. And most of the vegetables we do get are fried potatoes cooked in hydrogenated vegetable oil. Children are often picky eaters and their eating habits are usually worse.

It's bad enough that most of the foods we eat are nutritionally poor, but the problem is compounded even further by the fact that these same foods also destroy the nutrients we get from other foods. Sugar, for example, has no nutrients, yet it still uses up nutrients when it is metabolized. Eating sugary and starchy foods can drain the body of chromium, a mineral vital to making insulin. Without insulin, you develop blood sugar problems like a diabetic. The more processed our food is, the more nutrients we need in order to metabolize it. Polyunsaturated oils, another source of empty calories, eat up vitamins E and A and depletes zinc reserves; other food additives, including iron, burn up vitamins A, C, and E. A diet loaded with white flour products, sugar, and processed vegetable oil quickly depletes nutrient reserves, pushing us further toward malnutrition.

When we think of malnutrition, we usually think of emaciated drought victims in Africa or starving children in India. In more affluent countries, the problem is more insidious. Symptoms of malnutrition are not as evident. People don't look malnourished, and methods of diagnosing deficiency diseases require malnutrition to be in an advanced stage before they can be detected.

When a variety of foods are available, few people develop obvious symptoms of malnutrition, even when their diets are nutritionally poor. Instead, they suffer from subclinical malnutrition. The symptoms of subclinical malnutrition are subtle but have a definite effect on growth, development, and overall health. This condition can go on unnoticed indefinitely. In Western countries the problem of subclinical malnutrition is epidemic.

A diet that is loaded with sugar and refined carbohydrates, as is typical in our society today, is nutrient deficient. The best way to improve the diet is to reduce the total amount of carbohydrate consumed. Replace refined carbohydrates with more fat, protein, and complex carbohydrates (those accompanied by fiber). Although vegetables are considered carbohydrate-rich foods, most non-starchy vegetables, such as zucchini, tomatoes, and broccoli, are low in carbohydrate because they are around 90 percent water. These are also good sources of fiber, vitamins, minerals, antioxidants, and other phytonutrients.

THE BRAIN-GUT CONNECTION

Gastrointestinal disorders are among the most common symptoms associated with autism. The most likely cause is an imbalance in normal microflora. The over proliferation of certain potentially harmful organisms such as *Clostridium tetani* (tetanus) and candida can hamper the growth of friendly bacteria. Irritation and damage to the intestinal wall by these harmful microorganisms cause inflammation, often leading to Crohn's disease, ulcerative colitis, and other gastrointestinal disorders.

There are a number of possible explanations for abnormal microflora in infants. Intestinal populations can be influenced by the baby's diet (including bottle feeding and excessive sweets and grains), antibiotic use, cesarean delivery, and by drugs taken by the nursing mother. Vaccines can also have an influence. Viruses from vaccines using living organisms (MMR, influenza, polio, varicella/chickenpox, PPSV, BCG/tuberculosis) can infiltrate the digestive system infecting the intestinal wall.

Studies have shown that chronic constipation or diarrhea occur in 46 to 85 percent of children with autism, which is much higher than what is found in the general population.[8] For example, in one study a history of gastrointestinal symptoms including abnormal stool pattern, frequent constipation, frequent vomiting, and frequent abdominal pain was found in 70 percent of children with autism, but occurred in only 28 percent of normal children.[9]

Visual examination of the gastrointestinal tract using an endoscope has revealed a high incidence of colitis (inflammation of the colon) in autistic children as well as frequent inflammation in other areas of the gastrointestinal tract from the esophagus (throat) to the colon.[10-12]

Recently, celiac disease has become associated with autism in some cases. Eating foods containing gluten causes severe inflammation and destruction of the microvilli lining the intestinal wall that absorb nutrients from food. As the microvilli are damaged, they lose the ability to absorb nutrients, which can lead to vitamin, mineral, protein, and fat deficiencies. The association between celiac disease and brain disorders such as epilepsy, schizophrenia, ataxia, and dementia has been known for several decades.[13-14] In fact, many new cases of celiac disease are detected following a diagnosis of some type of neurological disorder.[15] As the incidence of autism has risen in recent years, it too, is being linked to celiac disease.[16] Associations between celiac disease and autism have been reported as early as 1971.[17] While not all children with celiac disease develop autism, a certain percentage do.

Some, but not all, autistic children seem to improve on a gluten-free, casein-free diet. It has been suggested that the reason these children improve is that during digestion some of the gluten and casein may be converted to opioid-like substances (gluteomorphin and casomorphin). It has been hypothesized that these substances can mimic the effects of opium-derived drugs like heroin and morphine. Leakage from the gut due to colitis, celiac disease, or some similar condition allows these opioid-like substances to pass into the bloodstream where they are carried to the brain, eliciting a morphine-like response. This has been proposed as the cause of the characteristic symptoms associated with autism. However, not all autistic children benefit from a GFCF diet and many that do benefit experience only slight improvement, so the theory does not provide a satisfactory solution. Microglia activation caused by a combination of factors including gastrointestinal inflammation, vaccines, allergic reactions, and other inflammatory stimulators provides a far better explanation. Neurosurgeon Russell Blaylock, MD states, "While the opioid effect exists, and in some cases may contribute to the problem, it appears that the recurrent immune stimulation of primed microglia is the primary mechanism causing most of the damage seen in autism."[18]

Gastrointestinal disorders can affect the brain in two major ways. First, when inflammation is involved in the gut, proinflammatory proteins are released that travel to the brain to ignite brain inflammation. Second, inflammation in the gut damages tissues and interferes with normal nutrient absorption, leading to vitamin and mineral deficiencies and malnutrition, which can adversely affect brain function as well as overall health. In some cases, the formation of opioids may compound the problem.

NUTRIENT DEFICIENCIES AFFECT THE BRAIN

The brain, like the rest of the body, needs good nutrition to develop and function properly. Vitamins and minerals are essential cofactors in hundreds of enzymatic reactions involving energy metabolism, protein and DNA synthesis, immune function, and cell growth and development. Some function as protective antioxidants, while others modulate neurotransmitters allowing the neurons to communicate with each other. A deficiency in just one nutrient can have serious consequences on brain and nerve function. While nutrient deficiencies don't cause autism, they can increase susceptibility and intensity.

Autistic children are often deficient in one or more essential nutrients, although there is wide variability from child to child. More than half of autistic children have low levels of vitamins A, B_1, B_3, and B_5, and biotin; minerals selenium, zinc, and magnesium; and essential amino acids and fatty acids.[19] Investigators have also reported frequent deficiencies in vitamins C, B_6, B_{12}, D, folate, and the mineral calcium. Adding these vitamins and minerals to the diet does not cure autism, but in many cases this has brought about remarkable improvements, such as better eye contact, less self-stimulatory behavior, more interest in surroundings, fewer tantrums, and better speech.[20-22]

One of the hallmark features of autism is runaway oxidative stress and free radical destruction. The brain is particularly vulnerable to lipid peroxidation of polyunsaturated fatty acids because of its relatively high concentration of these fats.[23] Chronic oxidative stress severely depletes protective antioxidants. The only way to boost brain antioxidant levels is by eating foods rich in antioxidant nutrients. The major dietary antioxidants include vitamins A, C, D, E, and K, the minerals zinc and selenium, alpha-lipoic acid, CoQ10, and flavonoids such as beta-carotene, alpha-carotene, lutein, and lycopene.

Zinc is found in every cell in the body and is needed for about 100 enzyme reactions. It's vital for antioxidant enzyme activity and is essential for a healthy brain, digestive tract, and immune function. Some investigators have found zinc deficiencies in 90 percent of autistic cases studied.[24]

Vitamin C functions as one of the body's major antioxidant nutrients. It participates as a cofactor in virtually hundreds of enzyme reactions, including neurotransmitter synthesis. Autistic children are almost always deficient in this nutrient and when given supplemental vitamin C have shown improvement in total symptom severity and sensory motor scores.[25] Vitamin C is quickly depleted in diets that are high in processed foods containing sugar and other refined carbohydrates (i.e., cold breakfast cereal, toaster pastries, pancakes and syrup, fruit juice, soda, cookies, etc.)

Blood tests that measure antioxidant levels show that people who have high amounts of vitamin C, beta-carotene, lycopene, and vitamin E, score higher on cognitive tests in comparison to those with low antioxidant levels.[26] High blood levels of antioxidants are associated with a high daily intake of vegetables and fruits.

Taking a multiple vitamin and mineral supplement may help make up for some of the missing nutrients in the diet, but it is not a solution in itself. Studies have repeatedly shown that dietary supplements do not afford the same benefits obtained from eating whole foods.[27] Apparently there are benefits associated with whole foods that cannot be duplicated with dietary supplements alone.

EAT YOUR VEGETABLES

Eating plenty of fresh vegetables and fruits is the best way to incorporate a variety of essential vitamins and minerals into the diet. (Please note that vegetables are mentioned before fruits because vegetables are far more important to health.) Studies consistently show that eating plenty of vegetables and fruits can reduce the risk and severity of chronic disease, including brain disorders such as autism. For this reason, the US Department of Health and Human Services has set guidelines to help us improve our eating habits.

You may have heard the advice to get five servings (½ cup each) of vegetables and fruits every day; the latest dietary guidelines actually recommend that we should get at least five to 13 servings (2½ to 6½ cups) a day. The amount depends on your total caloric requirements.[28] An average sized adult female needs about 2,000 calories a day to maintain her weight and health; this translates into nine servings or 4½ cups per day.

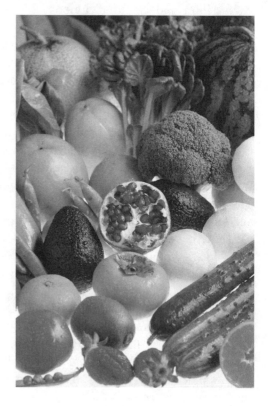

Children ages 2-3 years should get at least four to five servings (2-2½ cups) per day; ages 4-8 should get between five and seven servings, ages 9-13 should get seven to 10 servings, and those 14 and up should get eight to 13 servings.

What counts as a cup of vegetables and fruits? For most fresh or cooked vegetables and fruits, 1 cup is simply what you would put in a measuring cup. There are three exceptions to this rule: lettuce, dried fruit, and potatoes. You need 2 cups of lettuce and other raw leafy greens to get the equivalent of 1 cup of vegetables. For dried fruit, you only need to eat ½ cup to get the equivalent of 1 cup of fruit. Potatoes are not counted as vegetables, since they are mostly starch and should be used sparingly.

Technically, vegetable and fruit juices would count as part of the daily serving requirement. However, juices are very high in sugar and devoid of fiber that would ordinarily moderate sugar absorption. The sugar content of pure fruit juice is the same as an equal amount of cola—about 11 teaspoons per 12-ounce serving. While the juice may include some vitamins and minerals, it is really little more than just fruit flavored sugar water.

The average American adult gets a total of just three servings of vegetables and fruits a day. Children are often picky eaters and usually get less than this. If people are not eating vegetables and fruits, what are they eating? Most likely lots of processed, packaged foods loaded with sugar and refined carbohydrates that have been stripped of their nutrients.

The recommendation is to get *at least* five to 13 thirteen servings of vegetables and fruits in the diet. That is a minimum. If you could add more, that would be even better. These servings are not to be added on top of everything already consumed, but should replace less healthy foods like potatoes, white bread, and pasta in the diet. This would surely improve the nutrient content and reduce the amount of empty carbohydrate eaten. You are not adding more calories, but instead replacing empty calories with more nutritious foods.

WHOLE FOODS

Why are vegetables, fruits, and whole grains so good for us? The answer is because they contain the basic vitamins and minerals along with a myriad of phytonutrients that nourish our bodies, protect us from disease, and keep us healthy. Phytonutrients are chemicals produced in plants that have vitamin-like characteristics. One of these is beta-carotene. Beta-carotene acts as an antioxidant and helps protect us from cancer and heart disease. It can also be converted into vitamin A, if the body needs it. Beta-carotene gives carrots, squash, and other vegetables their characteristic yellow and orange colors. Lycopene is another phytonutrient that has gained recognition lately for its ability to lower the risk of some forms of cancer. It produces the red pigment in tomatoes, watermelon, and pink grapefruit. There are over 20,000 phytonutrients that have been identified in plant foods.

In the past, individual vitamins and minerals were thought to be adequate to cure various health problems. We now know that while a single nutrient may be helpful, a variety of nutrients working together provides the greatest benefit. Nutrients work together in concert, like how all the different instruments in a philharmonic orchestra together produce music. All of the instruments are needed to create the best harmony. Likewise, a wide variety of nutrients is needed in the proper proportion, like that found in whole foods, to provide the health benefits scientists see in nutritional studies.

We've been told for years to eat more calcium to protect our bones from osteoporosis. We eat more calcium than ever before, yet osteoporosis is still a growing problem. We now know that calcium alone isn't going to do it. You can eat calcium tablets until you choke and it won't have much effect on your bones unless you also include other nutrients. Researchers are now saying potassium, magnesium, boron, silicon, beta-carotene, and vitamins C, D, and K along with an adequate amount of fat are also necessary to avoid developing osteoporosis. A deficiency in any one of these could affect bone health.

This is why it is better to eat food containing hundreds of phytonutrients than to take a vitamin tablet which only has a dozen or so. This is why it is better to eat bread made from whole wheat flour rather than depleted white flour. This is why fresh vegetables and fruits are superior to processed, packaged foods containing refined carbohydrates.

Most people will admit that they need to add more vegetables into their diets. But some people just don't care for vegetables. They were raised on white bread, pasta, and junk foods and never developed a taste for vegetables. Too often, vegetables are served more or less plain—maybe with a squeeze of lemon and a dash of salt— but without butter or any other type of sauce in order to avoid adding fat into the diet. But vegetables become more nutritious when combined with a source of fat, which is necessary for optimal nutrient absorption. Adding sources of fat such as butter, cheese, cream, nuts, seeds, meat drippings, crumbled bacon, pieces of nitrite-free ham, and rich creamy sauces greatly improves both the nutritional value of the vegetables and their taste. When served this way, even the staunchest vegetable haters will love to eat their veggies. As you begin to add more vegetables into your diet, you and your children will develop a greater liking for them, especially when they are prepared this way.

GOOD QUALITY MEATS ARE IMPORTANT

As good as vegetables and other plant-based foods are, they don't provide all the nutrients necessary for optimal nutrition. Meat, fish, eggs, and dairy are the best sources of vitamins A, B_6, and B_{12}. In fact, it is impossible to get adequate amounts of these vitamins from plant sources alone. Vitamin B_{12} is essential for the formation of myelin sheath that surrounds the nerve cells in the developing central nervous system, a process that is not complete until around the age of 10 years. The myelin covering surrounding the nerve cells aids in signal transmission. A lack of myelin can greatly reduce cell to cell communication, reducing cognitive ability. B_{12} deficiency has been suggested as a contributory factor in the developmental regression in children.[29]

Meats and dairy also supply fats which are required for the proper absorption and utilization of fat soluble vitamins. Vegetables can provide an abundance of vitamins and minerals, but if you don't consume them with an adequate source of fat, they are not going to be absorbed into the body and will do little good. Along with protein, fat supplies the basic building blocks for most of the body's tissues, including the brain.

Phosphatidylcholine is a fatty substance that makes up a major constituent of cell membranes and also plays a role in membrane-mediated cell signaling. Phosphatidylcholine is a source of choline, one the B vitamins important to human health—particularly brain health. Choline is one of the few substances able to penetrate the blood-brain barrier. It goes directly into the brain where it is used to produce the neurotransmitter acetylcholine, which is important for cognitive function. A number of studies have shown that phosphatidylcholine improves cognitive function. Evidence suggests it may also be helpful in maintaining the myelin coating on the nerve cells. For these reasons, it is gaining recognition as a valuable dietary supplement to support brain health. Egg yolk is the richest natural source of phosphatidylcholine. Eating one or two eggs a day provides a good source of this important substance.

A similar substance that also plays an important role in cell membrane function is phosphatidylserine. This substance enables the brain cells to metabolize glucose and to release and bind with neurotransmitters, all of which aid learning, memory formation and retention, and other cognitive functions. Phosphatidylserine enhances communication between cells in the brain by increasing the number of membrane receptor sites for receiving messages. Phosphatidylserine modulates the fluidity of the cell membranes—essential to the brain cells' ability to send and receive chemical communication. It restores the brains' supply of acetylcholine. It also stimulates the brain to produce dopamine. Dietary sources of phosphatidylserine come from meat and fish. Plants are very poor sources. The typical North American diet supplies about 130 mg of phosphatidylserine a day. Diets with optimal meat and fish consumption provide 180 mg, while low-fat diets supply only 100 mg and vegetarian diets less than 50 mg. Many people can benefit by adding more good quality meat to their diets.

NATURAL INFLAMMATION FIGHTERS

A common feature in neurological disease is chronic inflammation. Inflammation promotes much of the destructive action that takes place in the brain. Logically, calming the inflammation should relieve much of the stress and ease symptoms. Limited success has been achieved with this approach. Anti-inflammatory drugs carry the risk of adverse side effects, some of which may promote neurodegeneration.

An alternative to drugs are natural anti-inflammatory phytonutrients found in vegetables, fruits, herbs, and spices. Eating foods rich in these substances can help fight destructive free radicals and douse inflammation associated with neurodegeneration. Unlike drugs, these compounds are constituents of everyday foods that nourish the body without causing unwanted side effects. For example, luteolin, a plant flavonoid found in abundance in celery and bell peppers, has been shown to exert potent anti-inflammatory effects within the central nervous system.[30]

Many anti-inflammatory compounds are found only in certain plants. Some of the herbs and spices we use every day contain these unique compounds. One of these is thymol, the oil from the herb thyme. Another is gingerol, from ginger root. Gingerol is chemically very similar to capsicum, the spicy ingredient that gives chili peppers their bite.

One of the most potent natural anti-inflammatory compounds is curcumin—the pigment that gives the spice turmeric its distinctive yellow color. Turmeric is a popular spice used to make curry. The yellow color of curry powder comes from turmeric. Because of curcumin's potent antioxidant and anti-inflammatory action, investigators are actively studying its effect on neurological disorders. The spice has proven effective in reducing brain inflammation associated with Alzheimer's disease, Parkinson's disease, stroke, epilepsy, and other disorders.[31-34] Curcumin has been shown to be effective in reducing brain inflammation associated with neurotoxins such as aluminum and infectious microorganisms.[35-36] Curcumin is also useful for reducing inflammation in the gut and other areas of the body that may be associated with autism.

There are hundreds of phytochemicals that possess anti-inflammatory and antioxidant properties, most of which have not yet been studied in any significant detail. Eating a variety of plant foods can provide a great deal of protection against neurodegenerative disease.

Plant foods aren't the only sources of anti-inflammatory compounds. Fish, and more specifically fish oil, can also help ease runaway inflammation. Fish oil is a rich source of omega-3 fatty acids. These fatty acids are converted by the body into hormone-like substances known as prostaglandins that have potent anti-inflammatory properties. The best source of fish oil is from eating fresh fish. Another source is cod liver oil. The advantage of cod liver oil over fish oil supplements is that it has a higher antioxidant content and is an excellent dietary source of vitamin D.

Some people have expressed concern about eating fish or even cod liver oil due to possible contamination by mercury and other pollutants. This is a legitimate concern. Toxic levels of mercury can accumulate in fish as a result of biomagnification. The higher up on the food chain the fish is, the greater the risk of contamination (see table on the following page). For this reason, some people prefer to get their omega-3s

Mercury Levels in Fish and Shellfish

LEAST MERCURY

Anchovies	Butterfish	Catfish
Clam	Crab (domestic)	Crawfish/Crayfish
Croaker (Atlantic)	Flounder	Haddock (Atlantic)
Hake	Herring	Mullet
Mackerel (Atlantic, Chub)	Oyster	Perch (ocean)
Plaice	Pollock	Salmon (canned)
Salmon (fresh)	Sardine	Scallop
Shad (American)	Shrimp	Sole (Pacific)
Squid (calamari)	Tilapia	Trout (freshwater)
Whitefish	Whiting	

MODERATE MERCURY

Bass (striped, black)	Carp	Cod (Alaskan)
Croaker (white Pacific)	Halibut (Atlantic)	Halibut (Pacific)
Jacksmelt (silverside)	Lobster	Mahi Mahi
Monkfish	Perch (freshwater)	Sablefish
Skate	Snapper	Tuna (skipjack)
Tuna (canned chunk light)	Weakfish (sea trout)	

HIGH MERCURY

Bluefish	Grouper	Sea Bass (Chilean)
Mackerel (Spanish, Gulf)	Tuna (albacore)	Tuna (yellowfin)

HIGHEST MERCURY

Mackerel (king)	Marlin	Orange Roughy
Shark	Swordfish	Tilefish
Tuna (bigeye, ahi)		

Source: Natural Resources Defense Council http://www.nrdc.org/health/effects/mercury/guide.asp.

A concern about eating fish or taking fish oil supplements is the possibility of mercury contamination. This chart lists relative mercury levels in various fish. Those with the least amount of mercury are generally safe to eat.

from krill oil. Krill are tiny shrimp-like crustaceans that live in the arctic oceans and feed on microscopic plankton. They are near the bottom of the food chain, so mercury contamination is not an issue. Krill oil also contains a number of antioxidants, including vitamins E, A, and D and a super antioxidant called astaxanthin. You can find krill oil at your health food store or online.

Fish oils contain two important omega-3 fatty acids: docosahexaenoic acid (DHA) and eicosapentaenoic acid (EPA). Both can be converted into anti-inflammatory prostaglandins and help reduce runaway inflammation. DHA is the more important of the two because it is also used as a structural component for some brain tissues. So eating fish weekly or taking a dietary supplement can be beneficial.

Another popular source of omega-3 fatty acids is flaxseed oil. Some people prefer flaxseed oil because it comes from a plant source. The omega-3 fatty acid in flaxseed, as well as other plant sources, is called alpha-linolenic acid (ALA). Unlike DHA, ALA is not needed in brain tissue or converted directly into prostaglandins. However, the body, through a long series of chemical steps, can convert ALA into EPA. The process is not very efficient and only about 10 percent of the ALA ends up as EPA. Little if any is converted into DHA. Even with a very high consumption of ALA, DHA levels in the brain do not change.[37] Therefore, it is essential that you get your omega-3s from fish or other animal sources (i.e., eggs, grass-fed beef), rather than relying solely on flaxseed or other plant sources.

A DAILY DOSE OF ANTIOXIDANTS FROM A COOKING OIL

In recent years there has been a wealth of exciting research on a relatively little known class of nutrients called tocotrienols. Tocotrienols are super-potent forms of vitamin E, possessing up to 60 times the antioxidant power of ordinary vitamin E. Their effects on health are far beyond that of regular vitamin E. Research shows that tocotrienols reduce high blood pressure, dissolve arterial plaque, extend lives of stroke and heart disease patients, possess powerful anticancer properties, and protect the brain from degenerative disease.

Ordinary vitamin E can be found in many foods. Tocotrienols, on the other hand, are not as common. They can be found in small amounts in some nuts, seeds, and grains. By far the most abundant source of these super antioxidants comes from palm oil. Palm oil is one of the richest natural sources of vitamin E in general, and by far the richest source of tocotrienols.

Because tocotrienols are powerful antioxidants, they are being investigated as a possible treatment for heart disease. Heart disease is characterized by atherosclerosis— buildup of plaque in the arteries. A number of studies have demonstrated the ability of antioxidants to prevent fat and cholesterol oxidation and, thereby, arrest the development of atherosclerosis. Although ordinary vitamin E is a potent antioxidant, it has only shown modest benefit in this respect. Palm tocotrienols, however, have shown to be very effective in stopping and even reversing atherosclerosis, therefore protecting against heart attacks and strokes. Researchers can purposely induce heart attacks in lab animals by cutting off blood flow to the heart. This causes severe injury and death. However, if the animals are fed tocotrienol-rich palm oil beforehand, survival rate is greatly increased, injury is minimized, and recovery time is reduced.[38]

The antioxidant power of palm oil has also shown to help protect against neurological conditions as well. Two of the most significant factors that affect brain function are oxidative stress and poor circulation. Oxidative stress generates free radicals that damage brain and nerve tissue. Poor circulation affects the brain by restricting oxygen and glucose vital for proper brain function. Tocotrienols aid the brain by reducing oxidative stress and improving blood flow. Studies show that palm oil increases blood circulation in arteries that feed the brain, thus helping to maintain brain health and prevent strokes.[39-40]

Palm tocotrienols are so effective in squelching free radicals and improving circulation that some doctors are prescribing palm oil supplements for the treatment of neurological disorders. For instance, one mother reports remarkable improvement in her son. "My 20-year-old son has intractable epilepsy. He did not develop seizures until the age of eight. At eleven they became uncontrollable and he suffered significant brain injury. He is now about 80 percent controlled with a regime of anticonvulsant medications and vitamins, including a tocotrienol complex from palm oil. The neurologist and I knew we are on to something with this supplement. His improvement has been remarkable. My son is even regaining cognitive skills!"[41]

Palm oil is also a rich source of beta-carotene, which the body converts into vitamin A. Autistic children are often vitamin A deficient. A study of 60 autistic children given natural vitamin A for three months or longer showed marked improvement. In some cases, substantial improvement was seen within days. Across the board, core autism symptoms such as language, eye contact, ability to socialize, and sleep patterns were consistently improved.[42]

Palm oil comes from the fruit of the oil palm. Palm fruit is about the size of a small plum. The oil is extracted from the fruit or pulp surrounding the seed. Palm fruit is a dark red color and produces an orange-red colored oil. This crude or virgin oil is called *red palm oil*. Red palm oil has undergone minimal processing and retains most of the naturally occurring fat soluble vitamins and other nutrients. The red color comes from the rich abundance of beta-carotene and other carotenes in the fruit.

Red palm oil is a virtual powerhouse of nutrition. It contains far more nutrients than any other dietary oil. Besides being the richest natural source of tocotrienols, it is also the richest dietary source of beta-carotene. It has 15 times more beta-carotene than carrots and 300 times more than tomatoes. In addition, it contains lycopene, alpha-carotene, gamma-carotene, and at least 20 other carotenes along with vitamin E, vitamin K, CoQ10, squalene, phytosterols, flavonoids, phenolic acids, and glycolipids. There are four tocotrienols—palm oil contains all of them. The combination of vitamin E, tocotrienols, carotenes, and other antioxidants makes red palm oil a natural super-antioxidant supplement. In fact, it is currently being encapsulated and sold as a vitamin supplement. The oil is also available in bottles, like other vegetable oils, for kitchen use.

One teaspoon for young children and one tablespoon for adults supplies more than enough to meet daily requirements of vitamins E and A. The best way to take red palm oil is to incorporate it into daily food preparation and use it like you would any other cooking oil. It is very heat tolerant and makes an excellent cooking oil.

Because of its distinctive orange-red color, red palm oil is easy to spot on store shelves. At room temperature it is semisolid, somewhat like soft butter. If refrigerated, it will harden. On the countertop on a warm day, it will liquefy. Red palm oil doesn't need to be refrigerated because it is very resistant to oxidation. You can use the oil when it is hard or soft. Nutritionally, there is no difference.

Red palm oil has a distinctive flavor and aroma. In cultures where palm oil is produced, it is an important ingredient in food preparation and gives the food much of its characteristic flavor. The oil has a pleasant, somewhat savory taste that enhances the natural flavor of meats and vegetables. This flavor complements soups, sauces, sautéed vegetables, eggs, and meats. In recipes that call for vegetable oil, butter, or margarine, you can usually replace them with red palm oil.

Please note that red palm oil is not the same as coconut oil. Besides the obvious difference in color, red palm oil does not contain any MCTs. Therefore, it does not produce the ketones needed by the brain. The benefit of red palm oil is its excellent cooking properties and its rich vitamin and antioxidant content.

Palm fruit produces two types of oil; one from the fleshy fruit and the other from the seed or kernel. Red palm oil comes from the soft fruit. *Palm kernel oil* is extracted from the seed. The two are not alike. Palm kernel oil is almost identical to coconut oil, containing about 53 percent MCTs, and like coconut oil is colorless.

Red palm oil is available at most good health food stores and online. To learn more about the health benefits of tocotrienols and palm oil, I recommend the book *The Palm Oil Miracle* by Bruce Fife.

13 | The Coconut Ketogenic Diet

A LOW-CARBOHYDRATE KETOGENIC DIET

When we eat a meal, the carbohydrates in the food (and to a much lesser extent some of the proteins) are reduced to glucose and released into the bloodstream. Glucose is the primary source of fuel for the brain. It is what keeps the brain alive and functioning. However, microglia over-activation and chronic inflammation disrupt the brain's ability to properly metabolize glucose. As a consequence, brain cells are unable to produce enough energy to function properly. Development is stunted. Healing and repair is hampered. Mental and emotional skills can regress.

In addition, if brain cells cannot effectively utilize glucose, there is nowhere for the glucose to go, so blood glucose levels in the brain rise. This is not a good thing. It promotes AGE accumulation that interferes with brain function and can also initiate seizures, which can cause further damage.

By restricting the amount of carbohydrate consumed, brain blood glucose levels are reduced. When blood levels of glucose are low, the body produces more ketones. Ketones bypass the defect in glucose metabolism, providing the brain with an alternative source of energy. Diets that are very low in carbohydrate become ketogenic, meaning that the levels of ketones in the blood increase to therapeutic levels. This is referred to as being in ketosis. Ketogenic diets reduce potentially troublesome glucose, replacing it with brain-boosting ketones, thus maintaining energy levels and normalizing brain function.

The ketogenic diet has been used successfully for 90 years to treat epilepsy. Recent research has shown that it can also be of benefit in treating other neurological disorders, including autism. The problem with the classic ketogenic diet (90 percent fat, 8 percent protein, and 2 percent carbohydrate), is that it is too difficult for most children and parents to adhere to for any length of time. Fortunately, such a strict diet isn't necessary in order to limit carbohydrate consumption or boost ketone levels. A modified MCT ketogenic diet using coconut oil, called the coconut ketogenic diet, has shown to provide a similar degree of protection while allowing a much greater variety of foods and even a higher, yet still restricted, intake of carbohydrate.

KETONE THERAPY

Ketone therapy is the process of increasing blood levels of ketones to therapeutic levels. This can be accomplished through a ketogenic diet or the administration of coconut oil, MCTs, or ketone-producing medications.

Some investigators have assumed that the higher the blood ketone levels are, the better. Research is being done to develop drugs that can increase ketone levels 10 times higher than what is possible from eating coconut or MCT oils. While some level of ketosis is necessary in order to supply the brain with the energy it needs, excessively high blood ketone levels have not been shown to be that much more effective than lower levels. The idea that "more is better" isn't necessarily true. This is apparently the case with seizure control in epileptics. Measures of seizure protection and seizure incidence with ketones levels do not correlate.[1]

We always have measurable concentrations of ketones in our blood and urine regardless of our diet. The blood concentration of beta-hydroxybutyrate (BHB), the primary ketone, is typically around 0.1 mmol/l (millimoles per liter). During starvation or prolonged fasting, BHB levels increase to 2-7 mmol/l, which is also the same level achieved on the classic ketogenic diet. Therapeutic levels of ketosis can be achieved with blood levels of BHB less than 0.5 mmol/l.[2] This level can easily be achieved by consuming a 2 tablespoon dose of coconut oil. Blood levels of ketones at about this level have shown to be just as effective as those which are many times higher and typically associated with the ketogenic diet.[3] High ketone levels are not necessary.

You can think of it like filling the gas tank of your car. The tank can be filled to the top with fuel, but the engine can only burn a little at a time. The amount of gas in the tank has no effect on the rate at which the engine can burn the fuel. As long as enough gas is available to keep the engine continually running, it doesn't matter how full the tank is. The same is true with ketones. Pumping the body with more ketones than it needs will have no additional benefit. Excess ketones are not stored, like fuel is in the gas tank, or like glucose (which is stored as glycogen or fat). Ketones have a short life span in the blood. If they are not used within a few minutes, they are flushed out of the body in the urine. So a large influx of ketones into the bloodstream will end up being removed from the body and do absolutely no good.

Even when blood ketones are high, the addition of carbohydrate into the diet can initiate seizures, which demonstrates that blood glucose levels also have an influence on brain function. Ketone therapy (adding a source of ketones) alone is not the complete answer. Controlling blood glucose levels with a low-carb diet is also vitally important.

While excessive ketone levels are not necessary, therapeutic levels should be maintained constantly throughout the day and night. Medications or supplements that boost ketone levels only last a few hours and need to be retaken often. During the day this is not a big problem, but at night it can be. At night, ketosis tapers off, and by morning, it is gone.

It is kind of like being able to breathe for 16 hours of the day and then being denied oxygen for 8 hours at night. As long as you have oxygen you are alive and well, but take away your oxygen and you begin to suffocate and die. You need oxygen 24 hours a day, not just 16. The same is true for the brain. It needs energy—ketones—24 hours a day.

Coconut oil is better than MCT oil in that it produces ketones over a much longer period of time, up to eight hours. Taken just before bedtime, coconut oil keeps ketone levels elevated through the night. One drawback to this is that coconut oil also stimulates metabolism, so after eating it, a person may have so much energy that he or she may find it difficult to fall asleep.

The solution to this problem is to combine ketone therapy with a low-carb ketogenic diet. The diet will allow the body to produce ketones continually, 24 hours a day. Even a mild ketogenic diet, when combined with the coconut oil, can maintain ketosis at a therapeutic level. Coconut oil is consumed only at mealtime, so it doesn't interfer with sleep. The brain is never denied the energy it needs, and healing can continue night and day.

The coconut ketogenic diet described in this book is a modified version of the Atkins low-carb diet combined with the MCT ketogenic diet. The diet takes full advantage of the ketone-producing, brain-protecting power of MCTs from coconut oil. This dietary program produces enough ketones to supply the brain with the fuel it needs to function properly. In addition, it enhances insulin sensitivity, normalizes metabolic parameters, neutralizes neurotoxins, calms inflammation, stops runaway oxidative stress and destructive glycation, and subdues harmful microorganisms. In other words, it removes the underlying factors that lead to autism and provides the energy and the building materials needed for brain revitalization.

BASIC GUIDELINES FOR THE COCONUT KETOGENIC DIET

The coconut ketogenic diet consists of a low-carb diet combined with coconut oil in order to enhance ketogenesis. The low-carb portion of the coconut ketogenic diet is based on total carbohydrate intake. It is much easier to follow than the classic or MCT ketogenic diets and allows a little more carbohydrate and protein with better nutrition. You do not need to count calories, measure the amount of fat or protein consumed, or limit what your child eats, except for the carbohydrate.

Let your child eat until he or she is satisfied, but not stuffed. Overeating reduces the effectiveness of the diet. As much as 58 percent of the protein eaten can be converted into glucose, so you do not want them to over-consume high-protein foods either. Since fat produces very little glucose, your child can eat as much as he or she desires.

The amount of carbohydrate allowed is based on the weight of your child (see the Dietary Reference Chart in Chapter 14). Use the weight column to determine how much carbohydrate your child is allowed per day. The entries in the age column are just for reference and correspond to what is typical for each weight group. For example, if your 2-year-old son weighs 30 pounds, his total carbohydrate intake should be limited to 10 grams maximum. If your 14-year-old son is 150 pounds, limit him to 30 grams of carbs. If your 9-year-old daughter is 55 pounds, 15 grams of carbs is her limit.

Total carbohydrate intake should be strictly limited to the values given. Fat, protein, and fiber make up the rest of the diet and can be eaten as desired. At first glance, you might think that limiting carbohydrates would cause a dramatic increase in meat consumption. This is not so. Low-carb vegetables, rich in fiber, provide the bulk of this diet. More nutritious carbohydrates replace less nutritious carbohydrates. This is actually a high vegetable diet, with adequate meat or protein, and ample fat. While meat consumption may increase a little (a few grams), most of the carbohydrate calories are replaced by added fat calories.

A person can live indefinitely on this diet. It is not lacking in nutrients. It provides all the nutrients needed for good health. Consider the fact that the Eskimo traditionally thrived on a diet consisting totally of meat and fat. Carbohydrate from plant foods constituted less than 1 percent of their total calories. They were healthy, without autism, diabetes, cancer, or any other lifestyle disease common in our high-carb society today. This new diet allows many more plant foods, greater variety, and more nutrients then the traditional Eskimo diet. It is probably a far healthier diet than what you have right now.

You *do*, however, need to calculate every gram of carbohydrate your child eats. This is important. As you gain experience you will be able to prepare meals with the appropriate carbohydrate limit without too much difficulty.

Meats, fish, fowl, butter, and all fats are free foods; meaning there is no limit on the amount your child is allowed to eat. Use the Net Carbohydrate Counter in Appendix B to calculate the amount of net carbohydrate in the foods eaten. The term "net carbohydrate" refers to carbohydrate that is digestible, provides calories, and raises blood sugar. Dietary fiber is also a carbohydrate, but it does not raise blood sugar or supply calories, so it is not included in the net carbohydrate count. Most plant foods will contain both digestible carbohydrate and fiber. To calculate the net carbohydrate content, you subtract the fiber from the total. The Carbohydrate Counter in the Appendix lists net carbohydrate on various whole, natural foods. You can figure out the net carbohydrate content of packaged foods yourself. The Nutrition Facts label on packages show the amount of calories, fat, carbohydrate, protein, and other nutrients per serving. Under the "Total Carbohydrate" heading you will see "Dietary Fiber." To calculate the net carbohydrate content, subtract the grams of fiber listed from the grams of total carbohydrate.

Nutrition Facts

Serving Size 1 box (28g)

Amount Per Serving

Calories 110	
Calories from Fat	10

	% Daily Value*
Total Fat 1g	**2%**
Saturated Fat 0g	**0%**
Trans Fat 0g	
Polyunsaturated Fat 0g	
Monounsaturated Fat 0.5g	
Cholesterol 0mg	**0%**
Sodium 170mg	**7%**
Potassium 4mg	**1%**
Total Carbohydrate 24g	**8%**
Dietary Fiber 1g	**4%**
Sugars 10g	
Protein 1g	

Vitamin A 8%	•	Vitamin C 8%
Calcium 8%	•	Iron 20%
Vitamin D 8%	•	Thiamin 20%
Riboflavin 20%	•	Niacin 20%
Vitamin B$_6$ 20%	•	Folic Acid 20%
Vitamin B$_{12}$ 20%	•	Zinc 20%

*Percent Daily Values are based on a 2,000 calorie diet.

This product contains 24 grams of total carbohydrate and 1 gram of fiber. Total net carbs is 23 grams.

The Carbohydrate Counter lists the most common vegetables, fruits, dairy, grains, nuts, and seeds. To find foods not on the list, including many popular packaged and restaurant foods, go online to www.calorieking.com. On this website, all you have to do is type in the food you are looking for and you will get a listing of everything included on a Nutrition Facts label. To find the net carbohydrate content you must go through the same steps you do with any Nutrition Facts label and subtract the fiber from total carbohydrate listed. In addition to CalorieKing another good website that provides the carbohydrate count on various foods is www.carb-counter.org.

In order to stay under the carbohydrate limit for the day, you will want to eliminate or dramatically reduce all high-carb foods in our child's diet. For instance, a slice of white bread contains 12 grams of carbohydrate. This may account for almost all of the carbohydrate you child is allowed for the day. Since all vegetables and fruits contain carbohydrate, only meat and fat would be allowed for the rest of the day in order to stay under the limit—which is not a good idea. A single medium-size baked potato contains 33 grams of carbohydrate—far more than a day's allotment. An apple has 18 grams, an orange 12 grams, and a medium-size banana 24 grams. Breads and grains contain the highest amount of carbohydrate. A single 4-inch pancake without any syrup or sweeteners has 13 grams, a 10-inch tortilla has 34 grams, and a plain 4½-inch bagel has 57 grams. Candy and desserts are even higher in carbohydrate and provide almost no nutritional value, and should be completely eliminated from the diet. All breads and most fruits are very limited if not removed entirely.

Vegetables, however, have a much lower carbohydrate content. One cup of asparagus has 2 grams, a cup of raw cabbage 2 grams, and a cup of cauliflower 3 grams. Lettuces of all types are very low in carbohydrate: a cup of shredded lettuce has only about 0.6 grams. A child can easily fill up on green salad and other low-carb vegetables without worrying too much about going over his or her carbohydrate limit.

A limited amount of fruit can be consumed. Fruits with the lowest carbohydrate content are berries such as blackberries (½ cup 3.5 grams), boysenberries (½ cup 4.5 grams), raspberries (½ cup 3 grams), and strawberries (½ cup sliced 4.8 grams). Any fruit, vegetable, or even grain product can be eaten, as long as the portion size is not so big that it goes over your child's carbohydrate limit. Since most fruits, starchy vegetables, and breads are high in carbohydrate, it is best to simply avoid them altogether.

Let's look at a typical daily meal plan limited to 20 grams of carbohydrate. Net carbs for each item are listed in parentheses.

Breakfast
Omelet with 2 eggs (1.2 g), 1 ounce of cheddar cheese (0.4 g), ½ cup sliced mushrooms (1.2 g), 2 ounces of diced sugar-free, nitrite-free ham (0 g), and one teaspoon of chopped chives (<0.1 g), cooked in 1 tablespoon of coconut oil (0 g). Carbohydrate count 2.8 grams.

Lunch

Tossed green salad with 2 cups shredded lettuce (1.2 g), ½ cup shredded carrot (4 g), ¼ cup diced sweet bell pepper (1.1 g), ½ medium tomato (1.7 g), ¼ avocado (0.9 g), 3 ounces chopped roasted chicken (0 g), 1 tablespoon roasted sunflower seeds (1 g), topped with 2 tablespoons of Italian dressing, without sugar (1.3 g). Carbohydrate count 11.2 grams.

Dinner

One pork chop (0 g), 1 cup cooked asparagus (2.4 g) with 1 teaspoon of butter (0 g), and ½ cup sliced cucumber (0.7 g) topped with ½ tablespoon sour cream with seasonings but no sugar (0.3 g). Carbohydrate count 3.4 grams.

Total net carbohydrate consumed in the above three meals is 17.4 grams, which is 2.6 grams under the 20 gram limit. As you see from this example, the diet provides a variety of nutritious foods.

In comparison, let's look at the carbohydrate content of some typical unrestricted meals. A typical breakfast might include a 1 cup serving of Frosted Flakes cereal (35 g) with ½ cup serving of 2% milk (12.5). Total carbohydrate count comes to 47 grams. A single serving of this cold cereal far exceeds the 20 gram limit. Obviously, cold cereals are not a good option for those following a low-carb eating plan.

Most people realize that cold breakfast cereals are not the healthiest of foods. People eat them because they are convenient, quick, and generally tasty. People certainly shouldn't eat them for their nutritional content. Hot whole grain cereal is considered a better choice. While a bowl of hot oatmeal is more nutritious than an equal portion of cold cereal, the carbohydrate content is about the same. A one cup serving of cooked oatmeal (21.3 g), with 1 tablespoon of sugar (12 g) and ½ cup of 2% milk (12.5 g) provides a total carbohydrate count of 45.8 grams.

A typical lunch might include a MacDonald's regular hamburger (29 g), one medium fries (43.3 g), and a 12-ounce soda (39.9 g) providing a whopping 112.2 grams of carbohydrate.

A typical dinner might include two medium-size slices of pepperoni pizza (64.8 g) and a 12-ounce soda (39.9 g), providing 104.7 grams of carbohydrate.

Our diet is overloaded with carbohydrates. Children learn to like carbohydrates because that is what they are served most often. Food preferences can and do change. As you serve your child more vegetables, especially when combined with butter, cheese, and rich sauces, they will become more satisfying than the junk foods he or she used to eat.

On this diet fresh, raw salads are recommend and should be eaten frequently. A variety of tossed green salads can be made by simply changing the type of vegetables, toppings, and dressings you use. Try a variety of different types of lettuce and other leafy green vegetables. Combine the leafy green vegetables with a mixture of other garden vegetables.

Homemade salad dressings are generally the best. If you use a store bought dressing, avoid those with added sugar. Check the Nutrition Facts label for carbohydrate content. See Chapter 15 for dressing recipes.

Very simple dinners may consist of a main course of meat—roast beef, roasted chicken, lamb chop, baked salmon, lobster, etc.—served along with a side dish or two of raw or cooked vegetables, such as steamed broccoli topped with butter and melted cheddar cheese.

You will find a few low-carb recipes in Chapter 15 to get you started. With the popularization of low-carb dieting, there has been an explosion of low-carb recipes. There are many dozens of low-carb cookbooks available at the bookstore or library and hundreds of low-carb recipes on the Internet. Just do a search for "low-carb recipes" and you will find a number of websites with free recipes. You must always check the total carbohydrate content of each recipe. Not all recipes that claim to be "low-carb" are really that low. Many are reduced-carb versions of standard favorites, but still deliver a substantial amount of carbohydrate.

Feel free to serve full-fat foods, butter, cream, coconut oil, the fat on meat, and chicken skin. Fat is good. Fat satisfies hunger and prevents food cravings, and even diminishes the desire for sweets. Because fat is filling, hunger can be satisfied with less food, so total calorie consumption may decline somewhat. Those who are overweight may even see a reduction in weight. Underweight and undernourished people usually don't have a problem with losing weight, but the added fat in their diet helps them to regain weight to a more healthy level.

Eating out can be a little challenging but has gotten much easier over the years. Because of the popularity of low-carbing, many restaurants now offer low-carb options. Most every restaurant that sells hamburgers, including all the popular fast food restaurants, offer bunless hamburgers. These hamburgers include everything you would expect in a regular hamburger but are wrapped in a blanket of lettuce without the bun. Even if this item isn't listed on the menu, most restaurants will be happy to make it for you on request.

BASIC FOOD CHOICES
Meats

All fresh meats—beef, pork, lamb, buffalo, venison, and game meats—can be eaten. All cuts of meat such as steaks, ribs, roasts, chops, and ground beef, pork, and lamb can be consumed. Red meat from organically raised, grass-fed animals without hormones and antibiotics is preferred. Leave the fat on the meat and eat it. Fat is necessary for proper protein metabolism and enhances the flavor of the meat.

Processed meats that contain nitrates, nitrites, MSG, or sugar should be avoided. This includes most lunch and processed meats like hot dogs, bratwurst, sausage, bacon, and ham. However, processed meats with only herbs and spices added are allowed. Read the ingredient labels. If they don't contain chemical additives or sugar they are likely okay to use. If they contain only a small amount of sugar and no other chemicals, you may still use them if you take the sugar into account and add it to your total carbohydrate allotment for the day. If you use breaded meats or meatloaf you must account for the carbohydrate content.

Unless you go the health food store it may be difficult to find sausage or bratwurst that is free from sugar, nitrites, and other additives. However, if the store has a meat department with a butcher, you can special order link sausages or bratwurst-type sausage without the additives. These sausages can be made using pork, chicken, turkey, beef, lamb, or some combination of ground meats with or without seasonings.

All forms of fowl are allowed—chicken, turkey, duck, goose, Cornish hen, quail, pheasant, emu, ostrich, and all others. Do not remove the skin; eat it along with the meat. It is often the tastiest part. All eggs are allowed.

All forms of fish and shellfish are allowed—salmon, tuna, sole, trout, catfish, flounder, sardines, herring, crab, lobster, oysters, mussels, clams, and all others. Wild-caught fish is recommended over farm raised. Fish roe or caviar is also allowed.

Most *fresh* meats do not have added carbohydrate. They are free foods, meaning you can eat them without doing any calculations on carbohydrate content. The only exceptions are some shell fish and eggs, which do contain a small amount of carbohydrate. A large chicken egg, for instance, contains about 0.6 grams of carbohydrate.

Processed meats are not free foods. They often have added carbohydrate, so you will need to calculate the carb content using the Nutrition Facts label on the package.

One of the things many people miss when they begin a low-carb diet is the crispy snacks they used to eat—the pretzels, chips, crackers. These, of course, are too high in carbohydrate and often contain unwanted additives such as high fructose corn syrup. A zero-carb alternative is fried pork rinds, sometimes also called pork skins. Pork rinds are made from the layer of fat under the animal's skin. As the fat is rendered off, only the protein matrix is left. These crispy treats can be eaten as snacks, used in place of croutons in salads, crushed and used as breading in frying fish or chicken, or as a topping on casseroles or other dishes.

Dairy

Some dairy products are relatively high in carbohydrate while others are low. A cup of whole milk contains 11 grams of carbohydrate; 2% has 11.4 grams and 1% has 12.2 grams. As you can see, as the fat content decreases, carbohydrate content increases.

A cup of full-fat plain yogurt contains 12 grams of carbohydrate and a cup of fat-free yogurt 19 grams. Sweetened vanilla low-fat yogurt has 31 grams and fruited low-fat yogurt 43 grams.

Most hard cheeses are very low in carbohydrate. Soft cheeses have a little higher carb count but are still not bad. Good cheese choices include cheddar, Colby, Monterey, mozzarella, gruyere, edam, Swiss, feta, cream cheese (plain), cottage cheese, and goat cheese. An ounce of cheddar cheese has only 0.4 gram of carbs. A full cup of cheddar cheese contains a mere 1.5 grams. A cup of cottage cheese has 8 grams; a tablespoon of plain cream cheese contains 0.4 grams. Whey cheese and imitation cheese products should be avoided.

Heavy cream has a little over 6 grams per cup. Half and half contains 10 grams per cup, so stick with full-fat cream. A tablespoon of sour cream has 0.5 grams.

You can use most cheeses and creams without overloading on carbs, but be careful with milk and yogurt. Sweetened dairy products like eggnog, ice cream, and chocolate milk should be avoided.

Fats and Oils

Fats and oils contain no carbohydrate, so they are free foods—they can be eaten as desired. Some fats are healthier than others. Choose fats from the "Preferred Fats" category below. All of these oils are safe for food preparation. Steer away from the "Non-Preferred Fats" and never use them in cooking. Completely avoid the "Bad Fats," all foods that contain them, and foods cooked in them such as fries and battered fish.

Preferred Fats

Coconut oil
Palm Oil/Palm Fruit Oil
Palm Shortening
Red Palm Oil
Palm Kernel Oil
Olive oil
Extra Virgin Olive Oil

Macadamia Nut Oil
Avocado Oil
Animal Fat (lard, tallow, meat drippings)
Butter
Ghee
MCT oil

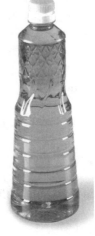

Non-Preferred Fats

Corn Oil
Safflower Oil
Sunflower Oil
Soybean Oil
Cottonseed Oil

Canola Oil
Peanut Oil
Walnut Oil
Pumpkin Seed Oil

Bad Fats

Margarine
Shortening
Hydrogenated Vegetable Oils

Vegetables

Vegetables are listed below according to their relative carbohydrate content. Vegetables with 6 grams of carbohydrate or less per cup are listed in the low-carb group. Some of these vegetables, particularly the leafy greens, have much less than 6 grams. The average carbohydrate content for the vegetables in the low-carb list is about 3 grams per cup. Most of the vegetables you use should come from this group.

The medium-carb vegetable group has between 7 and 14 grams of carbohydrate per cup. These vegetables should be eaten in moderation. Eating too many can easily go over your diet limit. A cup of chopped onions contains 14 grams of carbohydrate. However, it isn't often anyone would want to eat this much onion. A couple of tablespoons or less is more likely. A tablespoon of chopped onion has less than 1 gram.

High-carb starchy vegetables listed here have over 14 grams of carbohydrate per cup. While no vegetable is strictly off-limits, it makes sense that you would want to avoid using these types of vegetables as a general rule.

Most types of winter squash are high in carbohydrate. Two exceptions are pumpkin and spaghetti squash, which have about half the amount of carbohydrate as other squashes. Spaghetti squash gets its name from the fact that after it is cooked, it separates into strings resembling spaghetti noodles. These "noodles" can be used as a replacement for noodles in some pasta dishes. For example, a low-carb spaghetti dish can be made by topping the spaghetti squash noodles with meat and sauce.

Fresh corn is listed in the high-carb category. Technically, corn is not a vegetable; it is a grain, but it is typically eaten like a vegetable. Corn contains over 25 grams of carbohydrate per cup.

Fermented foods with live cultures, such a sauerkraut and pickles, are highly recommended as they supply a good source of friendly bacteria for a healthy digestive system. Make sure the fermented foods contain *living* or *active* bacteria cultures. Most store brands use vinegar in processing rather than fermentation. The best way to get fermented vegetables is by doing it yourself. For information on how to culture your own vegetables check out www.wildfermentation.com.

Low-Carb Vegetables (less than 6 g/cup)

Artichoke
Avocado
Asparagus
Bamboo Shoots
Bean Sprouts (mung bean)
Beet Greens
Bok Choy
Broccoli
Brussels Sprouts
Cabbage
Cauliflower
Celery
Celery Root/Celeriac
Chard
Chives
Collard Greens
Cucumber
Daikon Radish
Eggplant
Endive
Fennel
Green Beans
Herbs and Spices
Jicama
Kale
Lettuce (all types)
Mushrooms
Napa Cabbage
Okra
Kohlrabi
Peppers (hot and sweet)
Radish
Rhubarb
Sauerkraut
Scallions
Seaweed (nori, kombu, and wakame)
Sorrel
Spinach
Sprouts (alfalfa, clover, broccoli, etc.)
Snow Peas
Summer Squash
Taro leaves
Tomatillos
Tomato
Turnips
Water Chestnuts
Watercress
Wax Beans
Zucchini

Medium-Carb Vegetables (between 7-14 g/cup)

Beets

Carrot

Leeks

Onion

Parsnip

Pumpkin

Rutabaga

Soybean (edamame)

Spaghetti Squash

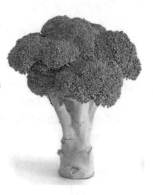

High-Carb Starchy Vegetables (over 14 g/cup)

Chickpeas (garbanzo)

Corn (fresh)

Dry Beans (pinto, black, kidney, etc.)

Jerusalem Artichoke

Lima beans

Lentels

Peas

Potato

Sweet Potato

Taro root

WinterSquash (acorn, butternut, etc.)

Yams

Fruits

A few fruits can be incorporated into the diet if eaten sparingly. Berries have the lowest carbohydrate content of all the fruits. Blackberries and raspberries contain about 7 grams per cup. Strawberries, boysenberries, and gooseberries have a little more, about 9 grams per cup. Blueberries, however, have a much higher carb content, nearly 18 grams per cup. Lemons and limes are also low in carbs, containing less than 4 grams per fruit. Most other fruits typically deliver about 15 to 30 grams of carbohydrate per cup.

With careful planning you can incorporate some low-carb fruits into the diet. Because of their high sugar content, fruits should always be eaten in moderation. Choose fresh fruits over canned or frozen. With fresh fruit you know exactly what you are getting. Canned and frozen fruits often have added sugar or syrup.

Dried fruit is extraordinarily sweet because the sugar is concentrated. For example, a cup of fresh grapes contains about 26 grams of carbohydrate while a cup of dried grapes (raisins) contains 109 grams. Dates, figs, currants, raisins, and fruit leathers are so sweet that they are really little more than candy.

Low-Carb Fruits

Boysenberries

Blackberries

Gooseberries

Lemon

Lime

Cranberries (unsweetened)

Raspberries

Strawberries

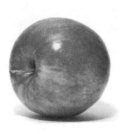

High-Carb Fruits

Apple

Apricot

Banana

Blueberries

Cherries

Currants

Dates

Elderberries

Figs

Grapefruit

Grapes

Guava

Kiwi	Orange	Pineapple
Kumquat	Papaya	Plum
Mango	Passion fruit	Prunes
Melons	Peach	Raisins
Mulberries	Pear	Tangerine
Nectarine	Persimmon	

Nuts and Seeds

At first, you might think of nuts and seeds as being high in carbohydrate, but surprisingly they are only a modest source. For example, one cup of sliced almonds contains only a little more than 7 grams of carbohydrate. A single whole almond supplies about 0.10 gram of carbohydrate.

Most tree nuts deliver about 6-10 grams of carbs per cup. Cashews and pistachios pack a higher carbohydrate punch of 40 and 21 grams per cup respectively. Seeds are generally more carbohydrate rich than nuts. Both sesame seeds and sunflower seeds contain about 16 grams per cup.

Black walnut, pecan, and coconut contain the lowest carbohydrate content of all the common nuts and seeds. One cup of shredded raw coconut has less than 5 grams of carbohydrate. One cup of dried, desiccated, unsweetened coconut has 7 grams. Canned coconut milk has about 6 grams per cup. In comparison, whole dairy milk with 11 grams per cup. Coconut milk can make a suitable lower carb substitute for dairy milk in most recipes.

All nuts and seeds can be used as toppings on vegetables and salads if the serving size is limited to a tablespoon or two. When eaten as a snack it is best to stick with the low-carb nuts. The nuts in the low-carb category below contain less than 10 grams of carbohydrate per cup. Those in the high-carb list have 11 grams or more per cup.

Low-Carb Nuts and Seeds

Almond	Coconut	Macadamia
Black walnut	English Walnuts	Pecan
Brazil nuts	Hazelnut (Filberts)	

High-Carb Nuts and Seeds

Cashew	Pumpkin Seed
Peanut	Sesame Seed
Pine nuts	Soy Nuts
Pistachio	Sunflower Seed

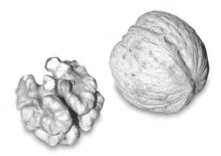

Breads and Grains

Breads and grains are among the 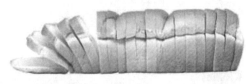 highest sources of carbohydrate. You will generally need to eliminate all breads, grains, and cereals. This includes wheat, barley, cornmeal, oats, rice, amaranth, arrowroot, millet, quinoa, pasta, couscous, cornstarch, and bran. A single serving can eat up all of the day's carbohydrate allotment. A large soft pretzel contains 97 grams of carbohydrate, a cup of Froot Loops breakfast cereal supplies 25 grams, and a cup of Raisin Bran cereal contains 39 grams. Hot cereals aren't any lower; a cup of Cream of Wheat with a half cup of milk and a spoonful of honey comes to 48 grams of carbohydrate.

Whole grain breads and cereals are more nutritious and have a much higher fiber content than refined breads; however, the carbohydrate content is about the same. A slice of whole wheat bread delivers about 11 grams of carbohydrate, while a slice of white bread has 12 grams. Not a big difference.

A small amount of flour or cornstarch can be used to thicken gravies and sauces. One tablespoon of whole wheat flour contains 4.5 grams of carbohydrate. A tablespoon of cornstarch contains 7 grams. This must be calculated into your daily total carbohydrate allotment, so you don't want to use too much. Cornstarch has greater thickening power than wheat or other flours so a smaller amount can be used to accomplish the same effect.

A non-carb thickening option is to use cream cheese, which will impart a cheesy flavor to the gravy or sauce. Another non-carb and tasteless thickener is xanthan gum, a soluble vegetable fiber commonly used as a thickening agent in processed foods. A similar product is ThickenThin not/Starch thickener. This product can be used to thicken sauces the way cornstarch or flour do, and since it is made from fiber it has no net carbs. Both ThickenThin not/Starch and xanthan gum powder are available at health food stores and online.

Beverages

Most beverages are loaded with sugar and provide little or no nutrition. Sodas and powdered drinks are nothing more than liquid candy. Even fruit juices and sports drinks are primarily sugar water. One cup of orange juice contains 25 grams of carbs. Vegetable juices are not much better. Many beverages contain caffeine, which is addictive and encourages the overconsumption of sugary beverages. Many people habitually down five, six, or 10 cups of coffee or cans of cola a day. Some people don't even drink water, relying solely on flavored beverages of one type or another for their daily fluid needs.

The absolute best beverage for the body is water. When the body is dehydrated and needs fluids, it requires water, not a Coke or a cappuccino. Water satisfies thirst better than any beverage without the added baggage of sugar, caffeine, or chemicals. Water is by far the best option and you should make it your first choice. You can spike the water—or club soda, which is basically carbonated water without sweetening or flavoring—with a little fresh lemon or lime juice to give it flavor. Another option is unsweetened essence-flavored seltzer water. Stay away from all artificially sweetened low-calorie soft drinks. Artificial sweeteners carry health risks and keep sugar cravings alive and active.

Condiments

Condiments include herbs, spices, garlic, salt, seasonings, salt substitutes, vinegar, mustard, horseradish, relish, hot sauce, soy sauce, and the like. Most condiments are allowed because they are used in such small quantities that the amount of carbohydrate consumed is insignificant. There are a couple of exceptions, however. Ketchup, sweet pickle relish, barbeque sauce, and some salad dressings are loaded with sugar. In many cases you can find low-carb versions. You need to read the ingredient and Nutrition Facts labels on all prepared foods.

Most salad dressings are made with polyunsaturated vegetable oil. A better choice is an olive oil-based dressing or a homemade dressing. See Chapter 15 for dressing recipes and ideas. Vinegar and olive oil or vinegar and water make excellent dressings.

Sugar and Sweets

It is best to avoid *all* sweeteners and foods that contain them. The so-called "natural" sweeteners such as honey, molasses, sucanat (dehydrated sugarcane juice), fructose, agave syrup, and such are no better than white sugar. All foods containing artificial sweeteners and sugar substitutes such as aspartame, Splenda, xyitol, and sorbitol should also be avoided. Stevia is an herbal extract that is used as a no-calorie sweetener. It is the only sweetener that is permitted.

In packaged foods, sugar and sugar substitutes can appear under a variety of names. Listed below are some of the different names for various types of sugar.

Agave		
Barley malt	Maple sugar	Sucrose
Brown rice syrup	Maple syrup	Treacle
Corn syrup	Molasses	Turbinado
Date sugar	Saccharose	Xylitol
Dextrin	Sorbitol	Xylose
Dextrose	Sorghum	
Dulcitol	Sucanat	
Fructose		
Fruit juice		
Glucose		
High fructose corn syrup		
Honey		
Lactose		
Levulose		
Maltodextrin		
Maltose		
Mannitol		

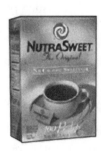 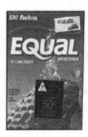 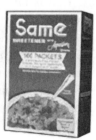

Snacks

Occasionally your child may want a snack between meals. Often when a person starts to feel hungry in the middle of the day, the reason isn't because of hunger but thirst. Simply drinking a glass of water is enough to satisfy these feelings.

If water isn't satisfying enough, there are some low-carb options. Vegetables such as cucumber, daikon radish, and celery make good snacks. Celery sticks can be filled with peanut butter or cream cheese. One tablespoon of peanut butter has 2 grams of carbs and a tablespoon of plain cream cheese 0.4 grams.

If you crave a crispy snack, pork rinds with zero carbs can fit the bill. Another crispy snack is nori—a seaweed. Nori is popular in Japanese cooking and is used as the wrapper for sushi. It is commonly sold dried and roasted in paper thin 8 x 8-inch (20 x 20-cm) sheets. Nori has a mild salty seafood flavor. It can be cut into bite-size squares and eaten like chips. It is usually purchased in a package containing 10 sheets. One sheet has essentially zero carbs.

Low-carb nuts such as almonds, pecans, and coconut make good snacks. A quarter of a cup of these nuts supplies about 2.5 grams of carbohydrate. A novel snack idea is coconut fries. Coconut fries are similar to toasted coconut but fried instead of toasted. Fresh or dried desiccated (unsweetened) coconut is fried in coconut oil until it turns a golden brown. This works best in a deep fryer, but coconut can be pan fried as well.

Meat, cheese, and eggs are other good snack foods. A 1-ounce slice of cheese has about 0.5 grams of carbs. Eggs have about the same. Meat has none, unless it is processed. Some simple snacks are sliced cheese and ham rolled together with a little mustard or sour cream or rolled around some fresh sprouts, deviled eggs, string cheese, and cucumber "boats" filled with tuna salad.

Store-bought protein bars are popular with low-carbers. I don't recommend them. They are nothing more than glorified candy bars and sweetened with artificial sweeteners or sugar substitutes. They are just a form of processed junk food.

DIETARY SUPPLEMENTS

At first glance, because many foods are restricted, including some healthy foods, it may seem that the diet could be lacking in nutrients. That is not the case. This diet supplies all the nutrition a person needs to be healthy.

For some reason, people tend to assume that meat and fat are nutritionally poor foods. That is far from the truth. Meat provides plenty of nutrition. In fact, it is an excellent source of many vitamins and minerals, supplying some essential nutrients not easily obtainable from plant sources, such as vitamins A, B_6, and B_{12} as well as CoQ10, zinc, and other nutrients. Fat, as discussed earlier, enhances the absorption of vitamins and minerals. In fact, this diet will supply more nutrients than your children had ever had when low-fat, empty calorie foods like sugar and refined grains made up the bulk of their diet.

This is *not* a "meat diet." It includes plenty of natural, whole plant foods, both raw and cooked. The amount of meat eaten on this diet may increase slightly (perhaps 5 percent of total calories) to replace some of the carbohydrate removed, but most of the added nutrition will come from a better quality, nutritionally dense source of carbohydrate—fresh vegetables. Your children will probably be eating more vegetables than they have in their entire lives. You could call this a vegetable-based diet supplemented with adequate protein and ample fat.

Your child does not need to take dietary supplements to make up for any missing nutrients because there aren't any that are missing. If you are already giving your child supplements and would like to continue them, you can.

Despite everything that has been said above, certain supplements are recommended *at the start of the diet*. This isn't a requirement, but it is strongly suggested. The reason for this is that that most children are deficient in many essential and supportive nutrients, especially those who have autism. Adding certain vitamins and minerals will help to make up for nutritional deficiencies and speed their progress. The supplements should be taken for the first two to three months of the program. By then, nutrient reserves should be restored and the foods in the diet should provide adequate nutrition, so supplementation should no longer be necessary.

Along with a vitamin and mineral supplement you should include a probiotic supplement. Probiotics are live bacteria, most notably bifidobacteria (e.g., *B. longum* and *B. bifidum*) and lactobacillus (e.g. *L. acidophilus, L. bulgaricus, L. casei,* and *L. reuteri*). These are the types of friendly bacteria that ordinarily inhabit the gut and keep it healthy. These bacteria compete for space in the digestive tract with other microflora, crowding out unfriendly bacteria and yeasts. They also produce essential nutrients such as some of the B vitamins and vitamin K as well as lactase (the enzyme that digests milk) and SCFAs needed to nourish the intestinal wall and keep it healthy. Adding a probiotic supplement will help to reestablish a healthy intestinal environment which will reduce inflammation, infection, leaky gut, food allergies, and digestive distress as well as improve nutrient absorption and bowel function.

14 | The Autism Battle Plan

In this chapter we sum up all the information discussed so far and lay out a plan of action—the Autism Battle Plan.

The Autism Battle Plan is divided into two sections. The first section offers advice for preventing autism, starting at pregnancy and going through birth, nursing, and into early childhood. This is the time when autism is often not yet diagnosed or is misdiagnosed. It is also the time when many children develop normally before suddenly regressing. This is the most critical time for children, when they are the most vulnerable to the conditions that can lead to autism. Taking these steps will not only greatly reduce your child's risk of developing autism, but will help your child develop to his or her full potential socially and intellectually.

The second part of the Battle Plan discusses what steps you should take if your child has already been diagnosed with autism or other neurodevelopmental disorder. This approach is based on the coconut ketogenic diet.

In prevention, the mother's diet is the major focus. In treatment, the child's diet takes center stage.

PREVENTION

Most parents have no idea what causes autism. Doctors keep telling us it is genetic and that there is nothing you can do about it. That is not true. Autism is an environmental disorder and what you do or don't do can have a very significant influence on whether your children develop autism or some other developmental disorder. Autism is preventable.

A recent study on twins by researchers at Stanford University found that in about 33 percent of fraternal twins both are autistic.[1] Fraternal twins are no more closely related genetically than other siblings, yet their rate of autism is higher. This is highly significant because it means that the *shared environment* of the twins had an influence on the development of autism. Their shared environment was primarily in the womb and to a lesser degree during nursing. Therefore, the mother's health, diet, lifestyle, and the quality of her milk appears to have a significant effect on her children's susceptibility to autism.

208

In the most detailed sibling study to date, researchers at the University of California-Davis found that parents with one autistic child have a 1 in 5 chance of having a second child with the same condition. The researchers followed 664 infants who had at least one older brother or sister with autism. Overall, 132 of the infants (19 percent) ended up being diagnosed with autism by their third birthdays.[2]

An interesting survey was conducted involving 378 families having a first born child with autism. Before the second child came along, each of the families initiated changes in their diet and lifestyle, similar to those recommended in this book, including the avoidance of all unnecessary vaccinations. According to the University of California-Davis study above, 75 of these second-born children should be expected to develop autism. Can you guess how many of these children were actually diagnosed with autism? Incredibly, none! Not a single second child developed autism, demonstrating that autism is an environmental disorder that *can* be controlled. If you have an autistic child, you can beat the odds with your next child. If you are having your first child you can be assured of a normal, happy, healthy baby free from developmental problems. By taking preventative action you can stop autism now.

Prevention starts before pregnancy. What the mother does has a considerable influence on the health of her children. Lifestyle, diet, oral health, overall health, and environmental factors during pregnancy and nursing all play a role in the health of the child. Let's look at the things you as the mother can do to assure your child has the best possible chance of developing to his or her fullest potential.

During Pregnancy

Take care of all dental issues. The healthier your gums and teeth are, the healthier your baby will be. Mercury in amalgam fillings is always leaching into the body and can affect the fetus. If you have mercury fillings consider having them replaced with composites *before* becoming pregnant.

When planning to become pregnant or as soon as possible thereafter, consume 2-3 tablespoons (30-45 ml) of coconut oil daily. Start off slowly with just ½ or 1 tablespoon daily with foods and gradually work up to 2-3 tablespoons. Divide the amount over each of the meals consumed during the day. Continue this throughout your pregnancy.

Eat healthfully. Cut down on sugar and refined carbohydrates. Add more fresh vegetables, fruits, and whole grains, supplemented with ample protein from good sources of meat, eggs, and dairy, preferably organic.

Get adequate vitamin D from sun exposure (preferred) or supplements (5,000-10,000 IU/day).

Take a prenatal multiple vitamin and mineral supplement.

Avoid exposure to environmental, industrial toxins (paint and gasoline fumes, smog, pesticides, tobacco, etc.).

Avoid all unnecessary drugs, including over-the-counter drugs.

Avoid drinking alcohol.

Avoid toxic food additives and all foods that contain them (aspartame, MSG, nitrites, nitrates, trans fatty acids/hydrogenated oils, caffeine, etc.).

Avoid all vaccines during pregnancy, including the flu vaccine, unless absolutely necessary.

After Delivery: Mother

Eat healthfully.

Avoid toxic food additives and all foods that contain them (aspartame, MSG, nitrites, nitrates, trans fatty acids/hydrogenated oils, caffeine, etc.).

Take a daily multiple vitamin and mineral supplement.

Get adequate vitamin D from sun exposure (preferred) or supplements while nursing (5,000-10,000 IU/day).

Nurse exclusively for at least the first 6 months. After this, foods may be added gradually, and continue nursing for as long as the baby and you feel comfortable, up to two years or more.

Nursing mothers should avoid alcohol, tobacco, and all drugs (unless absolutely necessary).

While nursing, continue to consume 2-3 tablespoons of coconut oil daily.

After Delivery: Child

The child should avoid all vaccinations unless absolutely necessary.

When weaning, start off with egg yolks, preferably organic, then gradually move on to puréed vegetables and meats, after which you can gradually add some unsweetened fruits. Grains and cereals should be introduced last and used sparingly. Egg whites can be added after the first year. Avoid desserts and sweets. Give ample water while avoiding fruit juices and other sweetened beverages.

After six months of age, when your child starts eating solid food, you can mix in a little coconut oil. The oil can also be added to warm formula. From six to 12 months of age, supplement the baby's diet with 1 teaspoon (5-ml) of coconut oil per day; between one to five years of age, 2 teaspoons (10 ml); after age five, you can increase this to 3 teaspoons or 1 tablespoon (15 ml). As long as the child is free from autism or other developmental disorders he or she can remain at 1 tablespoon daily indefinitely. A larger amount is recommended for those with diagnosed autism (see pager 212). A healthy maintenance dose for an adult is 1-3 tablespoons daily.

If your baby can't have mother's milk for some reason, use a dairy based formula, not soy based formula; preferably homemade (see www.westonaprice.org for formulas). Although these homemade formulas include some coconut oil, it would be better to add one additional teaspoon of coconut oil daily.

TREATMENT
Step 1: Ketone Therapy

The first step in the treatment plan is to raise ketone levels. You do this by having your child consume coconut oil every day. The amount depends on the child's weight (see the Dietary Reference Chart on page 212). Please note that a tablespoon is a unit of measurement and equals 15 ml of liquid. The tablespoon referred to here is not the same as the tablespoon commonly used for eating. The oil should be taken with food. It can be used in food preparation or taken separately by the spoonful like a dietary supplement. The total day's portion of coconut oil should be divided into three equal doses. One dose should be given at each meal. It is not necessary to give any coconut oil with snacks eaten between meals.

The dosages listed on the Dietary Reference Chart are the *minimum* amounts you should use. You can give your child a little more coconut oil without worry. There is no harm in it. Some parents have given their children nearly twice the amount recommended without experiencing any problems. Be aware, however, that consuming too much oil of any type can loosen the bowels, requiring multiple trips to the restroom. Over time the body builds a tolerance to oil and can handle more without this side effect.

Taking the required amount of coconut oil at one sitting can be difficult if it is not incorporated into a meal. Chapter 15 provides suggestions that make taking the oil relatively easy. See the Daily Dose of Coconut Oil section for ideas.

Step 2: Low-Carb Diet

The next step is to adopt a low-carb ketogenic eating plan. Using the Dietary Reference Chart, find the grams of carbohydrate that matches your child's weight, ages are listed only for reference. This is the maximum number of grams of carbohydrate he or she is allowed each day. There are no restrictions on fat and protein.

The carbohydrate gram count listed in the Dietary Reference Chart starts at 2 years of age or 25 pounds total body weight. Use the Net Carbohydrate Counter in Appendix B to calculate the number of digestible carbs in your meals. For children younger or smaller than this, don't count grams of carbohydrate but simply eliminate all grains, sweets, high carbohydrate vegetables (potatoes, winter squash, legumes), juices, and fruit.

Step 3: Dietary Supplements

Most people do not get the recommended amount of vitamins and minerals they need for optimal health. This is especially true for those with autism. Although the coconut ketogenic diet recommended here provides adequate nutrition, dietary supplements are recommended for the first two to three months to bring nutrient reserves up to normal.

A sugar-free, lactose-free children's multiple vitamin and mineral supplement containing vitamins A, B_1 (thiamin), B_2 (riboflavin), B_3 (niacin), B_6, and B_{12}, folic acid (folate), magnesium, zinc, and other basic nutrients should be taken daily. In addition to the multiple vitamin and mineral supplement, add the following even if they are already included in the supplement (see the Dietary Reference Chart for dosages).

- Vitamin C
- Zinc
- Curcumin/turmeric
- Probiotic

Curcumin should be divided into three equal doses with one dose taken at each meal. For example, a 2-3 year old should take 100-150 mg three times per day. You may need to break a capsule open and divide it evenly to get the correct amount for each dose. Curcumin is very safe, there have been no reported adverse side effects reported even in doses many times larger than these amounts.

Vitamin C should be taken once a day at mealtime. Vitamin C and curcumin are taken with meals because they are absorbed better when eaten with foods. The probiotic and zinc should be taken on an empty stomach, or one hour before or two hours after eating; a good time is just before going to bed.

Dietary fiber often binds tightly to zinc carrying it through the digestive tract and out of the body, thus providing the body little benefit. Taking the mineral between meals greatly improves absorption.

The probiotic supplement should contain various strains of bifidobacteria and lactobacillus bacteria. The reason why probiotics are taken on an empty stomach is so that they pass through the stomach as quickly as possible, when the stomach has the lowest acid level. The highest quality supplements are enteric coated. The stomach is filled with strong acids and digestive enzymes that will kill most of the bacteria in the supplement. Few survive to enter the intestinal tract, where they are needed most. So their effectiveness is greatly reduced. An enteric coating on the supplement prevents the capsule from disintegrating in the stomach, protecting the enclosed bacteria from the stomach's harsh environment. When the capsule passes down into the intestinal tract, the bacteria are released. After opening the bottle, store probiotic supplements in the refrigerator.

Young children often have difficulties swallowing pills. You can purchase non-enteric coated probiotics (they are less expensive) and break them open. Mix the contents with a glass of water or a little cream (approximately 1-2 tablespoons) and drink. The water will dilute the stomach acids allowing more of the bacteria to survive. Cream reduces stomach acidity, accomplishing the same thing. Follow with

Dietary Reference Chart

Age (years)	Weight lbs/kg	Carbs/Day (g)	Coconut Oil[1] (tbsp)	Red Palm Oil[1] (tsp)	Vitamin C (mg)	Zinc[2] (mg)	Curcumin[3] (mg)x3/d	Probiotic[2]
2-3	25-34/12-15	10	1	1	50-100	5-10	100-150	AD
4-8	35-60/16-27	15	2	1.5	100-200	10	200-250	AD
9-13	61-90/28-40	20	3	2	200-300	10	300-350	AD
14-18	91-140/41-63	25	4	3	300-400	12-15	450-500	AD
19+	141+/64+	30	5	3	500	15	450-500	AD

Dosage is based on the child's weight, not age.

AD = take as directed on bottle label.

1. Taking a little more than the amount recommended is not harmful.
   1 tablespoon (tbsp) = 15 ml; 1 teaspoon (tsp) = 5 ml.
2. Take on an empty stomach or at least 1 hour before or 2 hours after eating.
3. Take listed dose three times daily with meals. For example, a 2-year-old would take 100-150 mg three times per day. Taking a little more than the recommended amount is not harmful.

a glass of water. You must account for the carbs in the cream in your child's daily total carb intake. A serving of heavy cream has 0.4 grams of carbs per tablespoon.

Step 4: Red Palm Oil

Red palm oil is a food that supplies a rich source of vitamins, antioxidants, and other phytonutrients such as vitamin E (including the super potent tocotrienols), provitamin A, vitamin K, CoQ10, and numerous carotenes. It is heat stable and makes an excellent cooking oil. Use it in your cooking and baking or add it to dishes after cooking as a flavor enhancer. Taken by the spoonful it has a strong flavor that most people find difficult to tolerate, but when mixed with other foods or used to cook eggs, meat, or vegetables, it enhances the flavor of the foods. The amount of red palm oil listed on the Dietary Reference Chart is the *minimum* daily dosage. You can increase this somewhat if desired.

Step 5: Fish Oil

Fish oil is beneficial because it provides DHA, an important omega-3 fatty acid necessary for healthy brain function, and supplies precursors for the production of prostaglandins that help reduce inflammation. Fish oil can be obtained by eating fish or taking supplements. The best source of fish oil is from eating fresh fish. One fish meal a week is sufficient. Or you may also use cod liver oil or krill oil, 2-3 teaspoons per week. This is not a lot. Coconut oil improves the absorption of DHA into the brain, where it is needed most. If most of the fat in the diet comes from coconut oil, the need for omega-3 fatty acids is reduced by about half.

Fish oil supplements are vulnerable to oxidation. Do not use fish oil for cooking. Cooking temperatures seriously degrade the oil. Store the oil in the refrigerator. Do not use it after the expiration date.

Step 6: Vitamin D

Exposing the skin to direct sunlight, without sunscreen, is the most effective and the most natural way to get vitamin D. You don't want to use sunscreen because it blocks the UV rays that trigger vitamin synthesis. A lotion with a sun protection factor (SPF) of just 15 can cut vitamin D synthesis by 99 percent.[3] Contrary to overcautious recommendations to avoid sun exposure, we actually need some sun to produce vitamin D. For a light skinned person, about 10-15 minutes a day of full body exposure is usually adequate. More time is needed if the sun is not directly overhead, as in the early morning or late in the afternoon, or if it is cloudy, because the sun's intensity is decreased. A dark-skinned person may need two or three times this amount of exposure to produce the same amount of vitamin D.

If you have any reservations about sunburn, you can apply a thin coat of coconut oil over all exposed skin. The oil protects the skin from damage without interfering with vitamin D synthesis. Coconut oil will allow longer exposure under the sun without fear of burning. Other oils do not have this protective characteristic and are not recommended.

At latitudes greater than 35 degrees both north and south, sun exposure is greatly reduced in the winter. This would include US states north of Alabama and all of Europe. It is impossible to get enough sun exposure to produce sufficient amounts of vitamin D. Virtually everyone at a latitude greater than 35 has a chronic vitamin D deficiency during the winter no matter how much sun they get. In this case, vitamin D needs to come another way. One option is to eat foods that contain vitamin D. Foods, even those with the highest vitamin D levels, are generally insufficient, but the highest sources are found in milk, fish, eggs, Shitake mushrooms, and liver. Lard from pigs that have had ample exposure to sunlight is a modest source of vitamin D. Pigs get vitamin D just as humans do, from the sun. Pigs lack a thick covering of hair, so skin exposure to the sun produces the vitamin, which is stored in the animal's fat. The best dietary source of vitamin D, however, is cod liver oil.

One more source is from dietary supplements. If you take a supplement, make sure it contains vitamin D_3 (cholecalciferol), which is human vitamin D. Do not use the synthetic and inferior vitamin D_2. Vitamin D is a fat soluble vitamin and, therefore, requires an adequate amount of dietary fat for proper absorption. Vitamin D supplements should be taken with meals that contain fat. The recommended dietary allowance (RDA) for vitamin D is 10-15 micograms (400-600 IU) per day. These are minimum values set to prevent vitamin D deficiency diseases such as rickets. Based on the latest research, however, 5-10 times this amount appears to provide the best overall health benefit.[4] For a child up to 12 months of age that would equate to 50-100 mcg (2,000-4,000 IU) and for children 1-18 years of age 75-150 mcg (3,000-6,000 IU). Children with autism would do better with the higher values. Pregnant and lactating women should get 125-150 mcg (5,000-6,000 IU) daily.

The synthesis of cholesterol into vitamin D from sunlight is much more productive than that obtained from dietary sources. For example, 15 minutes of summer noonday sun on each side of the body will generate about 10,000 IU of vitamin D, which is the amount provided by consuming 100 glasses of milk (100 IU/8 oz glass) or taking 25 standard multivitamins (400 IU/tablet). You don't need to worry about getting too much vitamin D from the sun. It is impossible to get an overdose of vitamin D this way because the body has feedback mechanisms in place to prevent this. The best way to build up vitamin D reserves is to get out into the sun. Ten minutes of direct sun exposure on the arms and legs will produce about 3,000 IU.[2] Thirty minutes of full body sun exposure three to four times a week is adequate for most light skinned people. Dark skinned people need more.

BASIC DIETARY GUIDELINES

Focus on eating fresh, whole foods, preferably organically produced. Eat plenty of low-starch vegetables with adequate meats, fish, poultry, and eggs supplemented with full-fat dairy, nuts, fruits, and as allowed, a limited amount of higher starch vegetables.

Avoid as much as possible prepackaged, processed foods. Most packaged foods contain ingredients that are unhealthful and may contribute to neurological problems. Reading ingredient labels should become second nature to you. Ingredients that you should take special care to avoid are hydrogenated or partially hydrogenated vegetable oil, shortening, margarine, nitrites, nitrates, monosodium glutamate (MSG), aspartame, sodium aluminum phosphate, aluminum ammonium sulfate, calcium aluminum silicate, sodium aluminosilicate, and powdered or dehydrated milk, butter, cheese, and eggs. Additives that contain MSG include hydrolyzed vegetable protein, sodium caseinate, calcium caseinate, yeast extract, autolyzed yeast, soy protein isolate, textured protein, and often "natural flavors."

All products made with wheat flour contain gluten and are high in carbohydrate. This includes pizza, donuts, crackers, chips, cookies, pie crust, cake, pancake and muffin mixes, bread, rolls, egg rolls, hot and cold breakfast cereals, toaster pastries, pasta, pretzels, tortillas, canned soup, breaded fish, and macaroni and cheese, to mention just a few.

Sugar and artificial sweeteners of all types and especially aspartame, fructose, high fructose corn syrup, and agave syrup should be avoided. Look for different types of sugar such as sorbitol, dextrin, mannitol, or any ingredient ending in "-ose,' such as glucose, maltose, lactose, fructose, sucrose, dextrose, etc. All these sugars are converted into glucose—blood sugar, which will influence ketone production. Be aware that even non-food items can affect ketones levels. Some brands of sunscreen contain sorbitol. Enough sorbitol can be absorbed through the skin to lower ketone levels. Read ingredient labels on all skin lotions and creams your child uses. Many foods, gums, and candy that are advertised as being "sugar-free" are not carbohydrate free and may not be appropriate for this diet. Read nutrition facts labels for total carbohydrate content.

It is a good idea to avoid any product that contains refined vegetable oils, which would include corn, soybean, safflower, cottonseed, canola, sunflower, and peanut oils. If these oils are used in processed foods, they are probably rancid. They should never be used as cooking oils. Better choices for food preparation are olive, coconut, palm, and macadamia nut oils.

Avoid caffeinated beverages, sodas, powdered drink mixes, fruit and vegetable juices, and even zero calorie drinks sweetened with aspartame or other artificial sweetener. Water is the healthiest beverage.

Avoid aluminum cookware. Use aluminum-free salt or natural sea salt. Avoid all skin care products (e.g., deodorants) and drugs (e.g., antacids, buffered aspirin) that contain aluminum. Keep in mind that almost all commercially made non-yeast baked goods (available in grocery stores and restaurants) that use baking powder use aluminum-containing baking power. Boxed mixes, such a pancake mix, also contain aluminum. Even commercially made yeast breads, rolls, and sweetbreads are usually baked in aluminum pans. The fact that baked goods often contain preservatives, nitrates, dyes, and other potentially harmful additives provides further reasons to avoid them all.

TEST FOR ALLERGIES

A number of parents have reported significant improvement in their autistic children when put on gluten-free and casein-free diets. However, not all autistic children benefit. If the child is allergic to wheat/gluten or milk/casein, eliminating these foods will be of benefit. If there is no food sensitivity, eliminating these foods will likely have no effect. It is also possible for them to have allergies to other foods such as eggs, fish, soy, or corn. These foods need to be identified and eliminated as well.

Some parents put their children on a GFCF diet or eliminate other foods without any testing, hoping this might help. The problem with randomly eliminating foods is that it limits variety and may reduce nutrition. Dairy provides a good source of many nutrients, especially calcium. If your child is not allergic to milk or casein there is no need to eliminate all dairy products, which would include cream, cheese, and butter. Cheese and butter are wonderful foods that can spark up many vegetable dishes to make them more appetizing to your child. However, if your child is allergic to milk, he or she needs to eliminate all dairy. The only way to tell is by going to the doctor and having allergy tests done, including tests for celiac disease.

In some cases, children can be sensitive to certain foods even when no allergy can be detected. Food sensitivities can be identified by observation. After eating a suspect food does your child's symptoms become aggravated? Is there a deterioration in behavior, sleep patterns, or performance? Are digestive issues intensified?

Parents who keep food diaries can often associate the consumption of particular foods with an increased intensity of symptoms. If a particular food is suspected, it should be removed from the diet for a trial period of three weeks and any improvements noted. On being reintroduced into the diet, it will likely trigger an exacerbation of the symptoms. This way you can know for sure the food is causing problems and should be eliminated. If the food does not cause any noticeable changes when it is introduced back into the diet, it is probably not a problem. Often, the foods that your child likes the most and eats the most frequently cause the most problems. Be suspicious of any favorite foods.

Allergy testing should be done as soon as possible to identify and eliminate any troublemakers. It is important that you identify these foods, as they can keep inflammation alive and hamper progress. Not all children will have allergies or sensitivities. However, if digestive problems are present, chances are high that problems exist and allergy testing is warranted.

Some allergies are lifelong conditions and offending foods need to be eliminated for life. Other foods may cause problems for a period of time, but as intestinal health, immune function, and overall health improves these sensitivities diminish or fade away entirely. In time, some of these foods may be added back into the diet.

GETTING STARTED

If your child is old enough to get into the pantry, you may need to remove all forbidden foods or at least place them out of reach. You don't want to have all your efforts thwarted by a casual foray into the kitchen. If there are other people living in the house who have no dietary restraints, it will make the diet a bit harder. You might want to put restricted foods in a place where no one except you or those who eat them have access to them.

Next, you need to stock your refrigerator and cupboards with the types of foods that are allowed on the diet. Have them available at all times so that there is less of a temptation to resort to serving restricted foods. Purchase plenty of coconut oil. Have all your dietary supplements on hand.

Coconut oil, red palm oil, and the other items can all be purchased from your local health food store or online. It doesn't matter what brand or type of coconut oil you use. Most of the brands will be labeled as "Virgin," "Extra Virgin," or "Expeller Pressed." Any of them will do. Start using the oil in your everyday cooking now. In recipes that call for butter, margarine, vegetable oil, or shortening, use coconut oil instead. Start including some coconut oil in your cooking as soon as possible so that your child will become familiar with the taste.

Virgin coconut oil has had minimal processing so it always retains some coconut flavor and aroma. There are various ways to produce virgin coconut oil, so there is a wide variation in taste from one brand to the next. Some brands have a strong coconut flavor while others are more subtle. Try several different brands and stick with the ones that taste best to you and your family. If you don't like the taste of coconut, expeller pressed coconut oil would be more to your liking. It has undergone more processing and all of the coconut flavor and aroma has been removed, leaving it essentially tasteless. It's also a little less expensive.

Start immediately experimenting with preparing low-carb meals using coconut and red palm oils. Calculate the carb content for each serving, paying special attention to stay within your child's daily carbohydrate limit. Limiting carb intake is a primary feature of this program. Don't just guess: *calculate the carbs*. This is very important. With experience over time you will be able to judge fairly accurately the carb content of frequently eaten meals, and this task will become less of a chore.

It will be helpful to compile a file of tested low-carb recipes and meal plans that your children enjoy. Get into the habit of planning meals and snacks before going to the grocery store so you have everything on hand when preparing meals. If you shop for groceries once a week, it is a good idea to plan each meal for the week before shopping.

Meal planning isn't as difficult as it may seem at first. Once you find meals your child likes, use them often. You can do just fine with seven basic dinners and repeat them. You do the same with breakfast and lunch. Once you have these down, meal planning and preparation become relatively easy. As you become more comfortable with this schedule you can add variations into the meals or try entirely new meals now and again for a change of pace.

While the daily total carbohydrate amount consumed is strictly limited, there is no limit on other types of foods. At mealtimes your child should be allowed to eat until he or she is satisfied, but not stuffed. Eating too much can reduce blood ketones. Although you need not keep a count on the protein consumed, some of the protein will be converted into glucose. Eating too much meat can raise blood glucose levels. If portion sizes are reasonable, overeating is not usually a problem since the fat in the diet provides a feeling of satiety.

Instruct all members of the family, including grandparents, not to give your autistic child anything to eat that is off-limits. Grandparents are often tempted to give kids treats, thinking there is no harm in just a little. But there is. It can dramatically decrease ketone levels and cause seizures in those who are prone to seizures or affect behavior. Teachers and babysitters also need to know about your child's dietary restrictions.

WHAT TO EXPECT

Autistic children are often fussy eaters and resist changes to their diet. Depending on how different the new meals are, you may face some heavy opposition at first. This may involve tantrums and otherwise bad behavior. Don't succumb to your child's demands. It may take a few days, but in time hunger will rule out and he or she will begin eating what you serve. In time your son or daughter will even begin to enjoy your low-carb meals.

Seeing other members of the family eat favorite foods that are off limits will cause problems. Keep these foods out of sight. Don't allow other members of the family to eat these foods in his or her presence.

This program will improve not only brain health but overall health as well. Poor quality empty calorie foods are replaced by higher quality nutrient dense foods. This may have a dramatic affect on the body. Many people notice a marked increase in energy and vitality as they adopt the new eating regimen. Others experience a variety of changes, some good and some not so good, but all of them will ultimately result in improved health. Knowing what to expect will help prepare you for the transformation that will occur.

As you change your child's eating habits and the types of foods eaten, you will be increasing the amount of fiber consumed and reducing easily digestible starch and sugar. Fat consumption will be higher than it was previously. All this can have a marked impact on digestive function. The frequency and consistency of bowel movements may change. If your child is normally constipated, you can expect stools to be softer and more frequent. A healthy digestive tract should evacuate between one to three times daily. Any less than that indicates constipation. Doctors may say that one bowel movement every one to three days is average or normal, but *average* does not mean *healthy*. Whether your child suffers from constipation or diarrhea or both, as he or she eats healthier foods, bowel movements will become more regular.

Coconut oil's antimicrobial effects, along with improved immune efficiency due to the diet, may cause what is called a "die-off" reaction, also known as a Herxheimer reaction. This occurs when large numbers of bacteria or other microorganisms are killed and their toxins are dumped into the bloodstream for elimination. The death of the bacteria and associated toxins occurs faster than the body can remove them. In response, the body shifts into a heightened state of detoxification and elimination. As a consequence, symptoms resembling illness may become manifest. Symptoms may include one or more of the following: nausea, diarrhea, vomiting, fever, chills, headache, muscle or joint pain, skin outbreaks, itchiness, anxiety, irritability, insomnia, fatigue, and nasal congestion. In fact, any symptom or combination of symptoms can arise.

This cleansing reaction is often misdiagnosed as an illness or an allergic reaction. While the symptoms may be discomforting, they are not indications of an illness and do not need any special treatment or medications. The body is simply doing what it needs to do to cleanse itself. For example, if the sinuses are eliminating a great deal of mucus, they are doing so in order to rid the body of toxins. Taking a decongestant stops the removal of these toxins, preventing them from exiting the body. Likewise, anti-diarrhea medications prevent the elimination of toxins from the bowel. Antibiotics won't do any good because the bacteria are already dead; these drugs may actually depress the immune system and slow down the cleansing process. These symptoms are temporary. Just let the process run its course. Cleansing reactions can last anywhere from one day to two weeks, and sometimes even longer. Three to four days is typical. This die-off reaction usually occurs during the first few weeks on the diet, if it occurs at all. Not all children will experience these symptoms.

Since this new eating plan is probably far healthier than anything your child has ever experienced, you will begin to see many positive changes in his or her health. Better social interaction, improved speech, clearer thinking, happier mood, improved digestion, better eyesight, fewer and less severe infections, deeper and more restful night's sleep, and an overall feeling of better health will follow.

How long will it take to see improvement? It depends. Improvement may be noticeable within just a few weeks or it may take months. The success you achieve with the program depends on several factors.

The severity of the condition is a major factor. Mild forms of autism may show dramatic improvement within weeks. Such children may improve so rapidly that they can be integrated into regular school classrooms after just a few months on the program. Those with severe disabilities will take longer. If seizures occur frequently you may need to maintain the diet a couple of years or longer. In the treatment of epilepsy, children are usually kept on a ketogenic diet for two years. If seizures are controlled by that time they are gradually allowed more carbohydrate in their diet until they are eating the same foods as other children. If seizures come back then a modified or less restrictive ketogenic diet is usually instigated for a period of time, perhaps for another one or two years, or however long it takes. The coconut ketogenic diet is a healthy food plan that can be sustained indefinitely if needed.

Age of the child is a major factor too. Up to two years of age a child's brain is still in its growth spurt and most easily affected by treatment. As children mature, the brain gradually becomes hardwired and changes become more difficult. The brain continues to mature and develop throughout the teenage years. Progress can occur at any age but the younger the child is, the quicker the response and the more complete the healing. However, even adults with autism can see significant improvements with this program.

The child's overall health is another factor. Frequent infections mean multiple episodes of systemic inflammation, which adversely affect the brain. Multiple infections are also an indication of poor immune function. When immune function is low, healing is slowed.

Hidden food allergies can hamper progress as well. Being aware of your child's behavior and keeping a diet diary is helpful in spotting hidden allergies. Environmental allergies to pollen or mold may also cause a problem if not identified.

Total compliance to the program is very important. Are the recommended supplements and coconut oil taken daily? Are carbohydrate grams calculated for each meal and are they within the guidelines of the program? Are treats or other forbidden foods kept strictly off-limits? If you follow the program as directed your son or daughter will show improvement.

If your child is not progressing as quickly as you would expect, a possible problem could be heavy metal intoxication. While the Autism Battle Plan can help clear out a lot of mercury, aluminum, and other toxic metals from the body, oral chelation therapy can speed the process along.

Chelators such as DMSA (2,3-dimercaptosuccinic acid) and DMPS (2,3-dimercapto-1-propanesulfonic acid) pull toxic metals out of the tissues and remove them from the body through the urinary tract. DMSA is approved by the FDA for the treatment of lead poisoning in children. Mercury, cadmium, arsenic, antimony, and other metals are also chelated by these agents. To be conducted safely and effectively, oral chelation is best supervised by a qualified physician. Serious adverse side effects are rare but can occur, so professional monitoring is essential.

The coconut ketogenic diet can continue for as long as you like. If symptoms are completely resolved, you can start adding more carbohydrate into the diet. Don't abruptly stop the diet and start feeding your child bread and sweets. Carbohydrates should be gradually reintroduced into the diet. Care should be taken at this time to spot any regression in behavior. If there is a change for the worse, tighten back on the diet. Starchy vegetables, such as white or sweet potatoes and even fresh fruits, can be added back first. If there are no issues with gluten or wheat allergies, whole grains might be added next. Hold off on white flour, sweets, and sugary juices and drinks. It is best that they be consumed sparingly, if at all. To maintain the best health, hydrogenated oils, vegetables oils, MSG, aspartame, and other detrimental food additives should remain off-limits. Coconut oil and overall fat intake can decrease as your child is gradually weaned off the diet.

CASE STUDY

The following case study was described in the *Journal of Child Neurology*.[5] The case involved a young boy, who we will call Tyler, living in Alberta, Canada. For the first two years of his life Tyler progressed normally both physically and mentally. Before reaching his third birthday, however, Tyler began exhibiting unusual behavior. His language skills slowly began to regress and he developed an unconscious habit of repeating words just spoken by others—echolalia, a characteristic usually considered a symptom of autism. He also demonstrated a change in temperament, whining repeatedly and often screaming without provocation. He became an increasingly picky eater. Digestive problems became evident as he frequently experienced loose stools. There was no history of seizures, major illness, toxic exposure, or trauma which could have caused these dramatic changes.

Tyler received all of his vaccinations according to schedule. At the time, his mother did not suspect that vaccines would have any effect on his behavior or development, and later could not recall any noticeable changes immediately following the vaccinations. Since all vaccines contribute to inflammation in the body and the brain, however, they always have some effect whether they are immediately noticeable or not.

His symptoms continued to worsen and when Tyler was five years old he was officially diagnosed with autism spectrum disorder involving significant language disorder, scattered language development, and social communication impairment. Tyler displayed unexplained fatigue, confusion, and inability to tolerate bright lights in addition to his developmental delays. Like many other autistic children he experienced gastrointestinal symptoms including bloating, belching, and abdominal pain as well as frequent nausea, vomiting, and diarrhea. He experienced ringing in his ears and often put his fingers in his ears to deaden the noise. Along with recurrent upper respiratory tract infections and congestion, he had difficulty sleeping and often experienced nightmares. He often appeared depressed and became disproportionately angry at the slightest incident. His parents were told his condition was severe and incurable.

The doctors instituted a plan of treatment that involved speech-language therapy, individualized education programming, and support from a national autism society which followed conventional medical belief that autism was an incurable condition that must be managed for life. The parents were told that autism was a lifelong disorder, that there was no evidence for a relationship between vaccinations and autism, that there was no research to prove that any alternative therapies would be of any benefit, and that pursuing alternative treatments would be a waste of time and money.

Despite the doctor's warnings and since conventional medicine had no answers, the parents began looking to complementary and alternative medicine for help. Their search led them to a specialist in environmental medicine. A nutritional assessment revealed inadequate levels of fat-soluble vitamins, including notable deficiencies of vitamins A, D, and E, as well as CoQ_{10}, folate, and zinc. Blood levels of omega-3 fatty acids, specifically DHA, were also low. The biochemistry assessment also found his saturated fat status to be low despite regular consumption of saturated fats in his diet. All of these suggested difficulty with fat absorption. Additional testing revealed positive antiendomysial antibodies and extremely high antitissue transglutaminase antibodies which suggested he was suffering from celiac disease— a hypersensitivity to gluten. He frequently consumed wheat, which would cause severe intestinal inflammation, interfere with nutrient absorption, and likely was the cause of Tyler's gastrointestinal problems.

All sources of gluten (wheat, rye, barley, oats) were eliminated from Tyler's diet and a concerted effort to replenish deficient nutrients was undertaken. More fresh produce was added to his diet along with dietary supplements and fat.

Within one month, Tyler's gastrointestinal symptoms were gone and his behavior improved dramatically. His mother excitedly reported that her five-year-old boy was becoming progressively more communicative and for the first time he told her that he loved her. Within three months, he had improved so much that he no longer required an individualized learning program and was able to enter a normal classroom with no aide.

A follow-up examination revealed that there was no longer any evidence of autism. Tyler is now almost eight years old and is progressing normally for his age. "He is doing incredibly well and is so very happy," his mother delightfully exclaims.

A diagnosis of autism is *not* a life sentence. There is hope. There is an effective treatment. Autistic children can overcome this crippling disorder and reenter the world of normal happy childhood. The Autism Battle Plan offers that hope.

CONTINUED SUPPORT

The Internet has many websites offering low-carb advice, encouragement, and recipes that can be of tremendous benefit. One of the best resources is the Atkins website, www.atkins.com, which has numerous recipes, chat groups, and blogs for support, encouragement, a carb counter database so you can look up the net carbs for a variety of foods, the latest research on low-carb eating, and other aids. The recipes are numerous and creative and all include the net carb content. A couple of websites with a variety of recipes for a ketogenic diet are:

www.dietketogenic.com/ketogenic-diet-recipes.php
www.myketocal.com/recipes_kd.html

Not every recipe described on these websites is suitable for the coconut ketogenic diet. You may need to make some substitutions in ingredients and you must always calculate total carbohydrate content per serving.

For general autism support you may want to check out the following websites:

The Autism File, http://autismfile.com/
Autism One, http://www.autismone.org/
Autism Action Network, http://autismactioncoalition.org/
Elizabeth Birt Center for Autism Law and Advocacy, http://www.ebcala.org/
Generation Rescue, www.generationrescue.org
Talk About Curing Autism, http://www.tacanow.org/
Unlocking Autism, www.unlockingautism.org
National Autism Association New York, http://www.naanyc.org/naavrr.html
Defeat Autism Now, www.defeatautismnow.com
Autism Research Institute, www.autism.com
Developmental Delay Resources, www.devdelay.org
Resources for Children with Special Needs, www.resourcesnyc.org
Autism Network for Dietary Intervention, http://www.autismndi.com

Many additional useful websites can be found by doing a search for autism or ketogenic diets on the Internet.

15 | Recipes

At first, learning how to cook the low-carb way may seem like a daunting task. However, it isn't as hard as it may appear. While some low-carb recipes are complicated and time-consuming, much of the cooking is as simple as frying a lamb chop and steaming some zucchini. What could be easier than that?

If you are new to low-carb cooking, I strongly urge you to read this entire chapter. Whether you use any of the recipes or not, this chapter will show you how to make low-carb cooking simple and easy. It will also show you how to incorporate coconut oil into your family's everyday life. The recipes provided here are just a few examples of low-carb cooking. For more ideas, check out the many low-carb books and recipes available at your library, book store, and the Internet.

One of the biggest challenges to the program outlined in this book is consuming the amount of coconut oil recommended each day. The first part of this chapter provides numerous methods of consuming coconut oil in a palatable way. Recipes later on explain how to add the oil during meal preparation.

DAILY DOSE OF COCONUT OIL

The program in this book recommends consuming a fair amount of coconut oil daily, taken in divided doses during breakfast, lunch, and dinner. This is a lot of oil to consume during the day and often takes a little creative planning to accomplish in a palatable manner. The best way to take the oil is to use it in food preparation. Cook your foods in the oil or use it as a salad dressing or as a topping on vegetables. Below you will find a number of ideas to help you get that daily dose.

By the Spoonful

The simplest way to take the oil is by the spoonful, like a dietary supplement. Many people do this. However, others have a harder time because they find putting pure oil into their mouths difficult. They are not accustomed to the taste and texture. It does take some getting used to and over time most people can do it this way without problem. A good quality "virgin" coconut oil has a mild coconut flavor that tastes good enough to eat off the spoon. All brands are different however. Some brands have a much stronger flavor (sometimes tainted with smoke during processing), which can be overpowering. Choose the brand of coconut oil you use carefully. Try several brands and select the one that tastes best to you. If you don't like the taste of virgin coconut oil, you can use the tasteless "expeller pressed" coconut oil.

If consuming coconut oil by the spoonful is difficult for your child, one way to make it easier is to enhance the flavor using food extracts and flavorings. A little cinnamon oil mixed with the coconut oil gives it a remarkably pleasant taste that most children find very enjoyable. It's almost like candy. Here are some recipes. Adjust the quantities as needed.

- 1 tablespoon coconut oil mixed with 1-2 drops of cinnamon oil

- 1 tablespoon coconut oil mixed with 1-2 drops peppermint oil

- 1 tablespoon coconut oil mixed with 1-4 drops coconut flavoring

This last one may sound redundant, but the coconut flavoring gives the oil a richer, dessert-like coconut flavor. Experiment with other food flavorings available in the herb and spice section of the grocery store. You want to use only those products produced as flavorings for baking and food preparation, you don't want to use anything with added sugar. Oil-based extracts work better than alcohol-based flavorings. If you use an alcohol-based extract, combine the extract with the coconut oil in a small stovetop safe pan and heat for a minute or two to drive off the alcohol and leaving the flavor.

Meat Mix

Meat mixes provide a simple flavorful way to take a spoonful of coconut oil. By combining coconut oil with fresh meat and cooking it, the coconut oil takes on the flavor of the meat. One of the benefits of the meat mixes is that they combine coconut oil with red palm oil and turmeric/curcumin into one easy dish. This way you can get three of the nutrients from the Dietary Reference Chart (page 212) at once. You can use the turmeric sold for culinary use in these recipes.

Meat mixes are not meant to replace a meal, but to supplement it. The mixes can be eaten as is or, if desired, can be poured over cooked vegetables. They make good sauces. The recipes below are simple and basic. You can add or subtract ingredients as you desire. The red palm oil really enhances the flavor of the mixture and should not be deleted. You might even enjoy adding a little more than what is called for in the recipe. Use the following recipes but don't be afraid of experimenting using different herbs and spices to add a little diversity to the mixes.

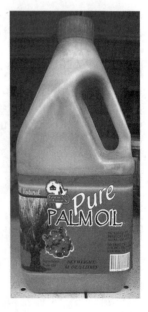

The following recipes are for one serving. You can make several servings at once and store the excess in the refrigerator for a day or two. Reheat and serve.

Basic Meat Mix

    1 tablespoon coconut oil
    ½ teaspoon red palm oil
    1 ounce meat*
    ¼ teaspoon turmeric powder
    ¼ teaspoon onion powder (optional)
    Salt and pepper to taste

In a small pan, heat coconut and red palm oils. Cook meat in hot oil over low heat until done. Add spices and cook for 1 minute. Remove from heat and let cool. Add salt and pepper to taste. Eat as is or use as a topping on vegetables. Makes one serving.

*Any type of meat can be used in this recipe: beef, pork, lamb, buffalo, chicken, turkey, pheasant, fish, shellfish, etc. Ground meat (beef, pork, turkey) can be used as is. Whole meat should be cut into small cubes. Only a small amount of meat is used—equivalent to about twice the volume of the oil used or about 1 ounce. The purpose of the meat is to flavor the oil, not to be a meal. Three ounces of meat is equivalent in size a stack of playing cards. One ounce would be a third of that.

Net Carbs 0 grams ser serving.

Curry Chicken Mix

Here is an example of the meat mix using additional spices.

    1 tablespoon coconut oil
    ½ teaspoon red palm oil
    1 ounce chicken, cut into small cubes*
    ¼ teaspoon turmeric powder
    ¼ teaspoon onion powder
    ¼ teaspoon curry powder
    Salt to taste

In a small pan, heat coconut and red palm oils. Cook chicken in hot oil over low heat until done. Add spices and cook for 1 minute. Remove from heat and let cool. Add salt to taste. Eat as is or use as a topping on vegetables. Makes one serving.

*Raw chicken is preferred, but leftover cooked chicken can be used as well.

Net Carbs 0 grams ser serving.

Chili Meat Mix

    1 tablespoon coconut oil
    ½ teaspoon red palm oil
    1 ounce ground beef

¼ teaspoon turmeric powder (optional)
¼ teaspoon onion powder
¼ teaspoon chili powder
Salt to taste

In a small pan, heat coconut and red palm oils. Cook ground beef in hot oil over low heat until done. Add spices and cook for 1 minute. Remove from heat and let cool. Add salt to taste. Eat as is or use as a topping on vegetables. Makes one serving.

Net Carbs 0 grams ser serving.

Mini Soups

Another way to incorporate coconut oil into your diet in a relatively easy manner is to make Mini Soups. I call them Mini Soups because only a small amount is consumed at any one time. This is basically a flavorful soup combined with coconut oil. The taste, texture, and smell of the soup make the oil easy to consume. Each serving amounts to only ¼ cup (60 ml) so it doesn't take the place of or interfere with meals. It is eaten before meals, much like an appetizer. The sole purpose of the Mini Soup is not to serve as a meal but to provide a tasty medium in which to consume the coconut oil. Red palm oil may be consumed like this too. If desired, however, any of these soups can be served as a full meal by increasing the serving size.

Multiple servings of the soup are made in advance and refrigerated or frozen. To each serving is added the amount of coconut oil needed for that meal. Over the course of several days the soup is gradually consumed. The soup is not eaten at every meal, but only when meals do not provide enough coconut oil to meet the daily minimum. The soups will keep in the refrigerator for several days and for several months when frozen.

Recipes for several soups are given below. Please note, coconut oil is not used in these recipes. *You add the oil to each serving just before consuming it.* This way you can add whatever amount of coconut oil you need for that particular meal. One serving is ¼ cup of soup, *plus* the added coconut oil. The number of net carbs is given in each recipe. You need to account for these carbs in your daily total.

Beef Soup

¼ pound (120 g) ground beef
½ cup (50 g) chopped vegetables*
1¼ cups (300 ml) water
¼ teaspoon onion powder
¼ teaspoon paprika
¼ teaspoon marjoram
Salt and pepper to taste

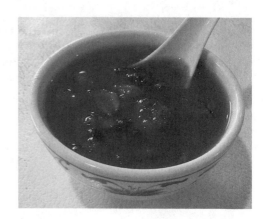

Put ground beef, vegetables and water in a quart saucepan. Bring to a boil, reduce heat and simmer for about 15 minutes. While cooking, break ground beef into small pieces. Add onion powder, paprika, and marjoram, cook for 1 minute and remove from heat. Add salt and pepper to taste. Let cool and store in an airtight container in the refrigerator. Makes six ¼ cup servings.

*Use two or more of the following vegetables: onion, carrot, mushroom, celery, green beans, bell peppers, okra, and asparagus.

Net carbs: 0.5 grams per ¼ cup serving.

Beef Salsa Soup

¼ pound (120 g) ground beef
½ cup (50 g) chopped vegetables*
1¼ (300 ml) cups water
2 tablespoons (30 ml) salsa
Salt and pepper to taste

Put ground beef, vegetables, water, and salsa in a quart saucepan. Bring to a boil, reduce heat and simmer for about 15 minutes. While cooking, break ground beef into small pieces. Remove from heat and add salt and pepper to taste. Let cool and store in an airtight container in the refrigerator. Makes seven ¼ cup servings.

*Use two or more of the following vegetables: onion, carrot, mushroom, celery, green beans, bell peppers, okra, and asparagus.

Net carbs: 0.6 gram per ¼ cup serving.

Pork Soup

¼ pound (120 g) ground or chopped pork
½ cup (50 g) chopped vegetables*
1¼ (300 ml) cups water
¼ teaspoon onion powder
¼ teaspoon thyme
Salt and pepper to taste

Put ground pork, vegetables, and water in a quart saucepan. Bring to a boil, reduce heat and simmer for about 15 minutes. Add onion powder and thyme, cook for 1 minute and remove from heat. Add salt and pepper to taste. Let cool and store in an airtight container in the refrigerator. Makes six ¼ cup servings.

*Use two or more of the following vegetables: onion, carrot, mushroom, celery, green beans, bell peppers, okra, and asparagus.

Net carbs: 0.5 grams per ¼ cup serving.

Chicken Soup

1 cup (120 g) chicken, chopped
½ cup (50 g) chopped vegetables*
1¼ (300 ml) cups water
⅛ teaspoon celery seed

¼ teaspoon ground sage
Salt and pepper to taste

Put chicken, vegetables, and water in a quart saucepan. Bring to a boil, reduce heat and simmer for about 15 minutes. Add onion powder and thyme, cook for 1 minute and remove from heat. Add salt and pepper to taste. Let cool and store in an airtight container in the refrigerator. Makes six ¼ cup servings.

*Use two or more of the following vegetables: onion, carrot, mushroom, celery, green beans, bell peppers, okra, and asparagus.

Net carbs: 0.5 grams per ¼ cup serving.

Clam Chowder

1 can (10 oz/300 ml) minced clams, with juice*
¼ cup (25 g) onion, chopped
⅛ teaspoon celery seed
⅛ teaspoon black pepper
1 cup (240 ml) heavy cream
2 teaspoons (10 ml) fish sauce

Drain juice from clams into saucepan and put the clams aside. Add onion, celery seed, and pepper to the juice in the saucepan and bring it to a boil, reduce heat and simmer for about 10 minutes or until onions are tender. Add cream, fish sauce, and clams. Cook for 2 minutes. Let cool and store in an airtight container in the refrigerator. Makes about 10 servings.

*Oysters may be substituted for the claims if desired.

Net carbs: 1 gram per ¼ cup serving.

Fish Chowder

¼ cup (25 g) onion, chopped
⅛ teaspoon celery seed
⅛ teaspoon black pepper
¼ pound (120 g) chopped fish*
1 cup (240 ml) heavy cream
2 teaspoons (10 ml) fish sauce

In a saucepan bring water to a boil. Add onion, celery seed, and pepper, reduce heat, and simmer for 8-10 minutes or until onions are tender. Add fish and cream and simmer for an additional 5 minutes. Let cool and store in an airtight container in the refrigerator.

*Use any type of low-mercury fish such as sole, catfish, salmon, trout, flounder, haddock, mackerel, perch, or tilapia. You can also use shellfish such as scallop, or crab.

Net carbs: 1 gram per ¼ cup serving.

Creamy Chicken Soup

> 1 cup (120 g) chicken, chopped
> ½ cup (50 g) chopped vegetables*
> ¾ cup (180 ml) chicken broth or water
> ½ cup (120 ml) heavy cream
> ⅛ teaspoon onion powder
> ⅛ teaspoon celery seed
> ¼ teaspoon thyme
> ⅛ teaspoon salt
> ⅛ teaspoon black pepper

Put chicken, vegetables, and water in a saucepan. Bring to a boil, reduce heat and simmer for about 15 minutes or until vegetables are tender. Add cream and seasonings, simmer for 1-2 minutes, and remove from heat. Let cool and store in an airtight container in the refrigerator. Makes six ¼ cup servings.

*Use two or more of the following vegetables: onion, carrot, mushroom, celery, green beans, bell peppers, okra, and asparagus.

Net carbs: 1 gram per ¼ cup serving.

Tomato Soup

> 1 cup (240 ml) water
> ½ cup (120 ml) tomato sauce
> ⅛ teaspoon celery seed
> ¼ teaspoon onion powder
> ⅛ teaspoon garlic powder
> ⅛ teaspoon paprika
> 1 teaspoon (5 ml) lemon juice
> Salt and black pepper to taste

Combine first six ingredients into a saucepan, bring to a boil, reduce heat, and simmer for three minutes to blend flavors. Remove from heat and add lemon juice, salt, and pepper. Makes six ¼ cup servings.

Net carbs: 1.3 grams per ¼ cup serving.

Creamy Tomato

> 1 cup (240 ml) water
> ½ cup (120 ml) tomato sauce
> ⅛ teaspoon celery seed
> ¼ teaspoon onion powder
> ⅛ teaspoon garlic powder
> ⅛ teaspoon paprika
> ½ cup (120 ml) heavy cream
> Salt and black pepper to taste

Combine first six ingredients in a saucepan, bring to a boil, reduce heat and simmer for three minutes to blend flavors. Remove from heat and add cream, salt, and pepper. Makes eight ¼ cup servings.

Net carbs: 1.3 grams per ¼ cup serving.

Tomato Beef Soup
¼ pound (120 g) ground beef
1 cup (120 ml) water
¼ cup (60 ml) tomato sauce
⅛ teaspoon celery seed
¼ teaspoon onion powder
⅛ teaspoon garlic powder
⅛ teaspoon paprika
¼ teaspoon salt
⅛ teaspoon black pepper
1 teaspoon (5 ml) lemon juice

Combine first nine ingredients into a saucepan, bring to a boil, reduce heat and simmer for 10 minutes. Remove from heat and add lemon juice. Makes seven ¼ cup servings.

Net carbs: 0.6 gram per ¼ cup serving.

Tomato Fish Soup
¼ pound (120 g) chopped fish*
1 cup (240 ml) water
¼ cup (60 ml) tomato sauce
⅛ teaspoon celery seed
¼ teaspoon onion powder
⅛ teaspoon paprika
⅛ teaspoon black pepper
2 teaspoons (10 ml) fish sauce

Combine all ingredients into a saucepan, bring to a boil, reduce heat and simmer for 5 minutes. Remove from heat and serve. Makes seven ¼ cup servings.

*Use any type of low-mercury fish such as sole, catfish, salmon, trout, flounder, haddock, mackerel, perch, whitefish, or tilapia. You can also use shellfish such as scallop, shrimp, or crab.

Net carbs: 0.5 gram per ¼ cup serving.

Cream of Asparagus
1 cup (240 ml) chicken broth
4 ounces (115 g) asparagus, chopped
½ cup (120 ml) heavy cream
¼ teaspoon basil
¼ teaspoon salt
⅛ teaspoon black pepper

½ teaspoon scallion, chopped

In a covered saucepan, simmer chicken broth and asparagus for 20 minutes until vegetables are soft. Remove from heat, put into a blender and blend until smooth. Add back to saucepan along with cream, basil, salt, and pepper. Heat to a simmer and cook 1 minute. Remove from heat. Serve with freshly chopped scallion sprinkled on top. Makes about six ¼ cup servings.

Net carbs: 1 gram per ¼ cup serving.

Cream of Broccoli with Cheese

    1 cup (240 ml) chicken broth
    1 cup (100 g) broccoli, chopped
    ½ cup (120 ml) heavy cream
    ¼ teaspoon salt
    ⅛ teaspoon black pepper
    ¼ cup (25 g) freshly grated Parmesan cheese
    1 teaspoon scallion, chopped

In a covered saucepan, simmer chicken broth and broccoli for 20 minutes until vegetables are soft. Remove from heat, put into a blender and blend until smooth. Add back to saucepan along with cream, salt, pepper, and cheese. Heat to a simmer and cook 1 minute. Remove from heat. Serve with freshly chopped scallion sprinkled on top. Makes about six ¼ cup servings.

Net carbs: 1.3 grams per ¼ cup serving.

Cream of Spinach with Chicken

    1 teaspoon (5 ml) butter
    1 cup (120 g) uncooked chicken cut into bite size pieces
    ¼ cup (60 ml) water
    ¾ cup (180 ml) heavy cream
    ¼ teaspoon onion powder
    ⅛ teaspoon garlic powder
    3 cups (80 g) spinach, chopped
    Salt and black pepper to taste

Melt butter in sauté pan over medium heat. Add chicken and cook, stirring frequently, until it turns white, about 3 minutes. Add all remaining ingredients and simmer until spinach is tender. Makes seven ¼ cup servings.

Net carbs: 0.9 grams per ¼ cup serving.

Creamy Cinnamon Soup

    1 cup (240 ml) heavy cream
    ½ cup (120 ml) water
    1 teaspoon cinnamon
    ¼ teaspoon nutmeg
    ½ teaspoon (3 ml) vanilla extract
    Stevia to taste (optinal)

In a small saucepan heat cream, water, cinnamon, and nutmeg to a low simmer, stir frequently, do not boil. Cook for about 5 minutes. Heating draws the flavors of the spices into the cream. Add vanilla and remove from heat. Add a little stevia to sweeten. Makes six ¼ cup servings.

Net carbs: 1.1 grams per ¼ cup serving.

Creamy Berry Soup
 1 cup (240 ml) heavy cream
 ¾ cup (75 g) berries (blackberries, boysenberries, or raspberries)
 ½ cup (120 ml) water
 ⅛ teaspoon vanilla
 Stevia to taste (optional)
 Combine all ingredients into a blender and blend until smooth. Add a little stevia to sweeten. Makes eight ¼ cup servings.

Net carbs: 1.5 grams per ¼ cup serving.

LOW-CARB SALAD DRESSINGS

Tossed green salads are the most popular types of salads because a variety of ingredients can be used to create them. Don't limit yourself to the common iceberg lettuce—try others such as butterhead lettuce, red leaf, romaine, and other varieties. Low-carb vegetables that go well with salads include cucumber, bell peppers, banana peppers, tomatoes, avocado, parsley, onion, shallots, scallions, radishes, jicama, parsley, cilantro, watercress, sprouts, celery, celery root (celeriac), bok choy (Chinese cabbage), napa cabbage, red and green cabbage, broccoli, cauliflower, spinach, chard, kale, carrots, Jerusalem artichoke, sauerkraut, chicory, endive, and snow peas.

Salads don't always have to include lettuce. You can make a variety of lettuce-free salads with all these vegetables. Toppings add spark to salads. Low-carb toppings can include hard boiled eggs, ham, crumbled bacon, beef, chicken, turkey, pork, fish (salmon, sardines, etc.), crab, shrimp, nori, hard cheeses (cheddar, Monterey, Munster, etc.), soft cheeses (feta, cottage, etc.), nuts, olives, and pork rinds.

The dressing is perhaps the most important part of the salad. It is what makes the salad stand out and gives the other ingredients zing. Most

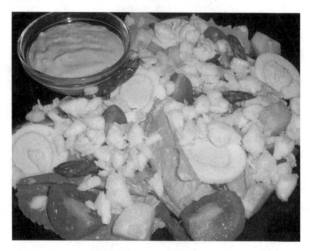

Crab Louie salad is typically made with crab meat, hard boiled eggs, romaine lettuce, tomato, bell pepper, asparagus, and cucumber and served with a mayonnaise based dressing such as the Thousand Island Dressing on page 237.

commercially prepared dressings are made using a base of soybean or canola oils and often include sugar, high fructose corn syrup, MSG, and other undesirable additives. Many of them are promoted as low-calorie or low-fat, but few are low-carb. A better choice is a homemade low-carb salad dressing using healthier ingredients. The following are a few such recipes.

Coconut Olive Mayonnaise

This recipe uses an equal mixture of extra virgin olive oil and coconut oil. You can make mayonnaise using only coconut oil but it must be used immediately because it does not store well. When put into the refrigerator it will harden. By combining coconut oil with another oil, such as extra virgin olive oil, you can refrigerate the mayonnaise and it will still remain soft and creamy. The olive oil gives the mayonnaise a slight olive oil flavor.

1 large egg yolk
2 teaspoons (10 ml) fresh lemon juice
1 tablespoon (5 ml) Dijon mustard
½ teaspoon salt
⅛ teaspoon black pepper
½ cup (240 ml) extra light olive oil
½ cup (240 ml) coconut oil (melted)

Have all ingredients at room temperature before beginning. Combine egg yolk, lemon juice, mustard, salt, pepper, and ¼ cup (60 ml) olive oil in blender or food processor. Blend for about 60 seconds. While machine is running, pour in the remaining olive oil and coconut oil *very slowly*, drop by drop at first and gradually building to a fine, steady steam. The secret to making good mayonnaise is to add the oil in slowly. Mayonnaise will thicken as oil is added. Taste and adjust seasonings as needed. Each tablespoon of coconut mayonnaise contains about ½ tablespoon of coconut oil.
Net carbs: 0.2 grams per 1 tablespoon serving.

Creamy Coconut Mayonnaise

For this recipe you use an equal mixture of coconut oil and MCT oil. If you use only MCT oil the mayonnaise will not thicken. Combining the two oils will allow the mayonnaise to thicken and will lower the melting point enough so that the mayonnaise will say soft when refrigerated.

2 egg yolks
2 tablespoons apple cider vinegar
½ tablespoon prepared mustard
⅛ teaspoon paprika
⅛ teaspoon salt
¾ cup coconut oil (melted)
¾ cup MCT oil

Combine egg yolks, vinegar, mustard, paprika, salt, and ¼ cup coconut oil into a blender or food processor. Blend for about 30 seconds. While machine is running pour in the remaining coconut oil followed by all of the MCT oil very slowly in a fine steady stream. The secret to making good mayonnaise is to add the oil slowly. Mayonnaise will thicken as oil is added. Taste and adjust seasoning as desired.

Net carbs: 0.2 grams per 1 tablespoon serving.

Balsamic Vinaigrette Dressing

¾ cup (180 ml) MCT oil
¾ cup (180 ml) balsamic vinegar
1 clove garlic, crushed
½ teaspoon dried oregano
2 teaspoons (10 ml) Dijon mustard
⅛ teaspoon salt
⅛ teaspoon black pepper

Combine all ingredients into a jar with a tight fitting lid, such as a Mason jar. Shake well and serve. Store in the refrigerator.

Net carbs: 1 gram per 1 tablespoon serving.

Vinegar and Coconut Oil Dressing

¼ cup (60 ml) coconut oil
¼ cup (60 ml) extra light olive oil
2 tablespoons (30 ml) water
¼ cup (60 ml) apple cider vinegar
⅛ teaspoon salt
⅛ teaspoon white pepper

Put all ingredients into a Mason jar or similar container. Cover and shake vigorously until well blended. Let stand at room temperature until ready to use. May be stored in cupboard for several days without refrigeration. If the dressing is to be stored for more than a week, put it into the refrigerator. When chilled, the oil will tend to solidify. To liquefy, take it out of the refrigerator at least 1 hour before using. Each tablespoon of dressing contains about ¼ tablespoon of coconut oil.

Net carbs: 0 grams per 1 tablespoon serving.

Simple Vinegar Dressing

¼ cup (60 ml) apple cider vinegar
½ tablespoon (8 ml) water
Dash of salt
Dash of pepper

Mix all ingredients together. That's all there is to it—simple and easy.
Net carbs: 0 grams per 1 tablespoon serving.

Toasted Almond Dressing
½ cup (120 ml) coconut oil
¼ cup (25 g) slivered almonds
1 tablespoon (15 ml) extra light olive oil
2 tablespoons (30 ml) tamari sauce
1 tablespoon (15 ml) apple cider vinegar
¼ teaspoon ground ginger
¼ teaspoon salt

Put coconut oil in small saucepan. At medium to low heat, sauté slivered almonds until lightly browned. Remove from heat and let cool to room temperature. Stir in remaining ingredients. As the dressing sits, the oil will separate to the top and the almonds will sink to the bottom. Stir just before using. Spoon dressing onto salad, making sure to include the almonds. May be stored in cupboard for several days without refrigeration. If the dressing is to be stored for more than a week, put it into the refrigerator. Each tablespoon of dressing contains about ½ tablespoon of coconut oil.
Net carbs: 0.3 grams per 1 tablespoon serving.

Vinaigrette
¼ cup (60 ml) red or white wine vinegar
¼ teaspoon salt
⅛ teaspoon white pepper
¾ cup (180 ml) extra virgin olive oil

In a bowl, mix vinegar, salt, and pepper with a fork. Add oil and mix vigorously until well blended. Makes 1 cup. MCT oil can be used in place of extra virgin olive oil if desired.
Net carbs: 0 grams per ¼ cup serving.

Garlic Vinaigrette
Place 1 peeled, bruised clove of garlic into ¾ cup extra virgin olive oil and let stand 2-3 days at room temperature. Remove garlic and use oil to make the Vinaigrette recipe above.
Net carbs: 0 grams per ¼ cup serving.

Spanish Vinaigrette
Prepare Vinaigrette dressing as directed and place in a Mason jar with 1 tablespoon minced green olives and 1 teaspoon each minced chives, capers, parsley, and gherkin, and 1 sieved hard-boiled egg yolk. Shake, let stand at room temperature for 30 minutes; shake again before using.
Net carbs: 0.2 grams per ¼ cup serving.

Herb Vinegar

2 cups (200 g) fresh herbs*
2 cups (480 ml) apple cider or white wine vinegar, heated to boiling

Place herbs in a quart-size wide-mouth Mason jar and crush lightly with the handle of a wooden spoon. Pour in hot vinegar and cool to room temperature. Screw on lid and let stand in a cool spot (not the refrigerator) for 10-14 days. Once every day shake the jar to stir contents. Taste vinegar after 10 days and, if strong enough, strain through several thicknesses of cheesecloth into a fresh pint jar. If too weak, let stand for the full 14 days.

*Choose any of the following herbs: tarragon, chervil, dill, basil, or thyme.

Net carbs: 0 grams per ¼ cup serving.

Fresh Herb Dressing

½ cup (120 ml) extra virgin olive oil
1 tablespoon fresh dill, minced
1 tablespoon fresh chives, minced
1 tablespoon fresh parsley, minced
½ teaspoon salt
⅛ teaspoon black pepper
¼ cup (60 ml) tarragon vinegar*

Place oil, herbs, salt, and pepper in a Mason jar and let stand at room temperature 2-4 hours. Add vinegar and shake or stir well to blend.

*Use store bought tarragon vinegar or home-made (see Herb Vinegar recipe above).

Net carbs: 0 grams per ¼ cup serving.

Garlic Herb Dressing

1 clove garlic, peeled and crushed
½ teaspoon tarragon
½ teaspoon marjoram
½ teaspoon powdered mustard
¼ teaspoon salt
⅛ teaspoon black pepper
¼ cup (60 ml) extra virgin olive oil
2 tablespoons (30 ml) red or white wine vinegar

Put all ingredients in a pint Mason jar or similar container. Screw on lid and shake contents to mix. Let stand at room temperature at least 1 hour. Shake again just before using.

Net carbs: 0 grams per ¼ cup serving.

Buttermilk Dressing

½ cup (120 ml) apple cider vinegar
1 tablespoon (15 ml) extra virgin olive oil

1 teaspoon salt
⅛ teaspoon white pepper
1 tablespoon scallions, minced
1 cup (240 ml) buttermilk

Put all ingredients in a Mason jar or similar container. Screw on lid and shake contents to mix. Makes 1½ cups.
Net carbs: 2.2 grams per ¼ cup serving.

Sour Cream Dressing

1 cup (240 ml) sour cream
3 tablespoons (45 ml) white or apple cider vinegar
¼ teaspoon dill
½ teaspoon salt
⅛ teaspoon black pepper

Mix all ingredients, cover, and chill. Makes 1¼ cups.
Net carbs: 2 grams per ¼ cup serving.

Blue Cheese Dressing

½ cup (120 ml) heavy cream
½ cup (120 ml) sour cream
¼ cup (60 ml) mayonnaise
2 tablespoons (30 ml) lemon juice
6 ounces (170 g) blue cheese, crumbled
Salt and black pepper to taste

In a bowl whisk cream, sour cream, mayonnaise and lemon juice. Add cheese and put into a blender or food processor and blend for 1 minute. Makes about 1¾ cups.
Net carbs: 2.5 grams per ¼ cup serving.

Thousand Island Dressing

1 cup (240 ml) mayonnaise
¼ cup (60 ml) sour cream
2 tablespoons dill pickle, chopped
2 tablespoons black olive, chopped
¼ cup (60 ml) low-sugar ketchup or tomato sauce
2 tablespoons (30 ml) lemon juice

Combine all ingredients together and a bowl and mix thoroughly. Makes about 1¾ cups.
Net carbs: 1.5 grams per ¼ cup serving.

SAUCES

Sauces and gravies make excellent complements to vegetables and meats and can enhance their flavor and add variety to meals. Adding a little butter, salt, and black pepper to boiled, baked, sautéed, stir-fried, steamed, or mashed vegetables tastes great, but adding a sauce creates a whole new flavor sensation. Ordinary vegetables take on new life when combined with a sauce. The following recipes can be used with vegetables, meat, fish, poultry, and even eggs.

Tartar Sauce

1 cup (240 ml) mayonnaise
3 scallions, minced
1 tablespoon parsley, minced
¼ cup dill pickle, chopped
2 tablespoons capers
1 teaspoon (5 ml) prepared Dijon-style mustard
2 tablespoons (30 ml) red wine vinegar

Mix all ingredients, cover, and chill. Serve with seafood. Makes about 1¼ cups. Net carbs: 0.1 grams per 1 tablespoon serving.

Creamy Cheese Sauce

2 tablespoons (30 ml) butter
½ cup (120 ml) heavy cream
1 cup (100 g) sharp cheddar cheese, shredded
⅛ teaspoon salt

In a saucepan, heat butter and cream until it begins to simmer and butter is melted. Turn off the heat, add cheese and salt stirring constantly until cheese is melted and mixture is thickened. Pour over cooked vegetables. Makes about 1 cup. Net carbs: 1.2 grams per ¼ cup serving.

Shrimp Cheese Sauce

Make the Creamy Cheese Sauce as directed but delete the salt and add 1½ cups (150 g) precooked baby shrimp and 1 teaspoon of fish sauce. Makes an excellent topping for cooked vegetables.
Net carbs: 0.7 grams per ¼ cup serving.

Tex-Mex Cheese Sauce

Make the Creamy Cheese Sauce as directed and add ½ cup (120 ml) salsa.
Net carbs: 1.5 grams per ¼ cup serving.

Hot Pepper Cheese Sauce

Make the Creamy Cheese Sauce as directed and add ¼ cup (25 g) chopped jalapeño chili pepper.
Net carbs: 1.2 grams per ¼ cup serving.

White Sauce

    2 tablespoons (30 ml) butter or coconut oil
    ½ cup 120 ml) heavy cream
    1 cup (100 g) Monterey cheese, shredded*
    ⅛ teaspoon salt
    ¼ teaspoon onion powder

In a saucepan, heat butter and cream until it begins to simmer and butter is melted. Turn off the heat and add cheese, salt, and onion powder, stirring constantly until cheese is melted and mixture is thickened. Pour over cooked vegetables, eggs, or meat. Makes about 1 cup.

    *May substitute Monterey Jack cheese if a spicier sauce is desired.

    Net carbs: 0.9 gram per ¼ cup serving.

White Fish Sauce

    2 tablespoons (30 ml) butter or coconut oil
    ½ cup 120 ml) heavy cream
    1 cup (100 g) Monterey cheese, shredded
    ½ teaspoon (3 ml) fish sauce

In a saucepan, heat butter and cream until it begins to simmer and butter is melted. Turn off the heat and add cheese and fish sauce, stirring constantly until cheese is melted and mixture is thickened. Pour over cooked vegetables. Makes about 1 cup.

    Net carbs: 0.9 gram per ¼ cup serving.

Sausage Cream Sauce

    ½ pound (240 g) ground pork sausage
    2 cloves garlic, minced
    ½ cup (120 ml) heavy cream
    ¼ teaspoon onion powder
    ½ teaspoon dried sage
    ¼ teaspoon paprika
    ⅛ teaspoon salt
    ⅛ teaspoon black pepper
    1 cup (100 g) Monterey cheese, shredded

In a saucepan, cook sausage and garlic until meat is browned and garlic is tender. Add cream and seasonings and bring to a simmer. Turn off the heat and add cheese, stirring constantly until cheese is melted and mixture is thickened. Pour over cooked vegetables, eggs, or meat.

    Net carbs: 0.9 grams per ¼ cup serving.

Chicken Cream Sauce

    2 tablespoons (30 ml) butter or coconut oil
    1 cup (120 g) chopped cooked chicken
    ½ cup (120 ml) heavy cream
    1 cup (100 g) Monterey cheese, shredded
    ¼ teaspoon dried sage
    ¼ teaspoon onion powder
    ⅛ teaspoon salt
    ⅛ teaspoon black pepper

Put butter, chicken, and cream in a saucepan and bring to a simmer. Turn off the heat and add cheese and seasonings, stirring constantly until cheese is melted and mixture is thickened. Pour over cooked vegetables, eggs, or meat.

Net carbs: 0.6 grams per ¼ cup serving.

Curry Sauce

    2 tablespoons (30 ml) butter or coconut oil
    ½ cup (120 ml) heavy cream
    1 cup (100 g) Monterey cheese, shredded
    ⅛ teaspoon salt
    ½ teaspoon curry powder or garam masala

In a saucepan, heat butter and cream until it begins to simmer and butter is melted. Turn off the heat and add cheese, salt, and curry powder, stirring constantly until cheese is melted and mixture is thickened. Pour over cooked vegetables, eggs, or meat. Makes about 1 cup.

Net carbs: 0.9 gram per ¼ cup serving.

MEALS FOR BREAKFAST, LUNCH, AND DINNER

Breakfast is often considered the most difficult part of the low-carb diet. Traditionally, breakfast consists of high-carb foods such as hot or cold cereal, pancakes, waffles, French toast, hash brown potatoes, muffins, bagels, donuts, toaster pastries, toast and jelly, orange juice, cocoa, and such. The only traditional low-carb breakfast foods are eggs, bacon, ham, and sausage. You can do a lot with eggs. Serve them fried, scrambled, poached, hard or soft boiled, deviled, or as omelets and soufflés, and you already have a great variety. Adding meats and vegetables increases the serving possibilities further. One of the advantages of egg-based meals is that a full meal along with meat and vegetables generally contains only a few grams of carbohydrate. This allows for a larger amount of carbohydrate to be eaten at lunch and dinner. Several egg dishes are provided below.

As tasty and nutritious as eggs are, it is still nice to have variety for breakfast. Therefore, you should experiment with eating foods not generally considered a part of the traditional breakfast such as salads, soups, beef, chicken, fish, and vegetables. The following recipes can be used for breakfast, lunch, or dinner.

Most of the recipes below specify the use of coconut oil, but you may use butter, bacon drippings, red palm oil, or any other cooking oil you desire. You may also use a combination of oils. Coconut oil is specified in most recipes since this is one of the best ways to add coconut oil into the diet.

Oils are used in cooking primarily to prevent foods from sticking to the pans. The anti-sticking properties of oil vary from oil to oil. Lard has a very good anti-sticking character. By comparison, coconut oil has very modest anti-sticking properties. Coconut oil works very well when frying most vegetables and meats, but not as well with eggs and bread products (such as pancakes). The anti-sticking properties of coconut oil can be improved by mixing in a small portion of another oil, such as butter, bacon or sausage drippings, red palm oil, or olive oil. If an egg recipe calls for 1 tablespoon of coconut oil, for example, you may add an additional teaspoon ($\frac{1}{3}$ tablespoon) or so of butter or some other oil. This isn't required, but it will make removing the egg from the pan a little easier.

Among the easiest lunch type meals are lettuce wraps. Lettuce wraps are sandwiches made without bread. In place of the bread a large leaf of lettuce is used and simply wrapped around the filling. For example, a tuna sandwich wrap is made by making the tuna filling (tuna, mayonnaise, pickle, onion, chopped celery, spices) and spreading it on a lettuce leaf and rolling it up. A hamburger wrap would be to place cooked hamburger meat along with a slice of cheese, tomato, onion, pickle, and mayonnaise inside the lettuce. The same can be done with deviled eggs, taco meat, chicken, roast beef, etc. for a variety of different sandwich wraps.

You don't have to be a gourmet chef to make delicious low-carb meals. The easiest low-carb meals consist simply of a piece of cooked meat (roasted, fried, baked, grilled, poached, stir-fried) and a vegetable or two. The vegetables can be sautéed, steamed, roasted, poached, or raw. Easier still is to combine the meat and vegetables into a single skillet, crock pot, or baking dish and cook them together. The advantage to this is that it simplifies cooking, requires less cleanup, and, best of all, the meat drippings, especially when combined with seasoned salt or other spices, give the vegetables a wonderful taste. Below you will find several single skillet recipes to show you how simple and tasty this way of cooking can be.

In most of the recipes provided below you can use more oil than indicated. If you want to make sure you get your daily dose, include enough coconut oil so that your child's portion of the meal includes full dose of coconut oil. Calculate this so that you know exactly how much coconut oil is in the dish. When meat is cooked in coconut oil, the oil takes on the flavor of the meat drippings. Use the cooked drippings like a sauce and pour it over the meat and vegetables before serving. Fatty cuts of meat and chicken with the skins on produce the best-tasting drippings.

Serving sizes listed in the following recipes are for adults. Depending on your child's size and appetite, serving size, and net carbs, will vary. Net carbs are given for each recipe so you can keep an accurate count.

Easy Omelet

Omelets are easy to make and with different ingredients can be made into a dozen or more variations. Omelets made in the traditional French manner can be a bit complicated. This recipe is a simplified version that tastes just as good and allows for multiple variations. These directions are for a plain omelet.

2 tablespoons (30 ml) coconut oil
4 eggs
¼ teaspoon salt
⅛ teaspoon black pepper

Melt coconut oil in skillet over medium heat. Whisk together eggs, salt and pepper in a bowl. Pour mixture into the hot skillet, cover, and cook without stirring until the top of the omelet is set, about five minutes. Remove omelet from pan and serve hot. Serves two.
Net carbs: 1.2 grams per serving.

Cheese Omelet

Follow the directions for making the Easy Omelet, but after pouring the egg mixture into the hot skillet, sprinkle 1 cup of shredded cheese over the top. Cover and cook without stirring until the omelet is set and the cheese is melted. Makes two adult servings.
Net carbs: 2 grams per serving.

Sausage, Mushroom, and Tomato Omelet

This is a good example of how to prepare an omelet that is combined with meats and vegetables. See the many variations below.

1 tablespoon (15 ml) coconut oil
¼ pound (120 g) sausage
2 mushrooms, sliced
4 eggs
¼ teaspoon salt
½ cup tomato, chopped

Heat coconut oil in a skillet. Add sausage and mushrooms and cook until browned. Whisk together eggs and salt in a bowl. Pour mixture into the hot skillet over the sausage and mushrooms, cover, and cook without stirring until the top of the omelet is set, about five minutes. Add tomato, cover, and cook 1 minute. Remove omelet from pan and serve hot. Makes two adult servings.
Net carbs: 2.8 grams per serving.

Variations: A variety of omelets can be made using many different ingredients including ham, bacon, chicken, sausage, ground beef, ground lamb, shrimp, crab, onions, eggplant, zucchini, garlic, sweet or hot peppers, tomatoes, avocado, asparagus, broccoli, cauliflower, spinach, and mushrooms. The meats and most of the vegetables are cooked before combining with the egg mixture. Tomato, avocado, and garnishes such as cilantro and chives are best used raw and added after cooking. Sour cream can be used as a garnish as well. Cheese can be melted on top during the cooking of the eggs. Any one or more of these ingredients can be combined. You need to make note of the quantities of each ingredient used so that you can calculate the net carbs.

Onion Frittata

This is an Italian omelet that is browned on both sides.

1 medium-size red onion, peeled and sliced very thin
2 tablespoons (30 ml) coconut oil
1 clove garlic, diced
4 eggs, lightly beaten
¾ teaspoon salt
⅛ teaspoon black pepper
1 teaspoon basil
2 tablespoons grated Parmesan cheese
1 tablespoon (15 ml) extra virgin olive oil

Using a skillet, sauté onion in coconut oil over medium heat for about 5 minutes until limp, but not brown. Add garlic and cook an additional 1 minute. In a bowl mix together eggs, seasonings, and cheese. Add extra virgin olive oil to the onions and garlic in the skillet. Pour the egg mixture into the hot skillet. Cook without stirring 3-4 minutes until browned underneath and just set on top. Cut in quarters, turn, and brown flip side 2-3 minutes. Serves two adults.

Net carbs: 6.6 grams per serving.

Ham and Tomato Frittata

This is a variation of the traditional Italian omelet described above.

1 clove garlic, diced
2 tablespoons (30 ml) coconut oil
4 eggs, lightly beaten
½ cup ham, diced
¾ teaspoon salt
⅛ teaspoon black pepper
1 teaspoon basil
2 tablespoons grated Parmesan cheese
1 medium tomato, chopped
1 tablespoon (15 ml) extra virgin olive oil

Using a skillet, sauté garlic in coconut oil over medium heat for 1-2 minutes, until lightly browned. In a bowl mix together eggs, ham, seasonings, cheese, and tomato. Add extra virgin olive oil to the garlic in the skillet. Pour the egg mixture into the hot skillet. Cook without stirring about 4 minutes until browned underneath and just set on top. Cut in quarters, turn, and brown flip side 2-3 minutes. Serves two adults.

Net carbs: 3.5 grams per serving.

Simple Soufflé

Soufflés are similar to omelets. This version starts on the stovetop like an omelet but is finished off in the oven, giving it a unique taste and texture. Use eggs at room temperature; this will give them better volume. It is important to use a pan that is both stovetop and oven safe.

4 eggs, separated
¼ teaspoon salt
⅛ teaspoon black pepper
2 tablespoons (30 ml) coconut oil

Preheat oven to 350 degree F (175 C). Beat egg yolks, salt, and pepper lightly with a fork. In a separate bowl beat egg whites until stiff peaks form. Gently mix one-fourth of the egg whites into the yolks. Fold remaining whites into the yolk mixture. Do not over mix. Heat oil in an oven safe pan on the stovetop. Pour egg mixture into hot pan and cook for 1 minute. Transfer pan to oven and cook uncovered for 15 minutes or until soufflé is puffy and delicately browned. Remove from oven, divide in half with a spatula, and serve. Serves two adults.

Net carbs: 1.2 grams per serving.

Cheese Soufflé

In this recipe you first make a cheese sauce which is then mixed into the egg whites. Use a pan that is both stovetop and oven safe.

2 tablespoons (30 ml) butter
½ cup (120 ml) heavy cream
1¼ cups (150 g) sharp cheddar cheese, shredded
3 eggs, separated
¼ teaspoon salt
⅛ teaspoon black pepper
2 tablespoons (30 ml) coconut oil

Melt butter in a saucepan over moderate heat. Add cream and cheese, stirring until cheese is melted. Beat egg yolks, salt, and pepper lightly with a fork. Blend about ¼ cup (60 ml) of hot cheese sauce into the yolks. Immediately stir the yolk mixture into the cheese sauce. Cook the sauce over low heat, stirring constantly, for 1-2 minutes. Remove from heat and let cool to room temperature. Meanwhile, preheat oven to 350 degree F (175 C). In a separate bowl, beat egg whites until stiff peaks form. Gently mix one-fourth of the egg whites into the sauce. Fold the remaining whites into the sauce. Do not over mix or your soufflé will become flat. Heat coconut oil in an oven safe pan on the stovetop. Pour egg mixture into hot pan and cook for 1 minute. Transfer pan to oven and cook uncovered for 18-20 minutes or until soufflé is puffy and delicately browned. Remove from oven, divide in half with a spatula, and serve. Makes two adult servings.

Net carbs: 3.2 grams per serving.

Variations: Prepare Cheese Soufflé as directed but before cooling cheese sauce, mix in any of the following: cooked ham or sausage, crisp crumbled bacon, minced sautéed chicken livers, deviled ham, minced sautéed mushrooms, minced cooked fish or shellfish, minced cooked vegetables (pimiento, asparagus, spinach, broccoli, cauliflower, cabbage, Brussels sprouts, or onions). Use ¼ to ½ cup (25-50 g) of any of these ingredients in the recipe. Adjust net cabs to account for additional ingredients.

Egg Foo Young
This egg dish is an interesting change from the traditional omelet or soufflé.

2 tablespoons (30 ml) coconut oil
2 eggs
½ cup (60 g) cooked meat (ham, chicken, pork, or shrimp)
1 medium mushroom, sliced
½ cup (50 g) bean sprouts
1 scallion, chopped
¼ cup (25 g) shredded Chinese cabbage (or green cabbage)
2 teaspoons (10 ml) tamari or fish sauce

Heat coconut oil in skillet. In a bowl, beat eggs. Stir in remaining ingredients. Pour mixture into hot skillet, cover, cook until eggs are firm, turning once to lightly brown both sides. Remove from heat and serve. Makes two adult servings.

Net carbs: 2.4 grams per serving.

Fried Egg and Ham with White Sauce
1 tablespoon (15 ml) coconut oil
1 egg
3-5 ounces (80-140 g) sliced ham
¼ cup (60 ml) White Sauce (page 239)

Heat oil in a skillet. Fry egg and ham to desired doneness. Place ham on serving plate with egg on top, cover with White Sauce. Makes one serving.

Net carbs: 1.5 grams per serving.

Deviled Eggs

Deviled eggs can be made in advance and eaten as an on-the-go lunch or as a snack. Combined with a small salad or other raw vegetables, they can make an entire meal.

6 hard boiled eggs, peeled and halved lengthwise
¼ cup (60 ml) mayonnaise
2 teaspoons (10 ml) lemon juice
¼ teaspoon powdered mustard or 1 teaspoon (5 ml) Dijon mustard
1 teaspoon grated yellow onion
1 teaspoon (5 ml) Worcestershire sauce
Pinch white pepper

Suggested Garnishes:
Parsley, watercress, tarragon, dill, or chervil
Pimiento strips
Sliced green olive
Capers
Rolled anchovy fillets
Paprika

Mash yolks well, mix in remaining ingredients, mound into whites, and chill at least ½ hour. Add garnish as desired and serve. Makes 12 servings.
Net carbs: 0.5 grams per serving.

Zucchini Delight

While the eggs in this recipe may make this sound like a good breakfast meal, it is suitable for dinner as well.

2 tablespoons (30 ml) coconut oil (more may be added)
4 eggs
1 small zucchini, sliced
½ cup (50 g) onions, chopped
¼ cup (25 g) bell pepper, chopped
2 tablespoons (12 g) hot pepper (optional)
½ cup (60 g) cheese, shredded
½ cup 50 g) tomato, diced
2 tablespoons (30 ml) coconut oil (more may use added)
Salt and pepper to taste

Heat oil in skillet and lightly sauté all vegetables except the tomatoes. In a bowl, beat eggs and pour over vegetables in the skillet. Cover and cook for about 5 minutes or until eggs are about half-cooked. Remove lid, sprinkle cheese on top, cover and cook until cheese is melted and eggs are thoroughly cooked. Uncover, sprinkle top with diced tomato, cover, and turn off heat. Let sit for 1-2 minutes to warm the tomato pieces without cooking them. Makes one adult serving.

Net carbs: 9.4 grams per serving.

Bratwurst and Cabbage

This delicious single skillet meal can be enjoyed for breakfast or for dinner.

2 tablespoons (30 ml) coconut oil (more may be added)
1 bratwurst
¼ cup (25 g) onion, chopped
¼ cup (25 g) bell pepper, chopped
1½ cups (125 g) cabbage, chopped
Salt and black pepper to taste

Heat coconut oil in skillet. Add bratwurst, onions, and bell pepper. Sauté until the vegetables are crisp and tender and bratwurst is lightly browned. Stir in cabbage, cover, and cook until tender. Add salt and black pepper to taste and serve. Pour meat drippings over vegetables. Makes one adult serving.

Net carbs: 9.2 grams per serving.

Rollups

Rollups can be prepared in advance and make an excellent lunch to go. They can also make tasty snacks or a quick breakfast.

1 slice meat (1 oz)
1 slice cheese (1 oz)

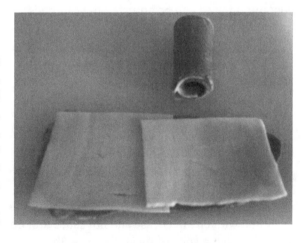

You can use most any type of thinly sliced meat (ham, beef, corned beef, chicken, turkey) and thinly sliced hard cheese (cheddar, Colby, Edam, Monterey jack, Swiss, mozzarella, Muenster). To make the basic rollup, layer one thinly sliced piece of cheese on top of a thinly sliced piece of meat. Roll both slices into a log. Eat and enjoy.

Net carbs: about 0.5 gram depending on the type of cheese used, one rollup per serving.

Variations: A variety of rollups can be created by wrapping other ingredients in the center of the log. You can use any one or more of the following: mustard, mayonnaise, sprouts, cream cheese, guacamole, avocado, pickle, chopped eggs, cucumber, sauerkraut, sweet or hot peppers, scallions, and sprouts with Vinaigrette Dressing (page 235).

Ruben Rollups

These rollups use a sauce that allows you to get a full tablespoon of coconut oil in one rollup. These rollups taste like a Ruben sandwich without the bread. You can adjust the recipe and add or subtract ingredients to suit your own taste.

1 slice (1 oz) nitrite-free corned beef or ham
1 slice (1 oz) Muenster or Swiss cheese (or cheese of your choice)
¼ slice pickle, cut lengthwise
2-3 tablespoons sauerkraut
Sauce
1 tablespoon coconut oil
1 tablespoon plain cream cheese
¼–½ teaspoon prepared mustard

Prepare the sauce first. Heat the coconut oil until it is soft or liquid, but not hot. Combine with cream cheese and mustard and mix thoroughly until creamy. Set aside. Lay out a slice of meat. Cover with a slice of cheese. Spread sauce evenly over the cheese. Top with a slice of pickle and the sauerkraut. Roll up and eat. Makes one rollup.

Net carbs 1.4 grams per serving.

Avocado Rollups

This is a delicious way to get a tablespoon of coconut oil. The amount of coconut oil used can be adjusted to your needs.

1 slice (1 oz) nitrite-free roast beef or pastrami
1 slice (1 oz) Monterey jack cheese (or cheese of your choice)
¼ avocado, cut lengthwise
2-4 tablespoons sprouts
Sauce
1 tablespoon coconut oil
1 tablespoon plain cream cheese
Dash hot pepper sauce (Tabasco Green Pepper Sauce is a good choice)*

Prepare the sauce first. Heat the coconut oil until it is soft or liquid, but not hot. Combine with cream cheese and hot sauce and mix thoroughly until creamy. Set aside. Lay out a slice of meat. Cover with a slice of cheese. Spread sauce evenly over the cheese. Top with a slice of avocado and sprouts. Roll up and eat. Makes one rollup.

*Salsa may be used instead of the hot pepper sauce if desired. If you use salsa do not mix it into the sauce. Instead, layer it on the rollup with the sprouts.

Net carbs 1.5 grams per serving.

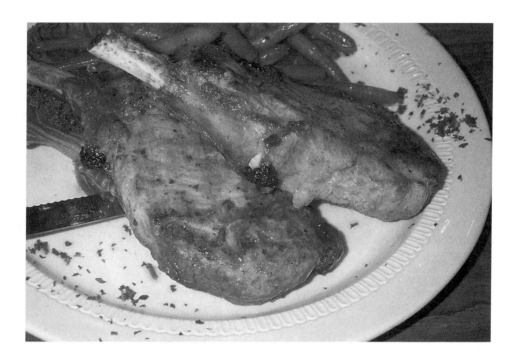

Pork Chops and Green Beans

2 tablespoons (30 ml) coconut oil (more may be added)
2 pork chops
½ cup (50 g) onion, chopped
3 cups (300 g) green beans
4 mushrooms, sliced
Salt and black pepper to taste

Heat coconut oil in skillet. Add pork chops and cook until browned on one side. Turn pork chops over and add onion and green beans. Cover and cook until chops are browned on second side and vegetables are tender. Stir in mushrooms and cook until tender, about 2 minutes. Remove from heat. Add salt and pepper and serve. Pour meat drippings over vegetables. Makes two adult servings.

Net carbs; 10.4 grams per serving.

Hamburger Steak, Mushrooms, and Onions

Ground beef is cooked like a steak with mushrooms and onions. Tastes fantastic with White Sauce, see page 239.

1 tablespoon (15 ml) coconut oil (more may be added)
1 pound (450 g) ground beef
8 ounces (230 g) mushrooms, sliced
1 medium onion, sliced and separated
Salt and black pepper to taste

Heat the oil in a skillet. Divide ground beef into four patties and place in the hot skillet. Add the onions. Cook the meat until one side is browned and flip over. Add mushrooms and continue to cook until second side of beef patty is cooked and mushrooms are tender. Add salt and pepper to taste. Pour drippings over meat and vegetables. Two beef patties with half the vegetables constitute one adult serving.

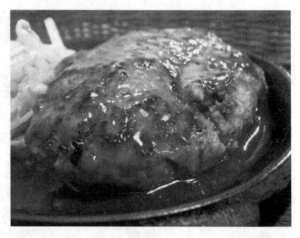

Net carbs: 7.2 grams per serving.

Variation: Serve with White Sauce (page 239) poured over the meat and vegetables.

Chicken and Broccoli

2 tablespoons (30 ml) coconut oil (more may be added)
1 pound (450 g) chicken parts (breast, thigh, or leg)
3 cups (200 g) broccoli, divided into stalks
Salt and black pepper to taste

Heat oil in a large skillet over medium heat. Place chicken, skin side down, in hot skillet, cover, and cook for 20-25 minutes. Turn chicken over, cover, and continue to cook for 15 minutes. Add broccoli, cover and cook another 10 minutes or until vegetables are tender and chicken is completely cooked. Add salt and pepper to taste. Pour meat drippings over broccoli. Makes two adult servings.

Net carbs: 4.5 grams per serving.

Lamb Chops and Asparagus

2 tablespoons (30 ml) coconut oil (more may be added)
2 lamb chops (may also use pork chops or steak)
4 cups (400 g) asparagus
Salt and black pepper to taste

Heat oil in a skillet, add chops, cover, and cook until one side is browned. Flip chops and add asparagus, cover and cook until asparagus is tender and chops thoroughly cooked. Remove from heat and add salt and pepper to taste. Pour meat drippings over asparagus. Serves two adults.

Net carbs: 5 grams per serving.

Variation: Serve with White Sauce (page 239) poured over the vegetables.

Chicken Stir-Fry

2 tablespoons (30 ml) coconut oil (more may be added)
1 pound (450 g) chicken, cut into bite size pieces
½ cup (50 g) onion, chopped
½ cup (50 g) snow peas, cut in half
½ cup (50 g) bok choy, chopped
½ cup (50 g) bell pepper, chopped
4 mushrooms, sliced
1 cup (100 g) bean sprouts
½ cup (50 g) bamboo shoots
2-3 teaspoons (10-15 ml) soy sauce
Salt to taste

Heat coconut oil in a skillet. Sauté chicken and vegetables until vegetables are tender and chicken is cooked. Turn off heat, add soy sauce and salt to taste. Serves two adults.

Net carbs: 9 grams per serving.

Stuffed Bell Peppers

1 bell pepper
½ pound (450 g) ground beef
¼ cup (25 g) onions, diced
2 mushrooms, chopped
1 tablespoon (15 ml) salsa
⅛ teaspoon salt
4 ounces (115 g) cheddar cheese

Preheat oven to 350 degrees F (175 C). Cut bell pepper in half lengthwise and remove stem, veins, and seeds. Place pepper halves aside. Mix together ground beef, onion, mushrooms, salsa, and salt. Fill each pepper shell with half of the mixture. Place the stuffed peppers on an oven safe pan or cookie sheet. Bake for 40 minutes. Divide the cheese in half and put half on each pepper. Cook another 10 minutes. Remove from the oven, cool, and enjoy. Makes two adult servings.

Net carb: 5.3 grams per serving.

Fillet of Sole in Coconut Milk

2 tablespoons (30 ml) coconut oil (more may be added)
½ medium onion, chopped
1 bell pepper, chopped
2 cups (200 g) chopped cauliflower
4 cloves garlic, chopped
4 sole fillets*
1 teaspoon garam masala**
1 cup (240 ml) coconut milk
Salt and black pepper to taste

Heat coconut oil in skillet and sauté onion, pepper, cauliflower, and garlic until tender. Push vegetable to side of skillet and add sole. Stir garam masala into coconut milk and add to skillet. Cover and simmer for about 8 minutes. Add salt and pepper. Makes four adult servings.

*You may use any type of fish in this recipe.

**Garam masala is a blend of spices commonly used in Indian cuisine and similar to curry powder. It's available in the spice section of most grocery stores. If you don't have garam masala, you can use curry powder.

Net carbs: 5 grams per serving.

Appendix A
Cholesterol in Some Common Foods

Cholesterol (mg) sorted by nutrient content

Description	Weight (g)	Common Measure	Content per Measure
Chicken giblets	145	1 cup	641
Turkey giblets	145	1 cup	419
Beef liver	85	3 oz	324
Egg, whole, extra large	58	1	245
Egg, whole, large	50	1	212
Duck, roasted	221	1/2 duck	197
Egg, whole, medium	44	1	186
Shrimp	85	3 oz	147
Salmon	155	1/2 fillet	135
Cheese, ricotta, whole milk	246	1 cup	125
Sardine, canned in oil	85	3 oz	121
Chicken breast, meat and skin	140	1/2 breast	119
Chicken, stewing, meat only	140	1 cup	116
Veal, leg (top round)	85	3 oz	114
Haddock	150	1 fillet	111
Chicken, liver	20	1 liver	110
Turkey, roasted	140	1 cup	106
Pork spareribs	85	3 oz	103
Lamb, trimmed to 1/4"fat	85	3 oz	103
Pork shoulder	85	3 oz	97
Veal, rib	85	3 oz	94
Beef, chuck roast	85	3 oz	90
Flounder	127	1 fillet	86
Sole	127	1 fillet	86
Lamb, loin	85	3 oz	85
Crab, fresh	85	3 oz	85
Ground turkey	82	1 patty	84
Pollock	85	3 oz	82
Chicken, dark meat	84	3 oz	81

Description	Weight (g)	Common Measure	Content per Measure
Ham	85	3 oz	80
Pork chops	85	3 oz	78
Beef, ground, 80% lean	85	3 oz	77
Beef, ground, 85% lean	85	3 oz	77
Beef, ground, 75% lean	85	3 oz	76
Cheese, ricotta, part skim milk	246	1 cup	76
Catfish	85	3 oz	69
Beef, rib, (ribs 6-12)	85	3 oz	68
Rockfish	149	1 fillet	66
Halibut	159	1/2 fillet	65
Beef, top sirloin	85	3 oz	64
Chicken, drumstick, meat and skin,	72	1 drumstick	62
Lobster	85	3 oz	61
Turkey, all classes, light meat	84	3 oz	58
Trout, rainbow	85	3 oz	58
Pollock, walleye	60	1 fillet	58
Clams	85	3 oz	57
Scallop	93	6 large	57
Swordfish	106	1 piece	53
Chicken, thigh, meat only	52	1 thigh	49
Tuna, yellowfin,	85	3 oz	49
Cod, Atlantic	85	3 oz	47
Ocean perch,	85	3 oz	46
Frankfurter, chicken	45	1 frank	45
Oyster,	84	6 medium	45
Hotdog, plain	98	1 sandwich	44

Source: USDA National Nutrient Database for Standard Reference, Release 17.

Appendix
B | Net Carbohydrate Counter

Units of Measure
1 tablespoon (tbsp) = ½ fl oz = 14.8 ml (approximately 15 ml)
3 teaspoons = 1 tbsp
4 tbsp = ¼ cup
16 tbsp = 1 cup
1 cup = 8 fl oz = 236.6 ml
1 inch (in) = 2.5 cm

Vegetables	Amount	Net Carbs (g)
Alfalfa sprouts	1 cup	0.4
Artichoke, boiled	1 medium	6.5
Arugula	1 cup	0.4
Asparagus, canned	1 cup	2.2
Asparagus, raw	1 cup	2.4
Asparagus, raw	5 in spear	0.2
Avocado (Haas)	1 each	3.5
Bamboo shoots, canned	1 cup	2.4
Beans, boiled		
black	1 cup	26.0
black-eyed peas	1 cup	25.0
garbanzo (chickpeas)	1 cup	32.0
great northern	1 cup	25.0
green beans	1 cup	4.1
kidney	1 cup	27.0
lentils	1 cup	24.0
lima	1 cup	24.0
navy	1 cup	36.0
pinto	1 cup	30.0
soybeans	1 cup	6.8
wax beans	1 cup	4.0

white beans	1 cup	34.0
Bean sprouts (mung)		
boiled	1 cup	4.2
raw	1 cup	4.4
Beets (sliced), raw	1 cup	9.3
Beet greens, boiled	1 cup	2.6
Broccoli, raw, chopped	1 cup	3.6
Brussels sprouts		
boiled	1 cup	7.0
raw	1 cup	4.6
Cabbage (green), shredded		
cooked	1 cup	3.2
raw	1 cup	2.2
Cabbage (red), shredded		
cooked	1 cup	4.0
raw	1 cup	2.8
Cabbage (savoy), shredded		
cooked	1 cup	3.8
raw	1 cup	2.0
Chinese cabbage (bok choy)		
cooked	1 cup	1.4
raw	1 cup	0.8
Carrot		
boiled, chopped	1 cup	11.2
raw, whole	1 medium	5.1
raw, shredded	1 cup	8.0
juice	1 cup	18.0
Cauliflower		
boiled	1 cup	1.6
raw, chopped	1 cup	2.8
Celery		
raw, whole	8 in long	0.8
raw, diced	1 cup	1.8
Chard		
boiled	1 cup	3.4
raw	1 cup	0.7
Chives, chopped	1 tbsp	<0.1
Collards		
boiled	1 cup	4.2
Cucumber, sliced		
raw with peel	1 cup	3.2
raw peeled	1 cup	1.8
Daikon, sliced	1 cup	2.0
Eggplant, raw	1 cup	3.0
Escarole, raw	1 cup	0.7
Garlic, raw	1 clove	0.9

Jerusalem artichokes, raw	1 cup	23.0
Jicama, raw	1 cup	5.0
Kale		
boiled, chopped	1 cup	4.7
raw, chopped	1 cup	5.4
Kohlrabi		
cooked, sliced	1 cup	9.0
raw, sliced	1 cup	3.5
Leeks,		
boiled	1 cup	6.8
raw	1 cup	11.0
Lettuce		
butterhead	1 leaf	0.1
iceberg	1 leaf	0.1
loose leaf, shredded	1 cup	0.6
Mushrooms (button)		
boiled	1 cup	4.8
raw, sliced	1 cup	2.4
raw	1 mushroom	0.4
Mustard greens, raw	1 cup	0.5
Okra, raw	1 cup	4.6
Onion		
raw, slice	¼ in thick	3.3
raw, chopped	1 tbsp	0.9
raw, chopped	1 cup	14.0
raw, whole medium	2½ in dia	9.6
Parsley		
raw, chopped	1 tbsp	0.1
Parsnips		
raw, chopped	1 cup	17.4
Peas		
edible-pod, cooked	1 cup	7.0
green, boiled	1 cup	7.0
split, boiled	1 cup	25.0
Peppers		
hot red chili, raw	1 cup	5.5
sweet (bell), raw	1 cup	4.4
sweet (bell), raw	1 medium	5.3
jalapeno, canned	1 pepper	0.4
Potatoes		
baked	1 small (4.9 oz)	26.0
baked	1 medium (6.1 oz)	33.0
baked	1 large (10.5 oz)	57.0
mashed, with milk	1 cup	31.0
hash brown	1 cup	30.0
Pumpkin, canned	1 cup	12.7

Radish, raw	1 medium	0.1
Rhubarb	1 cup	3.4
Rutabaga	1 cup	12.0
Sauerkraut	1 cup	2.4
Scallions,		
raw, chopped	1 tbsp	0.2
raw, chopped	4 in long	0.7
Shallots	1 tbsp	1.4
Spinach		
canned	1 cup	2.0
frozen, boiled	1 cup	4.6
raw	1 cup	0.4
Squash		
acorn, baked	1	20.8
butternut, baked	1 cup	21.4
crookneck, raw sliced	1 cup	2.8
Hubbard, baked	1 cup	22.0
scallop, raw sliced	1 cup	5.0
spaghetti, baked	1 cup	7.8
zucchini, raw sliced	1 cup	2.2
Sweet potatoes		
baked	1 small (2.1 oz)	10.4
baked	1 medium (4.0 oz)	19.8
baked	1 large (6.3 oz)	31.4
Taro		
root, cooked, sliced	1 cup	39.0
leaves, steamed	1 cup	3.0
Tofu	½ cup	2.5
Tomato		
cooked	1 cup	7.9
raw, chopped	1 cup	4.8
raw, sliced	¼ in thick	0.6
raw	1 small (3.2 oz)	2.4
raw	1 medium (4.3 oz)	3.3
raw	1 large (6.4 oz)	4.9
cherry	1 medium (0.6 oz)	0.5
Italian	1 medium (2.2 oz)	1.7
juice	1 cup	8.0
sauce	½ cup	7.0
paste	½ cup	19.0
Turnips, raw cubed	1 cup	6.0
Turnip greens, raw	1 cup	1.4
Water chestnuts	1 cup	14
Watercress, raw chopped	1 cup	0.2
Yam, baked	1 cup	32.2

Fruit	Amount	Net Carbs (g)
Apples		
raw	1 each	18.0
juice	1 cup	29.0
applesauce, unsweetened	1 cup	25.0
Apricots		
raw	1 each	3.1
canned, in syrup	1 cup	51.0
Banana	1 each	24.0
Blackberries, fresh	1 cup	7.1
Blueberries, fresh	1 cup	17.5
Boysenberries, frozen	1 cup	9.1
Cantaloupe		
small	1 each (4¼ in dia)	34.8
medium	1 each (5 in dia)	43.6
large	1 each (6½ in dia)	64.3
cubes	1 cup	12.8
Cherries		
Sweet, raw	10 each	9.7
Cranberry		
Raw	1 cup	11.6
Sauce, whole berry canned	1 cup	102.0
Dates, raw		
whole without pits	1 each	5.2
chopped	1 cup	98.5
Elderberries, raw	1 cup	16.4
Figs	1 each	10.5
Gooseberries, raw	1 cup	8.8
Grapefruit, raw	1 half	8.6
Grapes		
Thompson seedless	1 each	0.9
American (slip skin)	1 each	0.4
juice, canned	1 cup	37.0
juice, frozen concentrate	1 cup	31.0
Honeydew		
small	1 each (5 ¼-in dia)	83.0
large	1 each (6-7 in dia)	106.3
balls	1 cup	14.7
Kiwi, raw	1 each	8.7
Lemon, raw	1 each	3.8
Lemon Juice	1 tbsp	1.3
Lime, raw	1 each	3.2
Lime Juice	1 tbsp	1.3

Loganberries, frozen	1 cup	11.7
Mandarin orange,		
canned, juice pack	1 cup	22.0
canned, light syrup	1 cup	39.2
Mango, raw	1 each	31.5
Mulberries, raw	1 cup	11.2
Nectarines, raw	1 each	13.0
Olives, black		
large	1 each	0.2
jumbo	1 each	0.3
Oranges, raw	1 each	12.0
Juice, fresh	1 cup	25.0
Juice, frozen concentrate	1 cup	27.0
Papayas, raw	1 each	24.3
Peaches		
raw, whole	1 each	8.0
raw sliced	1 cup	14.2
canned, light syrup	½ fruit	16.4
Pears		
raw	1 each	20.0
raw, sliced	1 cup	20.5
halves, canned	1 cup	15.1
Persimmon, raw	1 each	8.4
Pineapple,		
fresh, cubed	1 cup	17.2
canned unsweetened	1 cup	35.0
Plantains, cooked	1 cup	44.4
Plums, raw	1 each	7.6
Prunes		
dried	1 each	4.7
juice	1 cup	42.2
Raisins	1 cup	109.0
Raspberries, raw	1 cup	6.0
Strawberries		
raw, whole	1 small	0.4
raw, whole	1 medium	0.7
raw, whole	1 large	1.0
raw, halves	1 cup	8.7
raw, sliced	1 cup	9.5
Tangerines, fresh	1 each	7.5
Watermelon		
sliced	1 inch	33.0
balls	1 cup	11.1

Nuts and Seeds	Amount	Net Carbs (g)
Almonds		
sliced	1 cup	7.2
slivered	1 cup	8.6
whole	1 each	0.1
whole	22 kernels (1 oz)	2.2
almond butter	1 tbsp	2.8
Brazil nuts	7 each	1.4
Cashew		
halves and whole	1 cup (4.8 oz)	40.7
whole	18 nuts (1 oz)	8.4
whole	1 each	0.5
cashew butter	1 tbsp	4.1
Coconut		
fresh	1 piece (2 x 2 in)	2.7
fresh, shredded	1 cup	5.0
dried, unsweetened	1 cup	7.0
dried, sweetened	1 cup	40.2
coconut milk, canned	1 cup	6.6
coconut water	1 cup	6.3
Filberts (hazelnuts)		
whole	10 nuts	0.9
whole	1 each	0.1
whole	1 cup	9.4
Macadamia		
whole	7 nuts	1.5
whole	1 each	0.2
whole or halves	1 cup	7.0
Peanuts		
raw	1 cup	11.1
dry roasted	1 cup	19.5
dry roasted	30 nuts	3.8
peanut butter	1 tbsp	2.1
Pecans		
halves, raw	20 halves	1.2
halves, raw	1 cup	4.3
chopped, raw	1 cup	4.7
Pine nuts		
whole	10 nuts	0.1
whole	1 cup	12.7
Pistachio		
whole	1 each	0.1
whole	49 kernels	5.0
whole	1 cup	21.4

Pumpkin seeds		
whole	10 seeds	1.8
whole	1 cup	22.5
Sesame seeds		
whole	1 tbsp	1.0
sesame butter (tahini)	1 tbsp	2.5
Soy nuts, roasted	1 cup	42.3
Sunflower seeds		
whole, hulled	1 tbsp	1.0
Walnuts		
black, chopped	1 tbsp	0.3
black, chopped	1 cup	3.9
English, chopped	1 cup	8.4
English, halves	10 halves	1.4

Grains and Flours	Amount	Net Carbs (g)
Amaranth		
grain	1 cup	99.4
flour	1 cup	108.4
Arrowroot flour	1 tbsp	6.8
Barley		
pearled, cooked	1 cup	36.4
flour	1 cup	95.4
Buckwheat		
grain, roasted	1 cup	34.2
flour	1 cup	72.8
Bulgur, cooked	1 cup	25.6
Corn		
whole kernel	1 cup	25.1
ear, small	5½ - 6½ in long	11.9
ear, medium	6¾ - 7½ in long	14.7
ear, large	7¾ - 9 in long	23.3
grits, dry	1 cup	121.7
grits, cooked with water	1 cup	30.5
cornmeal, dry	1 cup	84.9
corn starch	1 tbsp	7.0
popcorn, air popped	1 cup	5.0
hominy, canned	1 cup	18.8
Millet, cooked	1 cup	25.8
Oats		
oatmeal, cooked	1 cup	21.3
oatmeal, dry	1 cup	46.4
oat bran, cooked	1 cup	19.3
oat bran, dry	1 cup	47.7
Quinoa, cooked	1 cup	43.0

Rice

brown, cooked	1 cup	41.3
white, cooked	1 cup	43.9
instant, cooked	1 cup	40.4
wild rice, cooked	1 cup	32.0
brown rice flour	1 tbsp	7.1
white rice flour	1 tbsp	7.7
Rye flour, dark	1 cup	59.2
Semolina, enriched	1 cup	115.6
Soy flour	1 cup	21.6
Tapioca, pearl dry	1 tbsp	8.3

Wheat

white, enriched	1 cup	92.0
white, enriched	1 tbsp	5.8
whole wheat	1 cup	72.4
whole wheat	1 tbsp	4.5
wheat bran	1 tbsp	0.8

Bread and Baked Goods	Amount	Net Carbs (g)
Bagels		
white enriched	1 each (3.7 oz)	57.0
whole grain	1 each (4.5 oz)	64.0
Bread		
rye	1 slice	13.0
whole wheat	1 slice	10.7
raisin bread	1 slice	12.5
hamburger bun	1 roll	20.4
hot dog bun	1 roll	20.4
hard/Kaiser roll	1 roll	28.7
Crackers		
saltine	1 each	2.2
multigrain	1 each	2.0
cheese	1 each (1 in square)	0.6
English muffin	1 each	24.0
Pancake	1 each (4 in dia)	13.4
Pita		
white	1 each	32.0
whole wheat	1 each	30.5
Tortilla		
corn	1 each (6 in)	11.0
flour	1 each (8 in)	22.0
flour	1 each (10½ in)	33.8
Wonton wrappers	1 each (3½ in)	4.5

Pasta	Amount	Net Carbs (grams)
Macaroni, cooked		
white, enriched	1 cup	37.9
whole wheat	1 cup	33.3
corn	1 cup	32.4
Noodles, cooked		
cellophane (mung bean)	1 cup	38.8
egg	1 cup	38.0
soba	1 cup	37.7
rice	1 cup	42.0
Spaghetti, cooked		
white, enriched	1 cup	37.3
whole wheat	1 cup	30.9
corn	1 cup	32.4

Dairy	Amount	Net Carbs (grams)
Butter	1 tbsp	0
Buttermilk	1 cup	11.7
Cheese (hard)		
American, sliced	1 oz	0.4
Cheddar, sliced	1 oz	0.4
Cheddar, shredded	1 cup	1.5
Colby, sliced	1 oz	0.7
Colby, shredded	1 cup	2.9
Edam, sliced	1 oz	0.4
Edam, shredded	1 cup	1.5
goat milk cheese	1 oz	0.6
Gruyere, sliced	1 oz	0.1
Gruyere, shredded	1 cup	0.4
Monterey, sliced	1 oz	0.2
Monterey, shredded	1 cup	0.8
mozzarella, sliced	1 oz	0.6
mozzarella, shredded	1 cup	2.5
Muenster, sliced	1 oz	0.3
Muenster, shredded	1 cup	1.2
Parmesan, sliced	1 oz	0.9
Parmesan, grated	1 tbsp	0.2
Parmesan, shredded	1 tbsp	2.0
Swiss, sliced	1 oz	1.5
Swiss, shredded	1 cup	5.8
Cheese (soft)		
cottage, non-fat	1 cup	9.7

cottage, 2% fat	1 cup	8.1
cream cheese, plain	1 tbsp	0.4
cream cheese, low-fat	1 tbsp	1.1
feta, crumbled	1 oz	1.2
feta, crumbled	1 cup	6.1
ricotta, whole milk	1 oz	0.9
ricotta, whole milk	1 cup	7.4
ricotta, part skim	1 oz	1.4
ricotta, part skim	1 cup	12.5
Cream		
heavy, whipping	1 cup	6.7
half and half	1 cup	10.6
sour	1 tbsp	0.5
Goat milk	1 cup	11.0
Milk		
skim, non-fat	1 cup	12.3
1%	1 cup	12.2
2%	1 cup	11.4
whole, 3.3% fat	1 cup	11.0
Soy milk, non-fat	1 cup	9.5
Soy milk, low-fat	1 cup	12.0
Yogurt		
plain, fat-free	1 cup	18.9
plain, whole milk	1 cup	12.0
vanilla, low-fat	1 cup	31.0
fruit added, low-fat	1 cup	43.0

Meat and Eggs	Amount	Net Carbs (grams)
Beef	3 oz	0
Buffalo	3 oz	0
Eggs	1 large	0.6
Egg yolk	1 large	0.3
Fish	3 oz	0
Lamb	3 oz	0
Poultry	3 oz	0
Pork	3 oz	0
bacon, cured	3 pieces	0.5
Canadian-style bacon	2 pieces	1
fresh side (natural bacon)	3 oz	0
ham	1 oz	0.7
Shellfish		
oysters	1 oz	1.4
crab	1 oz	0
clams, canned	1 oz	1.4

lobster, cooked	3 oz	1.1
mussels, cooked	1 oz	2.1
scallops	1 oz	0.5
shrimp, cooked	3 oz	0
Venison	3 oz	0

Miscellaneous	Amount	Net Carbs (grams)
Baking soda	1 tsp	0
Catsup		
regular	1 tbsp	3.8
low-carb	1 tbsp	1.0
Fats and oils	1 tbsp	0
Gelatin, dry	1 envelope	0
Gravy, canned or dry mix	½ cup	6.5 (average)
Fish sauce	1 tbsp	0.7
Herbs and spices	1 tbsp	1 (average)
Honey	1 tbsp	17.2
Horseradish, prepared	1 tbsp	1.4
Maple syrup	1 tbsp	13.4
Mayonnaise	1 tbsp	3.5
Molasses	1 tbsp	14.9
Molasses, blackstrap	1 tbsp	12.2
Mustard		
yellow	1 tbsp	0.3
Dijon	1 tbsp	0
Pancake syrup	1 tbsp	15.1
Pickles		
dill, medium	1 pickle	3.1
dill, slice	1 (0.2 oz)	0.2
sweet, medium	1 pickle	11.0
pickle relish, sweet	1 tbsp	5.3
Tartar sauce	1 tbsp	2.0
Salsa	1 tbsp	0.8
Soy sauce	1 tbsp	1.1
Sugar		
white, granulated	1 tbsp	12.0
brown	1 tbsp	13.0
powdered	1 tbsp	8.0
Vinegar		
apple cider	1 tbsp	0
balsamic	1 tbsp	2.0
red wine	1 tbsp	0
rice	1 tbsp	0
white wine	1 tbsp	0
Worcestershire sauce	1 tbsp	3.3

References

Chapter 1: Is There a Cure for Autism?
1. Facts and statistics. http://www.autism-society.org/about-autism/facts-and-statistics.html. Accessed 10/25/2011.
2. Boyle, C.A, et al. Trends in the prevalence of developmental disabilities in US children, 1997-2008. *Pediatrics* 2011;127:1034-1042.

Chapter 2: The Vaccine Controversy
1. Wakefield, A.J., et al. Iieal-lymphoid-nodular hyper plasia, non-specific colitis, and pervasive developmental disorder in children. *Lancet* 1998;351:637-641.
2. The Other Side of the Story: The Vioxx Drug Case. http://www.maryalice.com/cases/Vioxx.asp.
3. First Fraud: Dr. Poul Thorsen and the original Danish Study. http://www.ageofautism.com/2010/03/first-fraud-dr-poul-thorsen-and-the-original-danish-study.html.
4. Poul Thorsen's Mutating Resume. http://www.ageofautism.com/2010/03/poul-thorsens-mutating-resume.html.
5. Kalb, C. Stomping Through A Medical Minefield. *Newsweek* Oct 25, 2008.
6. Klein, N.P., et al. Measles-mumps-rubella-varicella combination vaccine and the risk of febrile seizures. *Pediatrics* 2010;126:e1-8.
7. Jail for Belgians who reject polio shot. http://www.foxnews.com/wires/2008Mar12/0,4670,PolioVaccinePrison,00.html. Accessed 11/9/2011.
8. McNeil, D.G. Book is rallying resistance to the antivaccine crusade. *New York Times* Jan 12, 2009.
9. Handley, J.B. Dr. Paul Offit, The autism expert. Doesn't see patients with autism? www.whale.to/vaccine/handley56.html.
10. Inside the business of medical ghostwriting. http://www.cbc.ca/marketplace/pre-2007/files/health/ghostwriting/index.html.
11. Rapidly Increasing Criminal and Civil Monetary Penalties Against the Pharmaceutical Industry: 1991 to 2010. http://freepdfhosting.com/53888d5b53.pdf.

Chapter 3: Do Vaccines Cause Autism?

1. Hallmayer, J., et al. Genetic heritability and shared environmental factors among twin pairs with autism. *Arch Gen Psychiatry* 2011;68:1095-1102.

2. London, E.A. The environment as an etiologic factor in autism: a new direction for research. *Environ Health Perspect* 2000;108 Supple 3:401-404.

3.National Human Genome Research Institute. http://www.genome.gov/18016846. Accessed May 11, 2011.

4. Child Health Safety, June 30, 2010. http://childhealthsafety.wordpress.com/2010/06/30/vaccination-causes-autism-%E2%80%93-say-us-government-merck%E2%80%99s-director-of%C2%A0vaccines/ Accessed May 11, 2011.

5. Chouliaras, G., et al. Vaccine-associated herpes zoster ophthalmicus (correction of opthalmicus) and encephalitis in an immunocompetent child. *Pediatrics* 2010;125:e969-e972.

6. Wakefield, A.J., et al. Iieal-lymphoid-nodular hyper plasia, non-specific colitis, and pervasive developmental disorder in children. *Lancet* 1998;351:637-641.

7. Benjamin, C.M., et al. Joint and limb symptoms in children after immunisation with measles, mumps, and rubella vaccine. *British Medical Journal* 1992;304:1075-1078.

8. Mitchell, L.A., et al. Chronic rubella vaccine-associated arthropathy. *Archives of Internal Medicine* 1993;153:2268-2274.

9. Nussinovitch, M., et al. Arthritis after mumps and measles vaccination. *Arch Dis Child* 1995;72:348-349.

10. Ogra, P.L., et al. Rubella-virus infection in juvenile rheumatoid arthritis. *Lancet* 1975;24:1157-1161.

11. Pattison, E., et al. Environmental risk factors for the development of psoriatic arthritis: results from a case-control study. *Ann Rheum Dis* 2008;67:672-676.

12. Geier, D.A. and Geier, M.R. Rubella vaccine and arthritic adverse reactions: an analysis of the Vaccine Adverse Events Reporting System (VAERS) database from 1991 through 1998. *Clin Exp Rheumatol* 2001;19:724-726.

13. Mitchell, L.A., et al. Rubella virus vaccine associated arthropathy in postpartum immunized women: influence of preimmunization serologic status on development of joint manifestations. *J Rheumatol* 2000;27:418-423.

14. Valenzuela-Suarez, H., et al. A seventy-four-year-old man with bilateral conjunctival hyperemia, urinary symptoms, and secondary reactive arthritis following the administration of the BCG vaccine. *Gac Med Mex* 2008;144:345-347.

15. de Almeida, A.E., et al. Septic arthritis due to Haemophilus influenzae serotype a in the post-vaccination era in Brazil. *J Med Microbiol* 2008;57:1311-1312.

16. Dudelzak, J., et al. New-onset psoriasis and psoriatic arthritis in a patient treated with Bacillus Calmette-Guerin (BCG) immunotherapy. *J Drugs Dermatol* 2008;7:684.

17. Tinazzi, E., et al. Reactive arthritis following BCG immunotherapy for bladder carcinoma. *Clin Rheumatol* 2005;24:425-427.

18. Garyfallou, G.T. Mycobacterial sepsis following intravesical instillation of bacillus Calmette-Guerin. *Acad Emerg Med* 1996;3:157-160.

19. Hirayama, T., et al. Anaphylactoid purpura after intravesical therapy using bacillus Calmette-Guerin for superficial bladder cancer. *Hinyokika Kiyo* 2008;54:127-129.

20. Bruce, M.G., et al. Epidemiology of Haemophilus influenzae serotypea, North American Artic, 2000-2005. *Emerg Infect Dis* 2008;14:48-55.

21. Thoon, K.C., et al. Epidemiology of invasive Haemophilus influenzae type b disease in Singapore children, 1994-2003. *Vaccine* 2007;25:6482-6489.

22. Schattner, A. Consequence or coincidence? The occurrence, pathogenesis and significance of autoimmune manifestations after viral vaccines. *Vaccine* 2005;23:3876-3886.

23. Shoenfeld, Y. and Aron-Maor, A. Vaccination and autoimmunity-'vaccinosis': a dangerous liaison? *J Autoimmun* 2000;14:1-10.

24. Cutrone, R., et al. Some oral poliovirus vaccines were contaminated with infectious SV40 after 1961. *Cancer Res* 2005;65:10273-10279.

25. Giangaspero, M, et al. Genotypes of pestivirus RNA detected in live virus vaccines for human use. *J Vet Med Sci* 2001;63:723-733.

26. Johnson, J.A. and Heneine, W. Characteristics of endogenous avian leukosis virus in chicken embryonic fibroblast substrates used in production of measles and mumps vaccine. *J Virol* 2001;75:3605-3612.

27. Pastoret, P.P. Human and animal vaccine contaminations. *Biologicals* 2010;38:332-334.

28. Hewitson, L., et al. Influence of pediatric vaccines on amygdale growth and opioid ligand binding in rhesus macaque infants: A pilot study. *Acta Neurobiol Exp* 2010;70:147-164.

29. Baby death may be linked to toxic vaccine. http://www.whale.to/m/dpt1.html. Accessed 11/28/2011.

30. Cohly, H.H. and Panja, A. Immunological findings in autism. *Int Rev Neurobiol* 2005;71:317-341.

31. Singh, V.K., et al. Abnormal measles-mumps-rubella antibodies and CNS autoimmunity in children with autism. *J Biomed Sci* 2002;9:359-364.

32. Singh, V.K. and Jensen , R.L. Elevated levels of measles antibodies in children with autism. *Pediatr Neurol* 2003;28:292-294.

33. Sabra, A., et al. Ileal-lymphoid nodular hyperplasia, non-specific colitis, and pervasive developmental disorders in children. *Lancet* 1998;352:234-235.

34. Furlano, R.I., et al. Colonic CD8 and gamma delta T-cell infiltration with epithelial damage in children with autism. *J Pediatr* 2001;138:366-372.

35. Uhlmann, V., et al. Potential viral pathogenic mechanism for new variant inflammatory bowel disease. *Mol Pathol* 2002;55:84-90.

36. Kawashima, H., et al. Detection and sequencing of measles virus form peripheral mononuclear cells from patients with inflammatory bowel disease and autism. *Dig Dis Sci* 2000;45:723-729.

37. Blaylock, R.L. Central role of excitotoxicity in autism. *JANA* 2003;6(1):10-22.

38. Blaylock. R.L. Interaction of cytokines, excitotoxins, reactive nitrogen and oxygen species in autism spectrum disorders. *JANA* 2003;6(4):21-35.

39. Blaylock, R.L. The danger of excessive vaccination during brain development: the case for a link to Autism Spectrum Disorders (ASD). *Medical Veritas* 2008;5:1727-1741.

40. Gallagher, C.M. and Goodman, M.S. Hepatitis B vaccination of male neonates and autism diagnosis NHIS 1997-2002. *J Toxicol Environ Health* 2010;73:1665-1677.

41. Gallagher, C.M. and Goodman, M.S. Hepatitis B vaccine of male neonates and autism. *Annals of Epidemiology* 2009;19(9):659.

42. Kaye, J.A., et al. Mumps, measles, and rubella vaccine and the incidence of autism recorded by general practitioners: a time trend analysis. *BMJ* 2001;322:460-463.

43. Bernard, S., et al. Autism: a novel form of mercury poisoning. *Med Hypotheses* 2001;56:462-471.

44. Geier, M.R. and Geier, D.A. Thimerosal in childhood vaccines, neurodevelopment disorders, and heart disease in the United States. *JAPS* 2003:8:6-11.

45. Geier, D.A. and Geier, M.R. An assessment of the impact of thimerosal on childhood neurodevelopmental disorders. *Pediatr Rehabil* 2003;6:97 -102.

46. Geier, D.A. and Geier, M.R. Neurodevelopmental disorders following thimerosal-containing childhood immunizations: a follow-up analysis. *Int J Toxicol* 2004;23:369-376.

47. Young, H.A., et al. Thimerosal exposure in infants and neurodevelopmental disorderers: an assessment of computerized medical records in the Vaccine Safety Datalink. *J Neurol Sci* 2008;271:110-118.

48. Thimerosal content in some US licensed vaccines. http://www.vaccinesafety.edu/thi-table.htm. Accessed 10/28/11.

49. State of health of unvaccinated children. http://www.vaccineinjury.info/vaccinations-in-general/health-unvaccinated-children/survey-results-illnesses.html. Accessed 11/28/2011.

Chapter 4: Should Your Children Be Vaccinated?

1. Deforest, A., et al. Simultaneous administration of measles-mumps-rubella vaccine with booster doses of diphtheria-tetanus-pertussis and poliovirus vaccines. *Pediatrics* 1988;81:237-246.

2. CIA world factbook. www.cia.gov/library/publications/the-world-factbook/index.html. Accessed 3/2/ 2011.

3. Pertussis vaccination. http://www.cdc.gov/mmwr/preview/mmwrhtml/00048610.htm. Accessed 9/20/2011.

4. Doshi, P. Are US flu death figures more PR than science? *BMJ* 2005;331:1412.

5. Szilagyi, P.G., et al. Influenza vaccine effectiveness among children 6 to 59 months of age during 2 influenza seasons: a case-cohort study. *Arch Pediatr Adolesc Med* 2008;162:943-951.

6. Smith, S., et al. Vaccines for preventing influenza in healthy children. *Cochrane Database Syst Rev* 2006;Jan 25;(1):CD004879.

7. Black, S.B., et al. Effectiveness of influenza vaccine during pregnancy in preventing hospitalizations and outpatient visits for respiratory illness in pregnant women and their infants. *Am J Perinatol* 2004;21:333-339.

8. Thompson, W.W., et al. Influenza-associated hospitalizations in the United States. *JAMA* 2004;292:1333-1340.

9. Thompson, W.W., et al. Mortality associated with influenza and respiratory syncytial virus in the United States. *JAMA* 2003;289:179-186.

10. Jefferson, T., et al. Efficacy and effectiveness of influenza vaccines in elderly people: a systematic review. *Lancet* 2005;366:1165-1174.

11. Dr. J. Anthony Morris. http://www.whale.to/vaccines/morris_h.html. Accessed 3/3/2011.

12. Study: Whooping cough vaccination fades in 3 years. http://www.chron.com/news/article/Study-Whooping-cough-vaccination-fades-in-3-years-2177775.php. Accessed 9/20/2011.

13. http://www.vaccineinjury.info/vaccinations-in-general/health-unvaccinated-children/survey-results-illnesses.html. Accessed October 21, 2001.

14. Kristensen, I, et al. Routine vaccinations and child survival: follow up study in Guinea-Bissau, West Africa. *BMJ* 2000;321:1435-1441.

15. Immunisation Awareness Society. www.ias.org.nz. Accessed 4/3/2011.

16. Vaccinated kids 2-5 more diseases than unvaccinated. http://healthfreedoms.org/2011/10/14/big-study-vaccinated-kids-2-5-more-diseases-than-unvaccinated. Accessed 10/26/2011.

17. 50% of US children have chronic disease/disorders, 21% developmentally disabled. http://journal.livingfood.us/2011/05/26/alarming-new-studies-50-of-u-s-children-have-chronic-illnesses-21-developmentally-disabled/. Accessed 10/26/2011.

18. Blaylock, R.L. The danger of excessive vaccination during brain development: the case for a link to Autism Spectrum Disorders (ASD). *Medical Veritas* 2008;5:1727-1741.

19. Wegman, M.E. Sumposiuim: Accomplishments in child nutrition during the 20th century. Infant mortality in the 20th century, dramatic but uneven progress. *J Nutr* 2001;131:401S-408S.

20. McKinlay, J.B. and McKinlay, S.M. The questionable contribution of medical measures to the decline of mortality in the United States in the twentieth century. *Health and Society* 1977;55:405-429.

21. Menczer, J., et al. Possible role of mumps virus in the etiology of ovarian cancer. *Cancer* 1978;43:1375-1379.

Chapter 5: The Underlying Cause of Autism

1. Block, M.L., et al. Microglia-mediated neurotoxicity: uncovering the molecular mechanisms. *Nat Rev Neurosci* 2007;8:57-69.

2. Lull, M.E. and Block, M.L. Microglial activation and chronic neurodegeneration. *Neurotherapeutics* 2010;7:354-365.

3. Fife, B. *Stop Alzheimer's Now!: How to Prevent and Reverse Dementia, Parkinson's, ALS, Multiple Sclerosis, and Other Neurodegenerative Disorders.* Piccadilly Books, Ltd.:Colorado Springs, CO; 2011.

4. Blaylock, R.L. A possible central mechanism in autism spectrum disorders, part 1. *Altern Ther Health Med* 2008;14(6):46-53.

5. Blaylock, R.L. A possible central mechanism in autism spectrum disorders, part 2: immunoexcitotoxicity. *Altern Ther Health Med* 2009;15(1):60-67.

6. Blaylock, R.L. A possible central mechanism in autism spectrum disorders, part 3: the role of excitotoxins food additives and the synergistic effects of other environmental toxins. *Altern Ther Health Med* 2009;15(2):56-60.

7. Blaylock, R.L. Central role of excitotoxicity in autism. *JANA* 2003;6(1):10-22.

8. Vargas, D.L., et al. Neuroglial activation and neuroinflammation in the brain of patients with autism. *Ann Neurol* 2005;57:67-81.

9. Zimmerman, A.W., et al. Cerebrospinal fluid and serum markers of inflammation in autism. *Pediatr Neurol* 2005;33:195-201.

10. Chez, M.G., et al. Elevation of tumor necrosis factor-alpha in cerebrospinal fluid of autistic children. *Pediatr Neurol* 2007;36:361-365.

11. Li, X., et al. Elevated immune response in the brain of autistic patients. *J Neuroimmunol* 2009;207:111-116.

12. Sajdel-Sulkowska, E.M., et al. Increase in cerebellar neurotropin-3 and oxidative stress markers in autism. *Cerebellum* 2009;8:366-372.

13. Molloy, C.A., et al. Elevated cytokine levels in children with autism spectrum disorder. *J Neuroimmunol* 2006;172:198-205.

14. Chez, M.G. and Guido-Estrada, N. Immune therapy in autism: historical experience and future directions with immunomodulatory therapy. *Neurotherapeutics* 2010;7:293-301.

Chapter 6: Causes of Neuroinflammation
1. Okada, H., et al. Comparative analysis of host responses related to immunosuppression between measles patients and vaccine recipients with live attenuated measles vaccines. *Arch Virol* 2001;146:859-874.

2. Pukhalsky, A.L., et al. Cytokine profile after rubella vaccine inoculation: evidence of the immunosuppressive effect of vaccination. *Mediators Inflammation* 2003;12:203-207.

3. Daum, R.S., et al. Decline in serum antibody to the capsule of Haemophilus influenza type b in the immediate postimmunization period. *J Perdiatr* 1989;114:742-747.

4. Hussey, G.D., et al. The effect of Edmonston-Zagreb and Schwarz measles vaccines in immune response in infants. *J Infect Dis* 1996;173:1320-1326.

5. Abernathy, R.S. and Spink, W.W. Increased susceptibility of mice to bacterial endotoxins induced by pertussis vaccine. *Fed Proc* 1956;15:580.

6. Jang H., et al. Viral parkinsonism. *Biochim Biophys Acta.* 2008;1792:714–721.

7. MacDonald, A.B. Spirochetal cyst forms in neurodegenerative disorders…hiding in plain sight. *Med Hypoth* 2006;67:819-832.

8. Irkec, C., et al. The viral etiology of amyotrophic lateral sclerosis. *Mikrobivol Bul* 1989;23:102-109.

9. Volpi, A. Epstein-Barr virus and human herpesvirus type 8 infections of the central nervous system. *Herpes* 2004;11 Supple 2:120A-127A.

10. Honjo, K., et al. Alzheimer's disease and infection: do infectious agents contribute to progression of Alzheimer's disease? *Alzheimers Dement* 2009;5:348-360.

11. Itzhaki, R.F., et al. Infiltration of the brain by pathogens causes Alzheimer's disease. *Neurobiol Aging* 2004;25:619-627.

12. Chess, S. Autism in children with congenital rubella. *Journal of Autism and Childhood Schizophrenia* 1971;1:33-47.

13. Brown, A.S., et al. Nonaffective psychosis after prenatal exposure to rubella. *Am J Psychiatry* 2000;157:438-443.

14. Chess, S. Follow-up report on autism in congenital rubella. *J Autism Child Schizophr* 1977;7:69-81.

15. Bransfield, R.C., et al. The association between tick-borne infections, Lyme borreliosis and autism spectrum disorders. *Med Hypotheses* 2008;70:967-974.

16. Yamashita, Y., et al. Possible association between congenital cytomegalovirus infection and autistic disorder. *J Autism Dev Disord* 2003;33:455-459.

17. Gillberg, C. Onset at age 14 of a typical autistic syndrome. A case report of a girl with herpes simplex encephalitis. *J Autism Dev Disord* 1986;16:369-375.

18. Gillberg, I.C. Autistic syndrome with onset at age 31 years: herpes encephalitis as a possible model for childhood autism. *Dev Med Child Neurol* 1991;33:920-924.

19. DeLong, G.R., et al. Acquired reversible autistic syndrome in acute encephalopathic illness in children. *Arch Neurol* 1981;38:191-194.

20. Libbey, J.E., et al. Autistic disorder and viral infections. J Neurovirol 2005;11:1-10.

21. Nicolson, G.L., et al. Evidence for Mycoplasma ssp., Chlamydia pneumoniae, and human herpes virus-6 coinfections in the blood of patients with autistic spectrum disorders. *J Neurolscie Res* 2007;85:1143-1148.

22. Godbout, J.P., et al. Exaggerated neuroinflammation and sickness behavior in aged mice following activation of the peripheral innate immune system. *FASEB J* 2005;19:1329-1331.

23. Buttini, M., et al. Peripheral administration of lipopolysaccharide induces activation of microglial cells in rat brain. *Neurochem Int* 1996;29:25-35.

24. Cunningham, C., et al. Central and systemic endotoxin challenges exacerbate the local inflammatory response and increase neuronal death during chronic neurodegeneration. *J Neuroscie* 2005;25:9275-9284.

25. Lemstra, A.W. et al. Microglia activation in sepsis: a case-control study. *J Neuroinflammation* 2007;4:4.

26. Cunningham, C., et al. Systemic inflammation induces acute behavioral and cognitive changes and accelerates neurodegenerative disease. *Biol Psychiatry* 2009;65:304-312.

27. Holmes, C., et al. Systemic inflammation and disease progression in Alzheimer disease. *Neurology* 2009;73:768-774.

28. Cohly, H.H. and Panja, A. Immunological findings in autism. *Int Rev Neurobiol* 2005;71:317-341.

29. Singh, V.K., et al. Abnormal measles-mumps-rubella antibodies and CNS autoimmunity in children with autism. *J Biomed Sci* 2002;9:359-364.

30. Singh, V.K. and Jensen , R.L. Elevated levels of measles antibodies in children with autism. *Pediatr Neurol* 2003;28:292-294.

31. Horvath, K., et al. Gastrointestinal abnormalities in children with autistic disorder. *J Pediatr* 1999;135:559-563.

32. Wakefield, A., et al. Enterocolitis in children with developmental disorders, *American Journal of Gastroenterology* 2000;95:2285-2295.

33. Horvath, K. and Perman, J.A. Autism and gastrointestinal symptoms. *Curr Gastroenterol Rep* 2002;4:251-258.

34. Adams, J.B., et al. Gastrointestinal flora and gastrointestinal status in children with autism—comparisons to typical children and correlation with autism severity. *BMC Gastroenterol* 2011;11:22.

35. Ling, Z.D., et al. Rotenone potentiates dopamine neuron loss in animals exposed to lipopolysaccharide prenatally. *Exp Neurol* 2004;190:373-383.

36. Ling, Z.D., et al. Combined toxicity of prenatal bacterial endotoxin exposure and postnatal 6-hydroxydopamine in the adult rat midbrain. *Neuroscience* 2004;124:619-628.

37. Carvey, P.M., et al Prenatal exposure to the bacteriotoxin lipopolysaccharide leads to long-term losses of dopamine neurons in offspring: a potential new model of Parkinson's disease. *Front Biosci* 2003;8:S826-S837.

38. Leon, R., et al. Detection of Porphyromonas gingivlis in the amniotic fluid in pregnant women with a diagnosis of threatened premature labor. *J Periodontal* 2007;78:1249-1255.

39. Krejci, C.B. and Bissada, N.F. Women's health issues and their relationship to periodontitis. *J Am Dent Assoc* 2002;133:323-329.

40. Urakubo, A. et al. Prenatal exposure to maternal infection alters cytokine expression in the placenta, amniotic fluid, and fetal brain. *Schizophr Res* 2001;47:27-36.

41. Rodier, P.M. The early origins of autism. *Sci Am* 2000;282:56-63.

42. Torres, A.R. Is fever suppression involved in the etiology of autism and neurodevelopmental disorders? BMC Pediatr 2003;3:9.

43. Meyer, U., et al. The time of prenatal immune challenge determines the specificity of inflammation-mediated brain and behavioral pathology. *J Neurosci* 2006;26:4752-4762.

44. Comi, A.M., et al. Familial clustering of autoimmune disorders and evaluation of medical risk factors in autism. *J Child Neurol* 1999;14:388-394.

45. Atladóttir, H.O., et al. Maternal infection requiring hospitalization during pregnancy and autism spectrum disorders. *J Autism Dev Disord* 2010;40:1423-1430.

46. Lucarelli, S., et al. Food allergy and infantile autism. *Panminerva Med* 1995;37:137-141.

47. Knivsberg, A.M., et al. A randomized, controlled study of dietary intervention in autistic syndromes. *Nutr Neurosci* 2002;5:251-261.

48. What is the autism diet? http://health.howstuffworks.com/autism-diet.htm. Accessed 5/19/ 2011.

49. Zelnik, N., et al. Range of neurologic disorders in patients with celiac disease. *Pediatrics* 2004;113:1672-1676.

50. Grandjean, P. and Landrigan, P.J. Developmental nurotoxicity of industrial chemicals. *Lancet* 2006;368:2167-2178.

51. Potentials for exposure to industrial chemicals suspected of causing developmental neurotoxicity. http://www.hsph.harvard.edu/faculty/grandjean/appendix.pdf. Accessed 5/30/2011.

52. Roberts, E.M., et al. Maternal residence near agricultural pesticide applications and autism spectrum disorders among children in the California Central Valley. *Environ Health Perspect* 12007;15:1482–1489.

53. Larsson, M., et al. Associations between indoor environmental factors and parental-reported autistic spectrum disorders in children 6-8 years of age. *Neurotoxicology* 2009;30:822-831.

54. Kim, B.N., et al. Phthalates exposure and attention-deficient/hyperactivity disorder in school-age children. *Biol Psychiatry* 2009;66:958-963.

55. Larsson, M., et al. Associations between indoor environmental factors and parental-reported autistic spectrum disorders in children 6-8 years of age. *Neurotoxicology* 2009;30:822-831.

56. Bandiera, F.C., et al. Secondhand smoke exposure and mental health among children and adolescents. *Arch Pediatr Adolesc Med* 2011;165:332-338.

57. Volk, H.E., et al. Residential proximity to freeways and autism in the CHARGE study. *Environ Health Perspect* 2010, Dec 13.

58. Windham, G.C., et al. Autism spectrum disorders in relation to distribution of hazardous air pollutants in the San Francisco Bay area. *Environ Health Perspect* 2006;114:1438-1444.

59. Palmer, R.F., et al. Environmental mercury release, special education rates, and autism disorder: An ecological study of Texas. *Health Place* 2006;12:203-209.

60. Griffiths, P.D., et al. Iron in the basal ganglia in Parkinson's disease. *Brain* 1999;122:667-673.

61. Altamura, S. and Muckenthaler, M.U. Iron toxicity in diseases of aging: Alzheimer's disease, Parkinson's disease and atherosclerosis. *J Alzheimers Dis* 2009;16:879-895.

62. Yokel, R.A. Blood-brain barrier flux of aluminum, manganese, iron and other metals suspected to contribute to metal-induced neurodegeneration. *J Alzheimers Dis* 2006;10:223-253.

63. Bernard, S., et al. Autism: a novel form of mercury poisoning. *Medical Hypotheses* 2001;56:462–471.

64. Windham, G.C., et al. Autism spectrum disorders in relation to distribution of hazardous air pollutants in the San Francisco Bay area. *Environmental Health Perspectives* 2006;114:1438–1444.

65. DeSoto, M.C. and Hitlan, R.T. Blood levels of mercury are related to diagnosis of autism: a reanalysis of an important data set. *Journal of Child Neurology* 2007;22:1308–1311.

66. Adams, J.B., et al. Mercury, lead, and zinc in baby teeth of children with autism versus controls. *Journal of Toxicology and Environmental Health, Part A* 2007;70(12):1046–1051.

67. Bradstreet, J., et al. A case-control study of mercury burden in children with autistic spectrum disorders. *Journal of American Physicians and Surgeons* 2003;8:76–79.

68. Adams, J.B., et al. The severity of autism is associated with toxic metal body burden and red blood cell glutathione levels. Journal of Toxicology 2009; http:// www.hindawi.com/journals/jt/2009/532640/

69. Deadly immunity. www.icnr.com/articles/thimerosalcoverup.html. Accessed 5/19/2011.

70. Mahaffey, K.R., et al. Blood organic mercury and dietary mercury intake: National Health and Nutrition Examination Survey, 1999 and 2000. *Environ Health Prospect* 2004;112:562-570.

71. Pendergrass, J.C., et al. Mercury vapor inhalation inhibits binding of GTP to tubulin in rat brain: similarity to a molecular lesion in Alzheimer diseased brain. *Neurotoxicology* 1997;18:315-124.

72. Huggins, H.A. *Solving the MS Mystery: Help, Hope and Recovery*. Matrix, Inc:Colorado Springs, CO; 2002.

73. 25 member advisory panel rejects FDA safety report on mercury fillings. www.mercurypoisoned.com/FDA_hearings/advisory_panel_rejects_amalgam_safety.html. Accessed 6/6/ 2011.

74. Echeverria, D., et al. Neurobehavioral effects from exposure to dental amalgam Hg(0): new distinctions between recent exposure and Hg body burden. *FASEB J* 1998;12:971-980.

75. Crapper, D.R., et al. Intranuclear aluminum content in Alzheimer's disease, dialysis encephalopathy and experimental aluminum encephalopathy. *Acta Neuropath* 1980;50:19-24.

76. Petrik, M.S., et al. Aluminum adjuvant linked to gulf war illness induces motor neuron death in mice. *Neuromolecular Med* 2007;9:83-100.

77. Vaccines show sinister side. http://www.straight.com/article/vaccines-show-sinister-side. Accessed 5/30/2011.

78. The American Society for Parenteral and Enteral Nutrition (A.S.P.E.N.) Aluminum Task Force, Charney, P.J. Statement on Aluminum in Parenteral Nutrition Solutions. *Nutr Clin Pract.* 2004;19:416-417.

89. Bishop, N.J., et al. Aluminum neurotoxicity in preterm infants receiving intravenous-feeding solutions. *N Engl J Med* 1997;336:1557-1561.

80. Sears, R.W. Is aluminum the new thimerosal? *Mothering* 2008 Jan/Feb;146. http://mothering.com/health/is-aluminum-the-new-thimerosal?page=0,0. Accessed 5/30/2011.

81. Nagore, E., et al. Subcutaneous nodules following treatment with aluminum-containing allergen extracts. *Eur J Dermatol* 2001;11:138-140.

82. Stromland, K., et al. Autism in thalidomide embryopathy: a population study. *Dev Med Child Neurol* 1994;36:351-356.

83. Torres, A.R. Is fever suppression involved in the etiology of autism and neurodevelopmental disorders? *BMC Pediatr* 2003;3:9.

84. Schultz, S.T. Can autism be triggered by acetaminophen activation of the endocannabinoid system? *Acta Neurobiol Exp (Wars)* 2010;70:227-231.

85. Ingram, J.L., et al. Prenatal exposure of rats to valproic acid reproduces the cerebellar anomalies associated with autism. *Neurotoxicol Teratol* 2000;22:319-324.

86. Nowaczyk, M.J.M. and Tierney, E. *Smith-Lemli-Opitz Syndrome: Demystifying Genetic Syndromes*. Kingston, NY:National Association for the Dually Diagnosed Publishing; 2004, pp. 207-223.

87. Konstantareas, M.M. and Homatidis, S. Ear infections in autistic and normal children. *J Autism Dev Disord* 1987;17:585-594.

88. Principi, N., et al. Prophylaxis of recurrent acute otitis media and middle-ear effusion: comparison of amoxicillin with sulfamethoxazole and trimethoprim. *Am J Dis Child* 1989;143:1414-1418.

89. Casselbraant, M.L., et al. Efficacy of antimicrobial prophylaxis and of tympanostomy tube insertion for prevention of recurrent acute otitis media: results of a randomized clinical trial. *Pediatr Infect Dis J* 1992;11:278-286.

90. Koopman, L., et al. Antibiotic therapy to prevent the development of asymptomatic middle ear effusion in children with acute otitis media: a meta-analysis of individual patient data. *Arch Otolaryngol Head Neck Surg* 2008;134:128-132.

91. Fallon, J. Could one of the most widely prescribed antibiotics amoxicillin/ clavulanate "Augmentin" be a risk factor for autism? *Medical Hypotheses* 2005;64:312-315.

92. Finegold, S.M., et al. Gastrointestinal microflora studies on late-onset autism. *Clinical Infectious Diseases* 2002;35(Suppl 1):S6-16.

93. Bolte, E.R. Autism and Clostridium tetani. *Med Hypotheses* 1998;51:133-144.

94. Song, Y., et al. Real-time PCR quantitation of clostridia in feces of autistic children. *Appl Environ Microbiol* 2004;70:6459-6465.

95. Rosseneu, S.L.M., et al. Aerobic throat and gut flora in children with autistic spectrum disorder and gastrointestinal symptoms. Conference Proceedings of the Defeat Autism Now! Fall 2003 conference, Portland, OR.

96. Wakefield, A. Enterocolitis, autism and measles virus. *Molecular Psychiatry* 2002;7:S44-S45.

97. Sandler, R.H., et al. Short-term benefit from oral vancomycin treatment of regressive-onset autism. *J Child Neurol* 2000;15:429-435.

98. Rowland, I.R., et al. The methylation of mercuric chloride by human intestinal bacteria. *Experientia* 1975;31:1064-1065.

99. Schab, D.W., et al. Do artificial food colors promote hyperactivity in children with hyperactive syndromes? A meta-analysis of double-blind placebo-controlled trials. *Journal of Developmental & Behavioral Pediatrics* 2004;25:423-434.

100. Bateman, B, et al. The effects of a double blind placebo controlled artificial food colourings and benzoate preservatives challenge on hyperactivity in a general population sample of pre-school children. *Archives of Disease in Childhood* 2004;89: 506-511.

101. McCann, D., et al., Food additives and hyperactive behaviour in 3-year-old and 8/9-year-old children in the community: a randomised, double-blinded, placebo-controlled trial. *Lancet* 2007;370:1560-1567.

102. Twin study reveals food additives effect. http://news.bbc.co.uk/2/hi/health/ 2984519.stm. Accessed 5/26/2011.

103. Blaylock, R.L. A possible central mechanism in autism spectrum disorders, part 1. *Altern Ther Health Med* 2008;14(6):46-53.

104. Blaylock, R.L. A possible central mechanism in autism spectrum disorders, part 2: immunoexcitotoxicity. *Altern Ther Health Med* 2009;15(1):60-67.

105. Blaylock, R.L. A possible central mechanism in autism spectrum disorders, part 3: the role of excitotoxins food additives and the synergistic effects of other environmental toxins. *Altern Ther Health Med* 2009;15(2):56-60.

106. Blaylock, R.L. Interaction of cytokines, excitotoxins, reactive nitrogen and oxygen species in autism spectrum disorders. *JANA* 2003;6(4):21-35.

107. Blaylock, RL.. Chronic microglial activation and excitotoxicity secondary to excessive immune stimulation: possible factors in Gulf war syndrome and autism. *JAPS* 2004;9:46-52.

108. de la Fuente-Sandoval, C., et al. Higher Levels of Glutamate in the Associative-Striatum of Subjects with Prodromal Symptoms of Schizophrenia and Patients with First-Episode Psychosis. *Neuropsychopharmacology* 2011 Apr 20.

109. Choi, D. Glutamate neurotoxicity and diseases of the nervous system. *Neuron* 1988;1:623-34.

110. Lipton, S. and Rosenberg, P. Excitatory amino acids as a final common pathway for neurologic disorders. *N Engl J Med* 1994;330:613-22.

111. Whetsell, W. and Shapira, N. Biology of disease. Neuroexcitation, excitotoxicity and human neurological disease. *Lab Invest* 1993;68:372-387.

112. Olney, J. Glutamate, a neurotoxic transmitter. *J Child Neurol* 1989;4:218-26.

113. Olney, J., et al. Excitotoxic neurodegeneration in Alzheimer's disease. *Arch Neurol* 1997;54:1234-1240.

114. Hynd, M.R., et al. Glutamate-mediated excitotoxicity and neurodegeneration in Alzheimer's disease. *Neurochem Int* 2004;45:583-595.

115. Caudle, W.M. and Zhang, J. Glutamate, excitotoxicity, and programmed cell death in Parkinson disease. *Exp Neurol* 2009;220:230-233.

116. Foran, E. and Trotti, D. Glutamate transporters and the excitotoxic path to motor neuron degeneration in amyotrophic lateral sclerosis. *Antioxid Redox Signal* 2009;11:1587-1602.

117. Arauz-Contreras, J. and Feria-Velasco, A. Monosodium-L-glutamate-induced convulsions—I. Differences in seizure pattern and duration of effect as a function of age in rats. *Gen Pharmacol* 1984;15:391-395.

118. Koenig, H., et al. Capillary NMDA receptors regulate blood-brain barrier function and breakdown. *Bran Res* 1992;588:297-303.

119. Van Westerlaak, M.G., et al. Chronic mitochondrial inhibition induces glutamate-mediated corticomotoneuron death in an organotypic culture model. *Exp Neurol* 2001;167:393-400.

120. del la Monte, S.M., et al. Epidemiological trends strongly suggest exposures as etiologic agents in the pathogenesis of sporadic Alzheimer's disease, diabetes mellitus, and non-alcoholic steatohepatitis. *J Alzheimers Dis* 2009;17:519-529.

121. Eaves, L. and Ho, H. Brief repot: stability and changes in cognitive and behavioral characteristics of autism through childhood. *J Autism Dev Disord* 1996;26:557-569.

122. Aisen, P.S. the potential of anti-inflammatory drugs for the treatment of Alzheimer's disease. *Lancet Neurol* 2002;1:279-284.

123. McGeer, P.L. and McGeer, D.G. NSAIDs and Alzheimer disease: epidemiological, animal model and clinical studies. *Neurobiol Aging* 2007;28:639-647.

Chapter 7: The Ketone Miracle

1. Liu, Y.M., et al. A prospective study: growth and nutritional status of children treated with the ketogenic diet. *J Am Diet Assoc* 2003;103:707-712.

2. Sharman, M.J., et al. A ketogenic diet favorably affects serum biomarkers for cardiovascular disease in normal-weight men. *J Nutr* 2002;132:1879-1885.

3. Dashti, H.M., et al. Long term effects of ketogenic diet in obese subjects with high cholesterol level. *Mol Cell Biochem* 2006;286:1-9.

4. Patel, A., et al. Long-term outcomes of children treated with the ketogenic diet in the past. *Epilepsia* 2010;51:1277-1282.

5. Kossoff, E.H., et al. Ketogenic diets: an update for child neurologists. *J Child Neurol* 2009;24:979-88.

6. Kinsman, S.L., et al. Efficacy of the ketogenic diet for intractable seizure disorders: review of 58 cases. *Epilepsia* 1992;33:1132-1136.

7. Nordli, D.R. Jr., et al. Experience with the ketogenic diet in infants. *Pediatrics* 2001;108:129-133.

8. Pulsifer, M.B., et al. Effects of ketogenic diet on development and behavior: preliminary report of a prospective study. *Developmental Medicine and Child Neurology* 2001;43:301-306.

9. Husain, A.M., et al. Diet therapy for narcolepsy. *Nuerology* 2004;62:2300-2302.

10. Nebeling, L.C., et al. Effects of a ketogenic diet on tumor metabolism and nutritional status in pediatric oncology patients: two case reports. *Journal of the American College of Nutrition* 1995;14:202-208.

11. Seyfried, T.N. and Mukherjee, P. Targeting energy metabolism in brain cancer: review and hypothesis. *Nutrition and Metabolism (London)* 2005;21:30.

12. Evangeliou, A., et al. Application of a ketogenic diet in children with autistic behavior: pilot study. *J Child Neurol* 2003;18:113-118.

13. Strahlman, R.S. Can ketosis help migraine sufferers? A case report. *Headache* 2006;46:182.

14. Murphy, P. et al. The antidepressant properties of the ketogenic diet. *Biological Psychiatry* 2004;56:981-983.

15. Kossoff, E.H., et al. Ketogenic diets: an update for child neurologists. *J Child Neurol* 2009;24:979-988.

16. Mavropoulos, J.C., et al. The effects of a low-carbohydrate, ketogenic diet on the polycystic ovary syndrome: a pilot study. *Nutrition and Metabolism (London)* 2005;2:35.

17. Yancy, W.S., et al. A low-carbohydrate, ketogenic diet to treat type 2 diabetes. *Nutrition and Metabolism (London) 2005*;2:34.

18. Minassian, B.A., et al. Mutations in a gene encoding a novel protein tyrosine phosphatase cause progressive myoclonic epilepsy. *Nat Genet* 1998;20:171-174.

19. Longo, N., et al. Progressive decline in insulin levels in Rabson-Mendenhall syndrome. *J Clin Endocrinol Metab* 1999;84:2623-2629.

20. Veech, R.L. The therapeutic implications of ketone bodies: the effects of ketone bodies in pathological conditions: ketosis, ketogenic diet, redox states, insulin resistance, and mitochondrial metabolism. *Prostaglandins, Leukotrienes and Essential Fatty Acids* 2004;70:309-319.

21. Lardy, H.A., et al. The metabolism of bovine epididymal spermatozoa. *Arch Biochem* 1945;6:41-51.

22. Beck, S.A. and Tisdale, M.J. Nitrogen excretion in cancer cachexia and its modification by a high fat diet in mice. *Cancer Res* 1989;49:3800-3804.

23. Nebeling, L.C. and Lerner, E. Implementing a ketogenic diet based on medium-chain triglyceride oil in pediatric patients with cancer. *J Am Diet Assoc* 1995;95:693-697.

24. Nebeling, L.C., et al. Effects of a ketogenic diet on tumor metabolism and nutritional status in pediatric oncology patients: two case reports. *J Am Coll Nutr* 1995;86:202-208.

25. Seyfried, T.N., et al. Role of glucose and ketone bodies in the metabolic control of experimental brain cancer. *British Journal of Cancer* 2003;89:1375-1382.

26. Mukherjee, P., et al. Dietary restriction reduces angiogenesis and growth in an orthotopic mouse brain tumour model. *Br J Cancer* 2002;86:1615-1621.

27. Fife, B. *Coconut Cures: Preventing and Treating Common Health Problems with Coconut.* Piccadilly Books, Ltd; Colorado Springs, CO, 2005.

28. Hasselbalch, S.G., et al. Changes in cerebral blood flow and carbohydrate metabolism during acute hyperketonemia. *Am J Physiol* 1996;270:E746-751.

29. Marie, C., et al. Fasting prior to transient cerebral ischemia reduces delayed neuronal necrosis. *Metab Bran Dis* 1990;5:65-75.

30. Prins, M.L., et al. Increased cerebral uptake and oxidation of exogenous âHB improves ATP following traumatic brain injury in adult rats. *J Neurochem* 2004;90:666-672.

31. Suzuki, M., et al. Effect of â-hydroxybutyrate, a cerebral function improving agent, on cerebral hypoxia, anoxia and ischemia in mice and rats. *Jpn J Pharmacol* 2001;87:143-150.

32. Twyman, D. Nutritional management of the critically ill neurologic patient. *Crit Care Clin* 1997;13:39-49.

33. Calon, B., et al. Long-chain versus medium and long-chain triglyceride-based fat emulsion in parental nutrition of severe head trauma patients. *Infusionstherapie* 1990;17:246-248.

34. Gasior, M., et al. Neuroprotective and disease-modifying effects of the ketogenic diet. *Behav Pharmacol* 2006;17:431-439.

35. Van der Auwera, I., et al. A ketogenic diet reduces amyloid beta 40 and 42 in mouse model of Alzheimer's disease. *Nutrition* 2005;2:28.

36. Zhao, Z., et al. A ketogenic diet as a potential novel therapeutic intervention in amyotrophic lateral sclerosis. *BMC Neuroscience* 2006;7:29.

37. Duan, W., et al. Dietary restriction normalizes glucose metabolism and BDNF levels, slows disease progression, and increases survival in huntingtin mutant mice. *Proc Natl Acad Sci USA* 2003;100:2911-2916.

38. Kashiwaya, Y., et al. D-beta-hydroxybutyrate protects neurons in models of Alzheimer's and Parkinson's disease. *Proc Natl Acad Sci USA* 2000;97:5440-5444.

39. Tieu, K., et al. D-beta-hydroxybutyrate rescues mitochondrial respiration and mitigates features of Parkinson disease. *J Clin Invest* 2003;112:892-901.

40. VanItallie, T.B., et al. Treatment of Parkinson disease with diet-induced hyperketonemia: a feasibility study. *Neurology* 2005;64:728-730.

41. Van der Auwera, I., et al. A ketogenic diet reduces amyloid beta 40 and 42 in a mouse model of Alzheimer's disease. *Nutr Metab (London)* 2005;2:28.

42. Studzinski, C.M., et al. Induction of ketosis may improve mitochondrial function and decrease steady-state amyloid-beta precursor protein (AAPP) levels in the aged dog. *Brain Res* 2008;1226:209-217.

43. Costantini, L.C., et al. Hypometabolism as a therapeutic target in Alzheimer's disease. *BMC Neuroscience* 2008;9:S16.

44. Suzuki, M., et al. Beta-hydroxybutyrate, a cerebral function improving agent, protects rat brain against ischemic damage caused by permanent and transient focal cerebral ischemia. *Jpn J Phamacol* 2002;89:36-43.

45. Suzuki, M., et al. Effect of beta-hydroxybutyrate, a cerebral function improving agent, on cerebral hypoxia, anoxia and ischemia in mice and rats. *Jpn J Phamacol* 2001;87:143-150.

46. Imamura, K., et al. D-beta-hydroxybutyrate protects dopaminergic SH-SY5Y cells in a rotenone model of Parkinson's disease. *J Neuroscie Res* 2006;84:1376-1384.

47. Haas, R.H., et al. Therapeutic effects of a ketogenic diet in Rett syndrome. *Am J Med Genet Suppl* 1986;1:225-246.

48. Evangeliou, A., et al. Application of a ketogenic diet in children with autistic behavior: pilot study. *Journal of Child Neurology* 2003;18:113-118.

49. Maalouf, M., et al. The neuroprotective properties of calorie restriction, the ketogenic diet, and ketone bodies. *Brain Res Rev* 2009; 59:293-315.

50. Koper, J.W., et al. Acetoacetate and glucose as substrates for lipid synthesis for rat brain oligodendrocytes and astrocytes in serum-free culture. *Biochim Biophys Acta* 1984;796:20-26.

51. Veech, R.L., et al. Ketone bodies, potential therapeutic uses. *IUBMB Life* 2001;51:241-247.

52. Kirsch, J.R., et al. Butanediol induced ketosis increases tolerance to hypoxia in the mouse. *Stroke* 1980;11:506-513.

53. Suzuki, M., et al. Effect of beta-hydroxybutyrate, a cerebral function improving agent, on cerebral hypoxia, anoxia, and ischemia in mice and rats. *Jpn J Pharmacol 2001*;87:143-150.

54. Chance, B., et al. Hydroperoxide metabolism in mammalian organs. *Physiol Rev* 1979;59:527-605.

55. Kashiways, Y., et al. D-â-hydroxybutyrate protects neurons in models of Alzheimer's and Parkinson's disease. *Proc Natl Acad Sci USA* 2000;97:5440-5444.

56. Schwartzkroin, P.A. Mechanisms underlying the anti-epileptic efficacy of the ketogenic diet. *Epilepsy Res* 1999;37:171-180.

57. Kossoff, E.H., et al. Efficacy of the ketogenic diet for infantile spasms. *Pediatrics* 2002;109:780-783.

58. Husain, A.M., et al. Diet therapy for narcolepsy. *Nuerology* 2004;62:2300-2302.

59. Evangeliou, A., et al. Application of a ketogenic diet in children with autistic behavior: pilot study. *J Child Neurol* 2003;18:113-118.

60. Strahlman, R.S. Can ketosis help migraine sufferers? A case report. *Headache* 2006;46:182.

61. Murphy, P. et al. The antidepressant properties of the ketogenic diet. *Biological Psychiatry* 2004;56:981-983.

62. Prins, M.L., et al. Increased cerebral uptake and oxidation of exogenous âHB improves ATP following traumatic brain injury in adult rats. *J Neurochem* 2004;90:666-672.

63. Reger, M.A., et al. Effects of beta-hydroxybutyrate on cognition in memory-impaired adults. *Neurobiol Aging* 2004;25:311-314.

64. VanItallie, T.B., et al. Treatment of Parkinson disease with diet-induced hyperketonemia: a feasibility study. *Neurology* 2005;64:728-730.

65. Duan, W., et al. Dietary restriction normalizes glucose metabolism and BDNF levels, slows disease progression, and increases survival in huntingtin mutant mice. *Proc Natl Acad Sci USA* 2003;100:2911-2916.

66. Zhao, Z., et al. A ketogenic diet as a potential novel therapeutic intervention in amyotrophic lateral sclerosis. *BMC Neuroscience* 2006;7:29.

67. Page, K.A., et al. Medium chain fatty acids improve cognitive function in intensively treated type 1 diabetic patients and support the in vitro synaptic transmission during acute hypoglycemia. *Diabetes* 2009;58:1237-1244.

68. Sokoloff, L. Metabolism of ketone bodies by the brain. *Ann Rev Med* 1973;24:271-280.

69. Yeh, Y.Y. and Zee, P. Relation of ketosis to metabolic changes induced by acute medium-chain triglyceride feeding in rats. *J Nutr* 1976;106:58-67.

70. Tantibhedhyangkul, P., et al. Effects of ingestion of long-chain and medium-chain triglycerides on glucose tolerance in man. *Diabetes* 1967;16:796-799.

71. Kashiwaya, Y., et al Substrate signaling by insulin: a ketone bodies ratio mimics insulin action in heart. *Am J Cardiol* 1997;80:50A-60A.

72. Seyfried, T.N., et al. Role of glucose and ketone bodies in the metabolic control of experimental brain cancer. *British Journal of Cancer* 2003;89:1375-1382.

73. Nebeling, L.C., et al. Effects of a ketogenic diet on tumor metabolism and nutritional status in pediatric oncology patients: two case reports. *J Am Coll Nutr* 1995;86:202-208.

74. Kashiwaya, Y., et al Substrate signaling by insulin: a ketone bodies ratio mimics insulin action in heart. *Am J Cardiol* 1997;80:50A-60A.

75. Suzuki, M., et al. Beta-hydroxybutyrate, a cerebral function improving agent, protects rat brain against ischemic damage caused by permanent and transient focal cerebral ischemia. *Jpn J Phamacol* 2002;89:36-43.

76. Alam, H.B., et al. Ketone Ringer's solution attenuates resuscitation induced apoptosis in rat lungs. 5th *World Congress on Trauma, Shock, Inflammation, and Sepsis* 2000, pp 63-66.

77. Hiraide, A., et al. Effect of 3-hydroxybutyrate on posttraumatic metabolism in man. *Surgery* 1991;109:176-181.

78. Mavropoulos, J.C., et al. The effects of a low-carbohydrate, ketogenic diet on the polycystic ovary syndrome: a pilot study. *Nutrition and Metabolism (London)* 2005;2:35.

79. Lardy, H.A. and Phillips, P.H. Studies of fat and carbohydrate oxidation in mammalian spermatozoa. *Arch Biochem* 1945;6:53-61.

80. Yancy, W.S., et al. A low-carbohydrate, ketogenic diet versus a low-fat diet to treat obesity and hyperlipidemia: a randomized, controlled trial. *Ann Intern Med* 2004;140:769-777.

81. Cahill, G.F. Jr. and Veech, R.L. Ketoacids? Good Medicine? *Transactions of the American Clinical and Climatological Association* 2003;114:149-163.

82. Fontana, L. Neuroendocrine factors in the regulation of inflammation: excessive adiposity and calorie restriction. *Exp Gerontol* 2009;44:41-45.

83. Kaunitz, H. and Johnson, R.E. Influence of dietary fats on disease and longevity. In: Chavez, A., Bourges, H., Basta, S., eds. Proceedings of the 9th International Congress on Nutrition, Mexico, 1972. Basel: Karger, 1975;1:362-373.

84. Ruskin, D.N., et al. Reduced pain and inflammation in juvenile and adult rats fed a ketogenic diet. *PLoS One* 2009;4(12):e8349.

Chapter 8: The Cholesterol Factor

1. Muldoon, M.F., et al. Immune system differences in men with hypo- or hypercholesterolemia. *Clin Immunol Immunopathol* 1997;84:145-149.

2. Weinstock, C., et al. Low density lipoproteins inhibit endotoxin activation of monocytes. *Arterioscler Thromb Vasc Biol* 1992;12:341-347.

3. Feingold, K.R., et al. Role for circulating lipoproteins in protection from endotoxin toxicity. *Infect Immun* 1995;63:2041-2046.

4. Pearson, A. Protecting fetuses from mothers who drink. *NewScientist* January, 22, 2007.

5. Bhakdi, S., et al. Binding and partial inactivation of Staphylococcus aureus a-toxin by human plasma low density lipoprotein. *J Biol Chem* 1983;258:5899-5904.

6. Perez-Guzman, C., et al. A cholesterol-rich diet accelerates bacteriologic sterilization in pulmonary tuberculosis. *Chest* 2005;127:643-651.

7. Sivas, F., et al. Serum lipid profile: its relationship with osteoporotic vertebrae fractures and bone mineral density in Turkish post-menopausal women. *Rheumatol Int* 2009;29:885-890.

8. Edison, R.J., et al. Adverse birth outcome among mothers with low serum cholesterol. *Pediatrics* 2007;120:723-733.

9. Pfrieger, F.W. Role of cholesterol in synapse formation and function *Biochem Biophy Acta* 2003;1610:271-280.

10. Klopfleisch, S., et al. Negative impact of statins on oligodendrocytes and myelin formation in vitro and in vivo. *J Neurosci* 2008;28:13609-13614.

11. Goritz, C., et al. Role of glia-derived cholesterol in synaptogenesis: new revelations in the synapse-gila affair. *J Physiol Paris* 2002;96:257-263.

12. Tong, J., et al. A scissors mechanism for stimulation of SNARE-mediated lipid mixing by cholesterol. *Proc Natl Acad Sci USA* 2009;106:5141-5146.

13. Bjorkhem, I. and Meaney, S. brain cholesterol: Long secret life behind a barrier. *Arteriosclerosis Thrombosis and Vascular Biology* 2004;24:806-815.

14. Glueck, C.J., et al. Hypocholesterolemia, hypertriglyceridemia, suicide, and suicide ideation in children hospitalized for psychiatric diseases. *Pediatr Res* 1994;35:602-610.

15. Modal, I., et al. Serum cholesterol levels and suicidal tendencies in psychiatric inpatients. *J Clin Psychiatry* 1994;55:252-254.

16. King, D.S., et al. Cognitive impairment associated with atorvastatin and simvastatin. *Pharmacotherapy* 2003;23:1663-1667.

17. Wagstaff, L.R., et al. Statin-associated memory loss: analysis of 60 case reports and review of the literature. *Pharmacotherapy* 2003;23:871-880.

18. Orsi, A., et al. Simvastatin-associated memory loss. *Pharmacotherapy* 2001;21:767-769.

19. Ciacci C., et al. Low plasma cholesterol: a correlate of nondiagnosed celiac disease in adults with hypochromic anemia. *Am J Gastroenterol* 1999;94(7):1888-1891.

20. Ciampolini M, Bini S. Serum lipids in celiac children. *J Pediatr Gastroenterol Nutr* 1991;12(4):459-460.

21. Rosenthal E, Hoffman R, Aviram M, et al. Serum lipoprotein profile in children with celiac disease. *J Pediatr Gastroenterol Nutr* 1990;11(1):58-62.

22. Abad-Rodriguez, J., et al. Neuronal membrane cholesterol loss enhances amyloid peptide generation. *Journal of Cell Biology* 2004;167:953-960.

23. Lepara, O., et al. Decreased serum lipids in patients with probable Alzheimer's disease. *Bosn J Basic Med Sci* 2009;9:215-220.

24. Lamperti, E. Decreased concentration of low density lipoprotein cholesterol in patients with parkinson's disease. In: Musanti R, Rocca N, Ghiselli G, Parati E, editors. *Clinical Research* 1991;39:401A.

25. Huang, X., et al. Lower low-density lipoprotein cholesterol levels are associated with Parkinson's disease. *Mov Disord* 2007;22:377-381.

26. Huang, X., et al. Low LDL cholesterol and increased risk of Parkinson's disease: prospective results from Honolulu-Asia Aging Study. *Mov Disord* 2008;23:1013-1018.

27. Dupuis, L., et al. Dyslipidemia is a protective factor in amyotrophic lateral sclerosis. *Neurology* 2008;70:1004-1009.

28. Garrett, H.E., et al. Serum cholesterol values in patients treated surgically for atherosclerosis. *JAMA* 1964;189:655-659.

29. Sachdeva, A., et al. Lipid levels in patients hospitalized with coronary artery disease: an analysis of 136,905 hospitalizations in Get With The Guidelines. *Am Heart J* 2009;157:111-117.

30. Al-Mallah, M.H., et al. Low admission LDL-cholesterol is associated with increased 3-year all-cause mortality in patients with non ST segment elevation myocardial infarction. *Cardio J* 2009;16:227-233.

31. Dayton, S., et al. A controlled clinical trial of a diet high in unsaturated fat in preventing complications of atherosclerosis. *Circulation* 1969;40:1-63.

32. Dorr, A.E., et al. Colestipol hydrochloride in hypercholesterolemic patients—effect on serum cholesterol and mortality. *Journal of Chronic Disease* 1978;31:5-14.

33. Muldoon, M.F., et al. Lowering cholesterol concentrations and mortality: a quantitative review of primary prevention trials. *British Medical Journal* 1990;301:309-314.

34. Lindberg, G., et al. Low serum cholesterol concentration and short term mortality from injuries in men and women. *BMJ* 1992;305:277-279.

35. Elias PK, et al. Serum Cholesterol and Cognitive Performance in the Framingham Heart Study. *Psychosom Med* 2005; 67:24-30.

36. Lepara, O., et al. Decreased serum lipids in patients with probable Alzheimer's disease. *Bosn J Basic Med Sci* 2009;9:215-220.

37. Mason, R.P., et al. Evidence for changes in the Alzheimer's disease brain cortical membrane structure mediated by cholesterol. *Neurobiol Aging* 1992;13:413-419.

38. Ledesma, M.D., et al. Raft disorganization leads to reduced plasmin activity in Alzheimer's disease brains. *EMBO Rep* 2003;4:1190-1196.

39. Corrigan F.M., et al. Dietary supplementation with zinc sulphate, sodium selenite and fatty acids in early dementia of Alzheimer's Type II: Effects on lipids. *J Nutr Med* 1991; 2: 265-71.

40. Howland, D.S., et al. Modulation of secreted beta-amyloid precursor protein and amyloid beta-peptide in brain by cholesterol. *J Biol Chem* 1998;273:16576-16582.

41. Aneja, A. and Tierney, E. Autism: The role of cholesterol in treatment. *International Review of Psychiatry* 2008;20:165-170.

42. Deficient cholesterol. http://www.greatplainslaboratory.com/home/eng/cholesterol.asp. Accessed 6/15/2011.

43. Irons, M., et al. Treatment of the Smith-Lemli-Opitz syndrome: results of a multicenter trial. *Am J Med Genetics* 1997;68:311-314.

44. Tobin, C.J. and McMahon, A.P. Recent advances in hedgehog signaling. *Trends in Cell Biology* 1997;7:442-446.

45. Tierney, E., et al. Behavioral phenotype of RSHSmith-Lemli-Opitz syndrome. *Mental Retardation and Developmental Disabilities Research Reviews* 2000;6:131-134.

46. Irons, M., et al. Clinical features of the Smith-Lemli-Opitz syndrome and treatment of the cholesterol metabolic defect. *International Pediatrics* 1995;10:28-32.

47. Nwokoro, N.A. and Mulvihill, J.J. Cholesterol and bile acid replacement therapy in children and adults with Smith-Lemli-Opitz (SLO/RSH) syndrome. *Am J Med Genetics* 1997;68:315-321.

48. Opitz, J.M. RSH (so called Smith-Lemli-Opitz) syndrome. *Current Opinions in Pediatrics* 1999;11:353-362.

49. Ryan, A.K., et al. Smith-Lemli-Opitz syndrome: A variable clinical and biochemical phenotype. *Am J Med Genetics* 1998;35:558-565.

50. Tierney, E., et al. Behavior phenotype in the RSH/Smith-Lemli-Opitz syndrome. *Am J Med Genetics* 2001;98:191-200.

Chapter 9: The Facts on Fats

1. Brunner, J., et al. Cholesterol, omega-3 fatty acids, and suicide risk: empirical evidence and pathophysiological hypotheses. *Fortschr Neurol Psychiatr* 2001;69:460-467.

2. Colin, A., et al. Lipids, depression and suicide. *Encephale* 2003;29:49-58.

3. Wells, A.S., et al. Alterations in mood after changing to a low-fat diet. *Br J Nutr* 1998;79:23-30.

4. Life expectancy. http://en.wikipedia.org/wiki/Life_expectancy. Accessed 11/28/2011.

5. McGee, D., et al. The relationship of dietary fat and cholesterol to mortality in 10 years: the Honolulu Heart Program. *Int J Epidemiol* 1985;14:97-105.

6. Okamoto, K., et al. Nutritional status and risk of amyotrophic lateral sclerosis in Japan. *Amyotroph Lateral Scler* 2007;8:300-304.

7. Forsythe, C.E., et al. Comparison of low fat and low carbohydrate diets on circulating fatty acid composition and markers of inflammation. *Lipids* 2008;43:65-77.

8. Prior, I. A. Cholesterol, coconuts, and diet on Polynesian atolls: a natural experiment: the Pukapuka and Tokelau island studies. *Am J Clin Nutr* 1981;34:1552-1561.

9. Mendis, S., et al. Cardiovascular risk factors in a Melanesian population apparently free from stroke and ischaemic heart disease: the Kitava study. *J Intern Med* 1994;236:331-340.

10. Mendis, S. Coronary heart disease and coronary risk profile in a primitive population. *Trop Geogr Med* 1991;43:199-202.

11. Davis, G.P. and Park, E. *The Heart: The Living Pump.* Torstar Books: New York; 1983.

12. Aruoma, O.I. and Halliwell, B. eds. *Free Radicals and Food Additives.* Taylor and Francis, London, 1991.

13. Harman, D., et al. Free radical theory of aging: effect of dietary fat on central nervous system function. *J Am Geriatr Soc* 1976;24:301-307.

14. Seddon, J.M., et al. Dietary fat and risk for advanced age-related macular degeneration. *Arch Ophthalmol* 2001;119:1191-1199.

15. Ouchi, M., et al. A novel relation of fatty acid with age-related macular degeneration. *Ophthalmologica* 2002;216:363-367.

16. Sheddon, J.M., et al. Progression of age-related macular degeneration: association with dietary fat, transunsaturated fat, nuts, and fish intake. *Arch Ophthalmol* 2003;121:1728-1737.

17. Chauhan, A., et al. Oxidative stress in autism: increased lipid peroxidation and reduced serum levels of ceruloplasmin and transferring—the antioxidant proteins. *Life Sci* 2004;75:2539-2549.

18. Tewfik, I.H., et al. The effect of intermittent heating on some chemical parameters of refined oils used in Egypt. A public health nutrition concern. *Int J Food Sci Nutr* 1998;49:339-342.

19. Jurgens, G., et al. Immunostaining of human autopsy aortas with antibodies to modified apolipoprotein B and apoprotein(a). *Arterioscler Thromb* 1993;13:1689-1699.

20. Srivastava, S., et al. Identification of cardiac oxidoreductase(s) involved in the metabolism of the lipid peroxidation-derived aldehyde-4-hydroxynonenal. *Biochem J* 1998;329:469-475.

21. Nakamura, K., et al. Carvedilol decreases elevated oxidative stress in human failing myocardium. *Circulation* 2002;105:2867-2871.

22. Pratico, D. and Delanty, N. Oxidative injury in diseases of the central nervous system: focus on Alzheimer's disease. *The American Journal of Medicine* 2000;109:577-585.

23. Markesbery, W.R. and Carney, J.M. Oxidative alterations in Alzheimer's disease. *Brain Pathology* 1999;9;133-146.

24. Kritchevsky, D. and Tepper, S.A. Cholesterol vehicle in experimental atherosclerosis. 9. Comparison of heated corn oil and heated olive oil. *J Atheroscler Res* 1967;7:647-651.

25. Raloff, J. 1996. Unusual fats lose heart-friendly image. *Science News* 1996;150:87.

26. Mensink, R.P. and Katan, M.B. Effect of dietary trans fatty acids on high-density and low-density lipoprotein cholesterol levels in healthy subjects. *N Eng J Med* 1990;323(7):439-445.

27. Willett, W.C., et al. Intake of trans fatty acids and risk of coronary heart disease among women. *Lancet* 1993;341:581-585.

28. Booyens, J. and Louwrens, C.C. The Eskimo diet. Prophylactic effects ascribed to the balanced presence of natural cis unsaturated fatty acids and to the absence of unnatural trans and cis isomers of unsaturated fatty acids. *Med Hypoth* 1986;21:387.

29. Grandgirard, A., et al. Incorporation of trans long-chain n-3 polyunsaturated fatty acids in rat brain structures and retina. *Lipids* 1994;29:251-258.

30. Pamplona, R., et al. Low fatty acid unsaturation: a mechanism for lowered lipoperoxidative modification of tissue proteins in mammalian species with long life spans. *J Gerontol A Biol Sci Med Sci* 2000;55:B286-B291.

31. Cha, Y.S. and Sachan, D.S. Oppostie effects of dietary saturated and unsaturated fatty acids on ethanol-pharmacokinetics, triglycerides and carnitines. *J Am Coll Nutr* 1994;13:338-343.

32. Siri-Tarino, P.W., et al. Meta-analysis of prospective cohort studies evaluating the association of saturated fat with cardiovascular disease. *Am J Clin Nutr* 2010;91:535-546.

Chapter 10: The Ultimate Brain Food

1. Hawkins, R.A. and Biebuyck, J.F. Ketone bodies are selectively used by individual brain regions. *Science* 1979;205:325-327.

2. Wu, P.Y., et al. Medium-chain triglycerides in infant formulas and their relation to plasma ketone body concentrations. *Pediatr Res* 1986;20:338-41.

3. Veech, R.L. The therapeutic implications of ketone bodies: the effects of ketone bodies in pathological conditions: ketosis, ketogenic diet, redox states, insulin resistance, and mitochondrial metabolism. *Prostaglandins, Leukotrienes and Essential Fatty Acids* 2004;70:309-319.

4. Cahill, C.F. and Veech, R.L. Ketoacids? Good medicine? *Trans Am Clin Climatol Assoc* 2003;114:149-161.

5. Suzuki, M., et al. Beta-hydroxybutyrate, a cerebral function improving agent, protects rat brain against ischemic damage caused by permanent and transient focal cerebral ischemia. *Jpn J Pharm*acol. 2002;89:36–43.

6. Tieu, K., et al. D-beta-hydroxybutyrate rescues mitochondrial respiration and mitigates features of Parkinson disease. *J Clin Invest* 2003;112:892-901.

7. Suzuki, M., et al Effect of beta-hydroxybutyrate, a cerebral function improving agent, on cerebral hypoxia, anoxia and ischemia in mice and rats. *Jpn J Pharmacol* 2001;87:143-150.

8. Dardzinski, B.J., et al. Increased plasma beta-hydroxybutyrate, preserved cerebral energy metabolism, and amelioration of brain damage during neonatal hypoxia ischemia with dexamethasone pretreatment. *Pediatr Res* 2000;48:248-255.

9. Shadnia, S., et al. Successful treatment of acute aluminium phosphide poisoning: possible benefit of coconut oil. *Human & Experimental Toxicology* 2005;24:215-218.

10. Kono, H., et al. Medium-chain triglycerides enhance secretory IgA expression in rat intestine after administration of endotoxin. *Am J Physiol Gastrointest Liver Physiol* 2004;286:G1081-1089.

11. Medium-chain length fatty acids, glycerides and analogues as stimulators of erythropoiesis. http://www.wipo.int/patentscope/search/en/WO2004069237. Accessed 11/29/2011.

12. Nolasco, N. A., et al. Effect of Coconut oil, trilaurin and tripalmitin on the promotion stage of carcinogenesis. *Philipp J Sci* 1994;123(1):161-169.

13. Reddy, B. S. and Maeura, Y. Tumor promotion by dietary fat in azoxymethane-induced colon carcinogenesis in female F344 rats: influence of amount and source of dietary fat. *J Natl Cancer Inst* 1984;72(3):745-750.

14. Cohen, L. A. and Thompson, D. O. The influence of dietary medium chain triglycerides on rat mammary tumor development. *Lipids* 1987;22(6):455-461.

15. Lim-Sylianco, C. Y., et al. A comparison of germ cell antigenotoxic activity of non-dietary and dietary coconut oil and soybean oil. *Phil J of Coconut Studies* 1992;2:1-5.

16. Lim-Sylianco, C. Y., et al. Antigenotoxic effects of bone marrow cells of coconut oil versus soybean oil. *Phil J of Coconut Studies* 1992;2:6-10.

17. Bulatao-Jayme, J., et al. Epdemiology of primary liver cancer in the Philippines with special consideration of a possible aflatoxin factor. *J Philipp Med Assoc* 1976;52:129-150.

18. Witcher, K. J, et al. Modulation of immune cell proliferation by glycerol monolaurate. *Clinical and Diagnostic Laboratory Immunology* 1996;3:10-13.

19. Projan, S. J., et al. Glyceryl monolaurate inhibits the production of â-lactamase, toxic shock syndrome toxin-1 and other Staphylococcal exoproteins by interfering with signal transduction. *J of Bacteriol* 1994;176:4204:4209.

20. Teo, T. C., et al. Long-term feeding with structured lipid composed of medium-chain and N-3 fatty acids ameliorates endotoxic shock in guinea pigs. *Metabolism* 1991;40(1):1152-1159.

21. Lim-Navarro, P. R. T. Protection effect of coconut oil against E coli endotoxin shock in rats. *Coconuts Today* 1994;11:90-91.

22. Liu, J., et al. Malnutrition at age 3 years and externalizing behavior problems at ages 8, 11, and 17 years. *Am J Psychiatry* 2004;161:2005-2013.

23. Upadhyay, S.K., et al. Influence of malnutrition on intellectual development. *Indian J Med Res* 1989;90:430-441.

24. Jiang, Z.M., et al. 1993. A comparison of medium-chain and long-chain triglycerides in surgical patients. *Ann. Surg.* 217(2):175.

25. Burke, V. and Danks, D.M. Medium-chain triglyceride diet: its use in treatment of liver disease. *Brit Med J* 1966;2:1050-1051.

26. Kuo, P.T. and Huang, N.N. The effect of medium chain triglyceride upon fat absorption and plasma lipid and depot fat of children with cystic fibrosis of the pancreas. *J Clin Invest* 1965;44:1924-1933.

27. Cancio, M. and Menendez-Corrrada, R. Absorption of medium chain triglycerides in tropical sprue. *Proc Soc Exp Biol (NY)* 1964;117:182-185.

28. Isselbacher, K.J., et al. Congenital beta-lipoprotein deficiency: an hereditary disorder involving a defect in the absorption and transport of lipids. *Medicine (Baltimore)* 1964;43:347-361.

29. Holt, P.R. Dietary treatment of protein loss in intestinal lymphangiectasia. *Pediatrics* 1964;34:629-635.

30. Greenberger, N.J., et al. Use of medium chain triglycerides in malabsorption. *Ann Internal Med* 1967;66:727-734.

31. Tantibhedhyangkul, P. and Hashim, S.A. Medium-chain triglyceride feeding in premature infants: effects on fat and nitrogen absorption. *Pediatrics* 1975;55:359-370.

32. Zurier, R.B., et al. Use of medium-chain triglyceride in management of patients with massive resection of the small intestine. *New Engl J Med* 1966;274:490-493.

33. Salmon, W.D. and Goodman, J.G. Alleviation of vitamin B deficiency in the rat by certain natural fats and synthetic esters. *Journal of Nutrition* 1936;13:477-500.

34. Intengan, C.L., et al. Structured lipid of coconut and corn oils vs. soybean oil in the rehabilitation of malnourished children—a field study. *Phil J Internal Medicine* 1992;30:159-164.

35. Vaidya, U.V., et al. 1992 Vegetable oil fortified feeds in the nutrition of very low birthweight babies. *Indian Pediatr.* 29(12):1519.

36. Tantibhedhyangjul. P. and Hashim, S.A. Medium-chain triglyceride feeding in premature infants: effects on fat and nitrogen absorption. *Pediatrics* 1975;55:359-370.

37. Roy, C.C., et al. Correction of the malabsorption of the preterm infant with a medium-chain triglyceride formula. *J Pediatr* 1975;86:446-450.

38. Wang, X., et al. Enteral nutrition improves clinical outcome and shortens hospital stay after cancer surgery. *J Invest Surg* 2010;23:309-313.

39. Ball, M.J. Parenteral nutrition in the critically ill: use of a medium chain triglyceride emulsion. *Intensive Care Med* 1993;19:89-95.

40. Smirniotis, V., et al. Long chain versus medium chain lipids in patients with ARDS: effects on pulmonary haemodynamics and gas exchange. *Intensive Care Med* 1998;24:1029-1033.

41. Wang, X.Y., et al. Effect of high amounts of medium chain triglyceride and protein enteral nutrition on nutritional status in patients after major abdominal operation. *Zhonghua Wei Chang Wai Ke Za Zhi* 2007;10:329-332.

42. Isaacs, C.E. and Thormar, H. The role of milk-derived antimicrobial lipids as antiviral and antibacterial agents, in *Immunology of Milk and the Neonate* (Mestecky, J., et al., eds). Plenum Press, 1991.

43. Isaacs, C.E. and Thormar, H. The role of milk-derived antimicrobial lipids as antiviral and antibacterial agents. *Adv Exp Med Biol* 1991;310:159-165.

44. Isaacs, C.E., et al. Antiviral and antibacterial lipids in human milk and infant formula feeds. *Arch Dis Child* 1990;65:861-864.

45. Bergsson, G., et al. In vitro inactivation of Chlamydia trachomatis by fatty acids and monoglycerides. *Antimicrobial Agents and Chemotherapy* 1998;42:2290- 2292.

46. Petschow, B.W., et al. Susceptibility of Helicobacter pylori to bactericidal properties of medium-chain monoglycerides and free fatty acids. *Antimicrobial Agents and Chemotherapy* 1996;40;302-306.

47. Holland, K.T., et al. The effect of glycerol monolaurate on growth of, and production of toxic shock syndrome toxin-1 and lipase by, Staphylococcus aureus. *Journal of Antimicrobial Chemotherapy* 1994;33:41-55.

48. Sun, C.Q., et al. Antibacterial actions of fatty acids and monoglycerides against Helicobacter pylori. *FEMS Immunol Med Microbiol* 2003;36:9-17.

49. Bergsson, G., et al. Killing of Gram-positive cocci by fatty acids and monoglycerides. *APMIS* 2001;109:670-678.

50. Bergsson, G., et al. In vitro susceptibilities of Neisseria gonorrhoeae to fatty acids and monoglycerides. *Antimicrob Agents Chemother* 1999;43:2790-2792.

51. Ogbolu, D.O., et al. In vitro antimicrobial properties of coconut oil on Candida species in Ibadan, Nigeria. *J Med Food* 2007;10:384-387.

52. Bergsson, G., et al. In vitro killing of Candida albicans by fatty acids and monoglycerides. *Antimicrob Agents Chemother* 2001;45:3209-3212.

53. Chadeganipour, M, and Haims, A. Antifungal activities of pelargonic and capric acid on Miscrosporum gypseum. *Mycoses* 2001;44:109-112.

54. Isaacs, E.E., et al. Inactivation of enveloped viruses in human bodily fluids by purified lipid. *Annals of the New York Academy of Sciences* 1994;724:465-471.

55. Bartolotta, S., et al. Effect of fatty acids on arenavirus replication: inhibition of virus production by lauric acid. *Arch Virol* 2001;146:777-790.

56. Thormar, H., et al. Inactivation of visna virus and other enveloped viruses by free fatty acids and monoglycerides. *Ann NY Acad Sci* 1994;724:465-471.

57. Hornung, B., et al. Lauric acid inhibits the maturation of vesicular stomatitis virus. *J Gen Virol* 1994;75:353-361.

58. Thormar, H., et al. Inactivation of enveloped viruses and killing of cells by fatty acids and monoglycerides. *Antimicrob Agents Chemother* 1987;31:27-31.

59. Vazquez, C., et al. Eucaloric substitution of medium chain triglycerides for dietary long chain fatty acids improves body composition and lipid profile in a patient with human immunodeficiency virus lipodystrophy. *Nutr Hosp* 2006;21:552-555.

60. Wanke, C.A., et al. A medium chain triglyceride-based diet in patients with HIV and chronic diarrhea reduces diarrhea and malabsorption: a prospective, controlled trial. *Nutrition* 1996;12:766-771.

61. Thormar, H., et al. Hydrogels containing monocaprin have potent microbicidal activities against sexually transmitted viruses and bacteria in vitro. *Sex Transm Infect* 1999;75(3):181-185.

62. Kabara, J.J. *The Pharmacological Effect of Lipids.* Champaign, IL: The American Oil Chemists' Society, 1978.

63. Coconut Oil: A New Weapon Against AIDS, www.coconutresearchcenter.org/hwnl_5-5.htm.

64. Gordon, S. Coconut oil may help fight childhood pneumonia. *US News and World Report*, Oct 30, 2008.

65. Medium-chain length fatty acids, glycerides and analogues as neutrophil survival and activation factors. http://www.freepatentsonline.com/y2010/0279959.html. Accessed 4/4/2011.

66. D'Eufemia, P., et al. Abnormal intestinal permeability in children with autism. *Acta Paediatr* 1996;85:1076-1079.

67. Mane, J., et al. Partial replacement of dietary (n-6) fatty acids with medium-chain triglycerides decreases the incidence of spontaneous colitis in interleukin-10-deficient mice. *J Nutr* 2009;139:603-610.

68. Jorgensen, J.R., et al. In vivo absorption of medium-chain fatty acids by the rat colon exceeds that of short-chain fatty acids. *Gastroenterology* 2001;120:1152-1161.

69. Kono, H., et al. Medium-chain triglycerides enhance secretory IgA expression in rat intestine after administration of endotoxin. *Am J Physiol Gastrointest Liver Physiol* 2004;286:G1081-G1089.

70. Kono, H., et al. Enteral diets enriched with medium-chain triglycerides and N-3 fatty acids prevent chemically induced experimental colitis in rats. *Transl Res* 2010;156:282-291.

71. Kono, H., et al. Dietary medium-chain triglycerides prevent chemically induces experimental colitis in rats. *Transl Res* 2010;155:131-141.

Chapter 11: Prenatal and Postnatal Nutrition

1. Hallmayer, J., et al. Genetic heritability and shared environmental factors among twin pairs with autism. *Arch Gen Psychiatry* 2011;68:1095-1102.

2. Conley, D. and Bennett, N.G. Is biology destiny? Birth weight and life chances. *American Sociological Review* 2000;65:458-467.

3. Reddy, U.M., et al. Term pregnancy: a period of heterogeneous risk for infant mortality. *Obstetrics and Gynecology* 2011;117:1279-1287.

4. Meyer, U., et al. The time of prenatal immune challenge determines the specificity of inflammation-mediated brain and behavioral pathology. *J Neurosci* 2006;26:4752-4762.

5. Atladottire, H.O., et al. Maternal infection requiring hospitalization during pregnancy and autism spectrum disorders. *J Autism Dev Disord* 2010;40:1423-1430.

6. Blaylock, R.L. The danger of excessive vaccination during brain development: the case for a link to Autism Spectrum Disorders (ASD). *Medical Veritas* 2008;5:1727-1741.

7. Brown, A.S., et al. Elevated maternal interleukin-8 levels and risk of schizophrenia in adult offspring. *Am J Psychiatry* 2004;161:889-895.

8. Buka, S.L., et al. Maternal cytokine levels during pregnancy and adult psychosis. *Brain Behav Immun* 2001;15:411-420.

9. Buka, S.L., et al. Maternal exposure to herpes simplex virus and risk of psychosis among adult offspring. *Biol Psychiatry* 2008;63:809-815.

10. Croen, L.A., et al. Antidepressant use during pregnancy and childhood autism spectrum disorders. *Arch Gen Psychiatry* 2011, July 4, published online ahead of print.

11. Srisuphon, W. and Bracken, M.B. Caffeine consumption during pregnancy and association with late spontaneous abortion. *American Journal of Obstetrics and Gynecology* 1986;154:14-20.

12. Stjernfeldt, M., et al. Maternal smoking during pregnancy and risk of childhood cancer. *Lancet* 1986;1350-1352.

13. Pregnancy and infant health, in *Smoking and Health*, a report of the surgeon general, January 1979.

14. Even moderate drinking may be hazardous to maturing fetus (Medical News). *JAMA* 1977;237:2535.

15. Edison, R.J. and Muenke, M. Central nervous system and limb anomalies in case reports of first-trimester statin exposure. *N Engl J Med* 2004;350:1579-1582.

16. Ab Rahman, A., et al. The use of herbal medicines during pregnancy and perinatal mortality in Tumpat District, Kelantan, Malaysia. *Southeast Asian J Trop Med Public Health* 2007;38:1150-1157.

17. Dong, Y.M., et al. High dietary intake of medium-chain fatty acids during pregnancy in rats prevents later-life obesity in their offspring. *J Nutr Biochem* 2011;22:791-797.

18. Rubaltelli, F.F. et al. Effect of lipid loading on fetal uptake of free fatty acids, glycerol and beta-hydroxybutyrate. *Biol Neonate* 1978;33:320-326.

19. Centers for Disease Control and Prevention (CDC). Transmission of yellow fever vaccine virus through breast-feeding – Brazil, 2009. *MMWR Morb Mortal Wkly Rep* 2010;59:130-132.

20. Jensen, R.G. Lipids in human milk. *Lipids* 1999;34:1243-1271.

21. Taha, A.Y. Dietary enrichment with medium chain triglycerides (AC-1203) elevates polyunsaturated fatty acids in the parietal cortex of aged dogs: implications for treating age-related cognitive decline. *Neurochem Res* 2009;34:1619-1625.

22. Cannell, J.J. Autism and vitamin D. *Med Hypotheses* 2008;70:750-759.

23. Kauffman, J.M. Benefits of vitamin D supplementation. *JAPS* 2009;14:38-45.

24. Rovner, A.J. and O'Brien, K.O. Hypovitaminosis D among healthy children in the United States: a review of the current evidence. *Arch Pediatr Adolesc Med* 2008;162:513-509.

25. Martinez-Costa, C., et al. Effects of refrigeration on the bactericidal activity of human milk: a preliminary study. *J Pediatr Gastroenterol Nutr* 2007;45:275-277.

26. Chan, G.M. Effects of powdered human milk fortifiers on the antibacterial actions of human milk. *Journal of Perinatology* 2003;23:620-623.

27. Cunningham, A.S., et al. Breast-feeding and health in the 1980s: a global epidemiologic review. *J Pediatr* 1991;118:659-666.

28. Lucas, A., et al. Randomized outcome trial of human milk fortification and developmental outcome in preterm infants. *Am J Clin Nutr* 1996;64:142-151.

29. Lozoff, B. and Georgieff, M.K. Neurodevelopmental delays associated with iron-fortified formula for healthy infants. http://www.medscape.org/medscapetoday. Accessed 6/23/2011.

30. Centers for Disease Control and Prevention. Enterobacter sakazakii infections associated with the use of powdered infant formula—Tennessee, 2001. *JAMA* 2002;287:2204-2205.

31. Riordan, J.M. The cost of not breastfeeding: a commentary. *J Hum Lact* 1997;13:93-97.

32. Ip, S., et al. Breastfeeding and maternal and infant health outcomes in developed countries. *Evidence Reports/Technology Assessments, No. 153* 2007.

33. Pratt, H.F. Breastfeeding and eczema. *Early Human Development* 1984;9:283-290.

34. Kramer M., et al. Breastfeeding and child cognitive development: new evidence from a large randomized trial. *Arch Gen Psychiatry* 2008;65:578-584.

35. Francois, C.A., et al. 1998. Acute effects of dietary fatty acids on the fatty acids of human milk. *Am. J. Clin. Nutr.* 67:301.

36. Geliebter, A., et al Overfeeding with medium-chain triglyceride diet results in diminished deposition of fat. *Am J Clin Nutr* 1983;37:1-4.

37. St-Onge, M.P. and Jones, P.J.H. Physiological effects of medium-chain triglycerides: potential agents in the prevention of obesity. *J of Nutr* 2002;132:329-332.

38. St-Onge, M.P. and Bosarge, A. Weight-loss diet that includes consumption of medium-chain triacylglycerol oil leads to a greater rate of weight and fat mass loss than does olive oil. *Am J Clin Nutr* 2008;87:621-626.

39. Benito, C., et al. Identification of a 7S globulin as a novel coconut allergen. *Ann Allergy Asthma Immunol* 2007;98:580-584.

40. Fries, J.H. and Fries, M.W. Coconut: a review of its uses as they relate to the allergic individual. *Ann Allergy* 1983;51:472-481.

41. Stutius, L.M., et al. Characterizing the relationship between sesame, coconut, and nut allergy in children. *Pediatr Allergy Immunol* 2010;21:1114-1118.

42. Teuber, S.S. and Peterson, W.R. Systemic allergic reaction to coconut (Cocos nucifera) in 2 subjects with hypersensitivity to tree nut and demonstration of cross-reactivity to legumin-like seed storate protein: new coconut and walnut food allergens. *J Allergy Clin Immunol* 1999;103:1180-1185.

43. Rhoads, J.M., et al. Altered fecal microflora and increased fecal calprotectin in infants with colic. *J Pedatr* 2009;155:823-828.

44. Savino, F., et al. Lactobacillus reuteri (American Type Culture Collection Strain 55730) versus simethicone in the treatment of infantile colic: a prospective randomized study. *Pediatrics* 2007;119:e124-e130.

45. Savino, F., et al. Lactobacillus reuteri DSM 17938 in infantile colic: a randomized, double-blind, placebo-controlled trial. *Pediatrics* 2010;126:e526-e533.

Chapter 12: Nutrition and Brain Health

1. Hu, F.B. and Malik, V.S. Sugar-sweetened beverages and risk of obesity and type 2 diabetes: epidemiologic evidence. *Physiol Behav* 2010;100:47-54.

2. Stranahan, A.M., et al. Diet-induced insulin resistance impairs hippocampal synaptic plasticity and cognition in middle-aged rats. *Hippocampus* 2008;18:1085-1088.

3. Cao, D., et al. Intake of sucrose-sweetened water induces insulin resistance and exacerbates memory deficits and amyloidosis in a transgenic mouse model of Alzheimer disease. *J Biol Chem* 2007;282:36275-36282.

4. Sasaki, N., et al. Advanced glycation end products in Alzheimer's disease and other neurodegenerative diseases. *American Journal of Pathology* 1998;153:1149-1155.

5. Catellani, R., et al. Glycooxidation and oxidative stress in Parkinson's disease and diffuse Lewy body disease. *Brain Res* 1996;737:195-200.

6. Kato, S., et al. Astrocytic hyaline inclusions contain advanced glycation endproducts in familial amyotrophic lateral sclerosis with superoxide dismutase 1 gene mutation: immunohistochemical and immunoelectron microscopical analysis. *Aca Neuropathol* 1999;97:260-266.

7. Sanchez, A., et al. Role of sugars in human neutrophilic phagocytosis. *Am J Clin Nutr* 1973;26:1180-1184.

8. Horvath, K. and Perman, J.A. Autism and gastrointestinal symptoms. *Curr Gastroenterol Rep* 2002;4:251-258.

9. Valicenti-McDermott, M., et al. Frequency of gastrointestinal symptoms in children with autistic spectrum disorders and associateion with family history of autoimmune disease. *J Dev Behav Pediatr* 2006;27(2 Suppl):S128-S136.

10. Horvath, K., et al Gastrointestinal abnormalities in children with autistic disorder. *J Pediatr* 1999;135:559-563.

11. Torrente, F., et al. Focal-enhanced gastritis in regressive autism with features distinct from Crohn's and Helicobacter pylori gastritis. *Am J Gastroenterol* 2004;99:598-605.

12. Erickson, C.A., et al. Gastrointestinal factors in autistic disorder: a critical review. *J Autism Dev Disord* 2005;35:713-727.

13. Luostarinen, L., et al. Coeliac disease presenting with neurological disorders. *Eur Neurol* 1999;42(3):132-135.

14. Cooke, W.T. and Smith, W.T. Neurological disorders associated with adult coeliac disease. *Brain* 1966;89:683-722.

15. Bushara, K.O. Neurologic presentation of celiac disease. *Gastroenterology* 2005;128 Suppl 1:S92-S97.

16. Genuis, S.J. and Bouchard, T.P. Celiac disease presenting as autism. *Journal of Child Neurology* 2009;000:1-6.

17. Goodwin, M.S., et al. Malabsorption and cerebral dysfunction: a multivariate and comparative study of autistic children. *J Autism Child Schizophr* 1971;1:48-62.

18. Blaylock. R.L. Interaction of cytokines, excitotoxins, reactive nitrogen and oxygen species in autism spectrum disorders. *JANA* 2003;6(4):21-35.

19. Vogelaar, A. studying the effects of essential nutrients and environmental factors on autistic behavior. *DAN! (Defeat Autism Now!) Think Tank,* San Diego, CA: Autism Research Institute; 2000.

20. Rimland, B., et al. The effects of high doses of vitamin B6 on autistic children: a double-blind crossover study. *Am J Psychiatry* 1978;135:472-475.

21. Dolske, M.C., et al. A preliminary trial of ascorbic acid as supplemental therapy for autism. *Prog Neuropsychopharmacol Biol Psychiatry* 1993;17:765-774.

22. Megson, M.N. Is autism a G-alpha protein defect reversible with natural vitamin A? *Med Hypotheses* 2000;l54:979-983.

23. Halliwell, B. Reactive oxygen species and the central nervous system. *J Neurochem* 1992:59:1609-1623

24. Bradstreet, J. and Kartzinel, J. Biological interventions in the treatment of autism and PDD. In: Rimland, B. ed. *DAN! (Defeat Autism Now!) Fall 2001 Conference.* San Diego, CA:Autism Research Institue;2001.

25. Dolske, M.C., et al. A preliminary trial of ascorbic acid as supplemental therapy for autism. *Prog Neuropsychopharmacol Biol Psychiatry* 1993;17:765-774.

26. Polidori, M.C., et al. High fruit and vegetable intake is positively correlated with antioxidant status and cognitive performance in healthy subjects. *J Alzheimers Dis* 2009;17:921-927.

27. Chan, A., et al. Apple juice concentrate maintains acetylcholine levels following dietary compromise. *J Alzheimers Dis* 2006;9:287-291.

28. 2005 Dietary Guidelines for Americans. Center for Nutrition Policy and Promotion, U.S. Department of Agriculture.

29. Dillon, M.J., et al. Mental retardation, megaloblastic anaemic, homocysteine metabolism due to an error in B12 metabolism. *Clin Sci Mol Med* 1974;47:43-61.

30. Jang, S., et al. Luteolin reduces IL-6 produciton in microglia by inhibiting JNK phosphorylation and activation of AP-1. *Proc Nati Acad Sci USA* 2008;105:7534-7539.

31. Reeta, K.H., et al. Pharmacokinetic and pharmacodynamic interactions of valproate, phenytoin, phenobarbitone and carbamazepine with curcumin in experimental models of epilepsy in rats. *Pharmacol Biochem Behav* 2011;99(3):399-407.

32. Khuwaja, G., et al. Neuroprotective effects of curcumin on 6-hydroxydopamine-induced Parkinsonism in rats: behavioral, neurochemical and immunohistochemical studies. *Brain Res* 2011;1368:254-263.

33. Scapagnini, G., et al. Therapeutic potential of dietary polyphenols against brain ageing and neurodegenerative disorders. *Adv Exp Med Biol* 2011;698:27-35.

34. King, M.D., et al. Attenuation of hematoma size and neurological injury with curcumin following hermorrhage in mice. *J Neurosurg* 2011;115(1):116-123.

35. Sood, P.K., et al. Curcumin attenuates aluminum-induced oxidative stress and mitochondrial dysfunction in rat brain. *Neurotox Res* 2011;20:351-361.

36. Mimche, P.N., et al. The plant-based immunomodulator curcumin as a potential candidate for the development of an adjunctive therapy for cerebral malaria. *Malar J* 2011;10 Suppl:S10.

37. Dell, C.A., et al. Lipid and fatty acid profiles in rats consuming different high-fat ketogenic diets. *Lipids* 2001;36:373-374.

38. Esterhuyse, A.J., et al. Dietary red palm oil supplementation protects against the consequences of global ischemia in the isolated perfused rat heart. *Asia Pac J Clin Nutr* 2005;14:340-347.

39. Tomeo, A.C., et al. Antioxidant effects of tocotrienols in patients with hyperlipidemia and carotid stenosis. *Lipids* 1995;30:1179-1183.

40. Mishima, K., et al. Vitamin E isoforms alpha-tocotrienol and gamma-tocopherol prevent cerebral infarction in mice. *Neurosci Lett* 2003;337:56-60.

41. Fife, B. *The Palm Oil Miracle.* Piccadilly Books, Ltd:Colorado Springs, CO; 2007.

42. Megson, M.N. Is autism a G-alpha protein defect reversible with natural vitamin A? *Med Hypotheses* 2000;54:979-983.

Chapter 13: The Coconut Ketogenic Diet

1. Dell, C.A., et al. Lipid and fatty acid profiles in rats consuming different high-fat ketogenic diets. *Lipids* 2001;36:373-374.

2. Reger, M.A., et al. Effects of beta-hydroxybutyrate on cognition in memory-impaired adults. *Neurobiol Aging* 2004;25:311-314.

3. Likhodii, S.S., et al. Dietary fat, ketosis, and seizure resistance in rats on the ketogenic diet. *Epilepsia* 2000;41:1400-1410.

4. Gordon, N. and Newton, R.W. Glucose transporter type 1 (GLUT) deficiency. *Brain Dev* 2003;25:477-480.

Chapter 14: The Autism Battle Plan

1. Hallmayer, J., et al. Genetic heritability and shared environmental factors among twin pairs with autism. *Arch Gen Psychiatry* 2011;68:1095-1102.

2. Ozonoff, S., et al. Recurrence risk for autism spectrum disorders: a baby siblings research consortium study. *Pediatrics* 2011, Aug 15. Published online ahead of print.

3. Holick, M.F. Vitamin D deficiency. *N Engl J Med* 2007;357:266-281.

4. Vitamin D Council. www.vitamindcouncil.org. Accessed 10/28/2011.

5. Genuis, S.J. and Bouchard, T.P. Celiac disease presenting as autism. *Journal of Child Neurology* 2009;000:1-6.

Index

Coconut Cures
Preventing and Treating Common Health Porblems with Coconut

Discover the amazing health benefits of coconut oil, meat, milk, and water. In this book you will learn why coconut oil is considered the healthiest oil on earth and how it can protect you against heart disease, diabetes, and infectious illnesses such as influenza, herpes, candida, and even HIV.

There is more to the healing power of coconut than just the oil. You will also learn about the amazing health benefits of coconut meat, milk, and water. You will learn why coconut water is used as an IV solution and how coconut meat can protect you from colon cancer, regulate blood sugar, and expel intestinal parasites. Contains dozens of fascinating case studies and remarkable success stories. You will read about one woman's incredible battle with breast and brain cancer and how she cured herself with coconut. This book includes an extensive A to Z reference with complete details on how to use coconut to prevent and treat dozens of common health problems.

Statements made in this book are documented with references to hundreds of published medical studies. The foreword is written by Dr. Conrado Dayrit, the first person to publish studies showing the benefit of coconut oil in treating HIV patients.

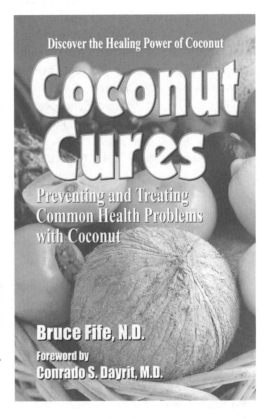

"As a doctor I have found coconut oil to be very useful. It has been of great help in treating hypertension, high cholesterol, and thyroid dysfunction as well as many other conditions. I highly recommend that you read this book."
—Edna Aricaya-Huevos, M.D.

"Coconut oil has an important medical role to play in nutrition, metabolism, and health care. Indeed, properly formulated and utilized, coconut oil may be the preferred vegetable oil in our diet and the special hospital foods used promoting patient recovery."
--Conrado S. Dayrit, M.D.

"Excellent book. It is very helpful for those seeking to improve their health using natural medicine. I am actively conducting clinical trials and medical research using coconut oil and have seen very positive results with my patients."
--Marieta Jader-Onate, M.D.

Piccadilly Books, Ltd.
www.piccadillybooks.com

The Palm Oil Miracle

Palm oil has been used as both a food and a medicine for thousands of years. it was prized by the pharaohs of ancient Egypt as a sacred food. Today palm oil is the most widely used oil in the world. In tropical Africa and Southeast Asia it is an integral part of a healthy diet just as olive oil is in the Mediterranean.

Palm oil possesses excellent cooking properties. It is more heat stable than other vegetable oils and imparts in foods and baked goods superior taste, texture, and quality.

Palm oil is one of the world's healthiest oils. As a natural vegetable oil, it contains no trans fatty acids or cholesterol. It is currently being used by doctors and government agencies to treat specific illnesses and improve nutritional status. Recent medical studies have shown that palm oil, particularly virgin (red) palm oil, can protect against many common health problems. Some of the health benefits include:

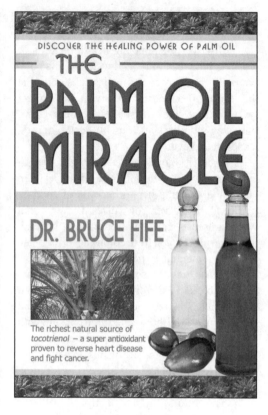

DISCOVER THE HEALING POWER OF PALM OIL

THE PALM OIL MIRACLE

DR. BRUCE FIFE

The richest natural source of *tocotrienol* – a super antioxidant proven to reverse heart disease and fight cancer.

- Improves blood circulation
- Protects against heart disease
- Protects against cancer
- Boosts immunity
- Improves blood sugar control
- Improves nutrient absorption and vitamin and mineral status
- Aids in the prevention and treatment of malnutrition
- Supports healthy lung function
- Supports healthy liver function
- Helps strengthen bones and teeth

- Supports eye health
- Highest natural source of health promoting tocotrienols
- Helps protect against mental deterioration, including Alzheimer's disease
- Richest dietary source of vitamin E and beta-carotene

"A fascinating guide to the healthful and nutritional properties of palm oil."
--Small Press Bookwatch

Visit us on the Web

 Piccadilly Books, Ltd.
www.piccadillybooks.com